# The Secrets, Struggles

## and

# Successes

## of an Alzheimer's Caregiver

## A daughter's twelve-year journey

### Ellen Pettijohn Stephens

TheWritersPorch.com

Edited by Terrie White

Interior Formatting by Carol Beth Anderson

Forward by Ethan Stephens

**Photo credits:**

Page VIII: Olin Mills Portrait Studio

Page 23: Burt Goode Photography

Pages 99 and 319: Meagan Swinney Gonzalez

**Scripture**: Unless otherwise indicated, all Scripture quotations are taken from the *Holy Bible,* New Living Translation, copyright © 1996, 2004, 2015 by Tyndale House Foundation. Used by permission of Tyndale House Publishers, Inc., Carol Stream, Illinois 60188. All rights reserved.

**Disclaimer:** This memoir is based on true events and personal experiences. To protect the privacy of individuals and maintain confidentiality, names and identifying details have been changed. While the essence of the story and the integrity of the journey remains true, certain events, timelines, and dialogue may have been modified or reconstructed for the sake of narrative coherence. This book is intended to share personal experiences and insights, not to provide professional medical advice, but instead my personal medical experience.

ISBN: 978-1-957925-02-8 Hardcover

ISBN: 978-1-957925-03-5 Paperback

ISBN: 978-1-957925-04-2 E-book

Dedicated to my sweetheart, James, my husband of 43 years. Your love, patience, genuine care, and support of me through this walk with Mama was nothing more than perfect. You never complained, judged, or doubted me. You held the torch at home while I ran the marathon with Mama. Together, we completed the race. Thank you for passing on these much-needed, admirable qualities to our children. ~ Elle

To my daughters, Mary Ellen and Chrissy –I realize I introduced you to the world of caregiving and Alzheimer's without your consent. You were both so young. I had so much guilt thinking I had ruined you, frightened you, or even scarred you being around that environment. But no, not you two. You are both now in health care professions. I've never been more thankful to be proven wrong by my kids. ~ Mama

# CONTENTS

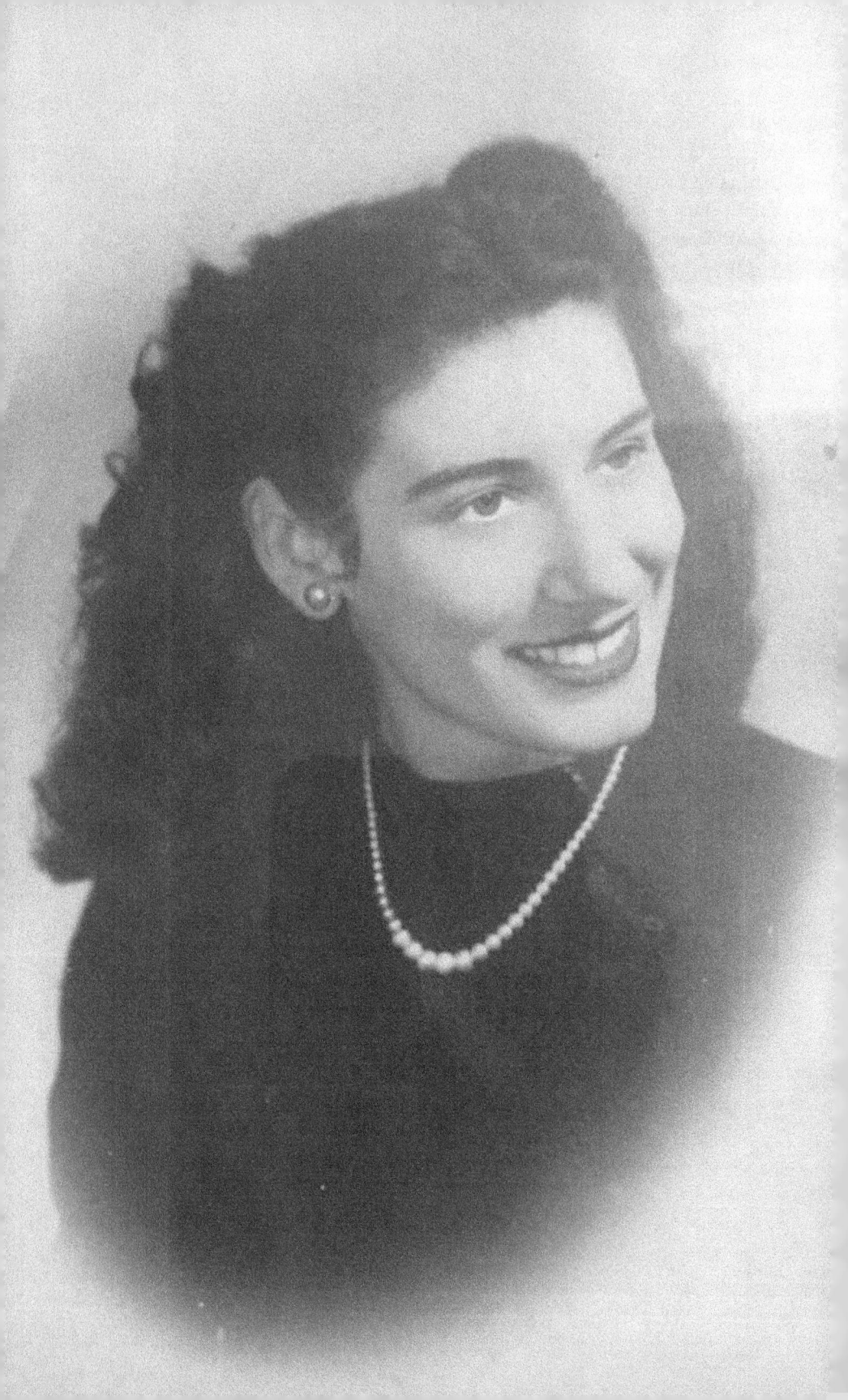

# FOREWORD

Every journey, no matter how profoundly challenging or deeply personal, holds within it universal truths. As readers, we are privileged to walk these paths alongside the author, not only exploring their experiences but also illuminating our own. *The Secrets, Struggles and Successes of an Alzheimer's Caregiver* takes us on one such journey—a journey that extends beyond the mere pages of this book.

This is a narrative that delves into the complexities of love and obligation, courage and resilience, despair and hope. It is a memoir of a daughter's twelve-year journey caring for her mother who slowly succumbs to Alzheimer's—a disease known for its cruel ability to erase memory, to blur identities, and to transform relationships. Each chapter represents a poignant time in this harrowing, heartfelt journey. We witness the relentless progression of the disease and its impact on both my mother and grandmother. We see my mother, Ellen, grappling with role reversal, navigating healthcare systems, advocating for her mother, managing the day-to-day care, and dealing with the emotional toll such responsibility brings. But amid the struggles, we also uncover secrets, resilience, triumphs, and an unparalleled love Alzheimer's could not diminish.

This memoir is not merely a chronicle of an Alzheimer's caregiver's journey but a testament to the human spirit's capacity to endure, adapt, and find hope in the most despairing of circumstances. It reflects our collective struggle with Alzheimer's and related dementia, providing a voice to millions of caregivers worldwide who shoulder a similar responsibility. *The Secrets, Struggles and Successes of an Alzheimer's Caregiver* is a tribute to all caregivers—honoring their courage, resilience, and the unspoken sacrifices they make. Above all, it is an invitation to understand, empathize with, and reflect upon a journey many of us may one day undertake.

In sharing this journey, the author provides us with an opportunity to explore our own capacity for resilience, to appreciate the complexity of the human condition, and to consider the far-reaching impact of our actions on those we love. As you turn the pages, remember this is not just a story—it is an experience. And as with any profound experience, we are all irrevocably changed by it.

With this in mind, I invite you to delve into this memoir—to share in the secrets, confront the struggles, and celebrate the successes of an Alzheimer's caregiver.

Ethan Stephens

## CHAPTER I

# STANDING STRONG IN THE STORM

ACT I OF THIS "PLAY" was jaw-dropping. The main character was the 78-year-old widowed mother of six adult children, beloved by all and affectionately called "Norma Jean" by her offspring, siblings, and friends when she wasn't being referred to as Mama or Mamaw.

She lost her dearly beloved sweetheart, our father, when she was only 51 years old but continued to carry the torch for our family. This journey took place in Southwest Louisiana. I am Ellen, the fifth child and the only one who lived near Mama. I won the prestigious role of caregiver in this family drama. There were no auditions, so I naively accepted the lead role.

In September, a Category 3 major hurricane reaching winds as high as 129 mph, slammed into our hometown and destroyed Mama's home. Thankfully, she had evacuated with my family to my brother's home in north Louisiana. After nearly a week, permission was granted from the parish for residents to return home for a "look and see" only. There was no power, which meant all stores were closed. It was a ghost town except for utility workers, police officers, and firefighters. I feared our town might never be the same.

Mama and I were unprepared for the catastrophic aftermath of this hurricane. My mother's neighbors who had stayed behind and weathered the storm reported her home had minimal damage from their vantage point, but those findings were grossly inaccurate. As we drove to Mama's home, the front of the house looked quite normal. However, we quickly noticed a large oak tree had fallen down in the backyard onto her shed. When we walked inside her home, the kitchen and living room were amazingly intact. Hopeful, we continued toward the dining room when Ralph, my brother, yelled, "Mama, we've got a tree in the dining room!" Branches filled the entire room. The dining room table she and my dad purchased decades ago at an auction now held the weight of this massive tree. Mama's face said it all; she didn't utter a single word and was barely able to breathe. I held her tightly as we continued the tour.

The first bedroom and entryway looked in fair shape. The second bedroom, however, was in disarray. It had been showered with insulation, and a gaping hole in the ceiling exposed the rafters. The beautiful, antique bedspread was ruined and held an accumulation of small branches. Glancing around the room, we noted a lamp lying on the floor with the lampshade several feet away. That 'ole hurricane had redecorated my Mama's home. We turned to survey the master bedroom and it was much, much worse. A giant oak tree had crashed through the roof and was lying across her bed, the bed she would have been sleeping in had she not evacuated. Tears welled up in our eyes. The furniture was broken into pieces. You could see outside, and I don't mean through the window. The heat and humidity weighed heavily in the room.

As we continued to take in the devastation, we noticed her ceramic statue of the Virgin Mary was unscathed. It was a gift to our family from dear friends. I don't recall a time when it wasn't prominently displayed in the living room of our childhood home. My mother, a life-long, devout Catholic, stared at her cherished statue in awe. Goosebumps surfaced on her arms with more tears freely falling. All told Mama's house had several trees fall on it, as well as through it. Our tour of the home concluded in the backyard, where we found yet another tree lying on top of her crushed patio awning. It was heartbreaking.

During the following twelve months, Mama lived in four different places. First, she stayed with my family, followed by a short time with her sister. She then secured a duplex apartment, and eventually, returned to our house while waiting to close on her new house.

Finally, after ten, long and frustrating months of dealing with countless insurance adjusters and two structural engineers, her house was ultimately declared "A TOTAL LOSS." I had handled all the insurance details while working, raising my family of four, and handling everything for Mama. In addition to my mountain of duties, I was worried sick about my sweet Mama. If a year of walking through the aftermath of a catastrophic event doesn't affect you, I applaud you. I was a certifiable basket case, and to protect Mama from unnecessary stress, I shared as little information with her as possible.

Although our house did not sustain significant damage, my elderly in-laws' home also succumbed to the high winds of this monstrous storm. My husband, their only child, was wheelchair-bound due to a recent surgery and couldn't help anyone.

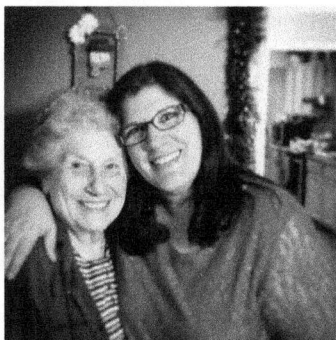

It was nearly a year before some semblance of normalcy returned to our lives. After Mama received her insurance money, we began the search for a new home and found a beautiful one just a hop, skip, and jump away from me. We were finally coming out of the storm, no pun intended.

With frequent phone calls to check on Mama, my siblings noticed how much our mother repeated herself. Her memory had always been remarkable, and now her reputation for being sharp was beginning to tarnish. Those days were long gone. The situation only grew worse.

3

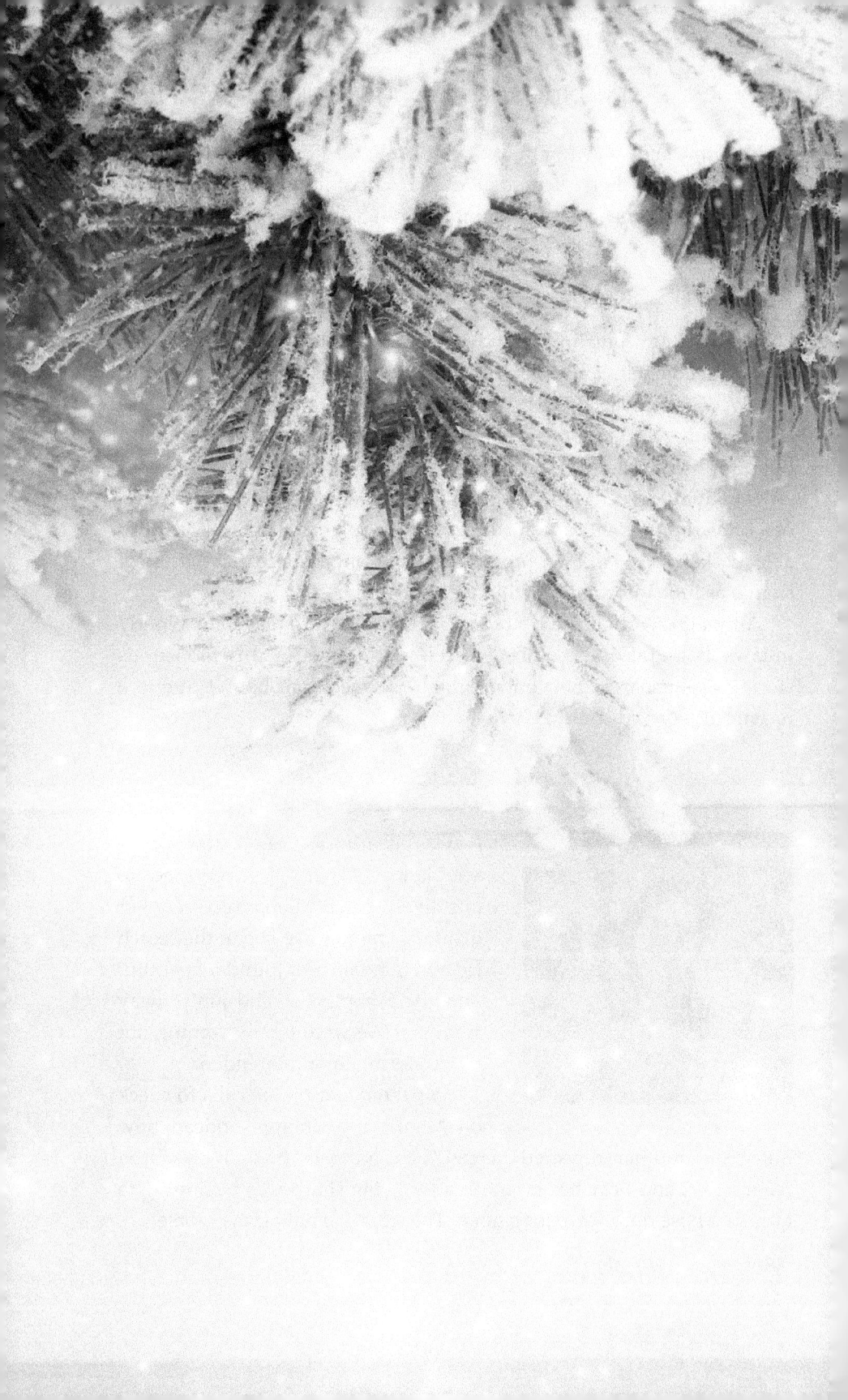

# CHAPTER 2
# A "RARE" CHRISTMAS

HISTORICALLY, with any approaching holiday like Christmas, most, if not all of my five siblings gathered in our hometown. Before the family arrived, Mama purchased her groceries and proudly prepared her delicious, signature dishes and yummy holiday treats like pralines, fudge, and pecan pies. She made it a priority to be actively present with her children and grandchildren once they arrived. This woman had her priorities right. This family gathering was the first Christmas in her new home and she couldn't be happier.

Holiday decorations adorned every inch of her home, a 'la Southern Living style, and the only missing ingredients to this perfect day were her children and grandchildren.

My family and I arrived a few hours before mealtime. My sister rushed to me as I entered the living room and said Mama had just driven to the store to purchase the roast. "What? Why? Did she burn the first roast?" It was so out of character for our mother not to plan ahead. Typically, everything was always done in a timely manner. *Hmmm. What was she thinking?*

Later, after Mama had "cooked" the roast on the stove, she placed her prized garlic roast on her holiday serving platter. The recipe for the garlic roast was everyone's favorite. The grandchildren still talk about how delicious it was as no other roasts held a candle to Mamaw's roast. The new dining room table was festive, with beautiful linens and an impressive flower arrangement made by Mama and placed as the centerpiece under the chandelier. Mama sliced the roast with chef-type culinary expertise anticipating accolades around the dinner table. We noticed right away the roast was RAW! She was nonchalant about the whole matter; it didn't seem to register with her that, "Houston, we have a problem!"

While the family sat around the table, we passed the Cajun dirty rice, vegetables, and fresh rolls. As Mama reached for a bowl, we noticed she had burned the palm of her hand. It was bright red with blisters! She was not alarmed or the least bit concerned. We were astonished, and we shared looks of concern with each other—some with furrowed brows, others with gaping mouths and wide eyes. Surely, someone must have been in the kitchen assisting her with the preparations. *Did she not moan, scream, or wince when her palm was scorched? Could it have been she was not even aware of what had transpired?* We tended to her wound immediately. These first two precursors at the dining table were very unusual and bewildering. Were these accidental or the beginning of some demise in her health? The atmosphere in the dining room changed dramatically that afternoon.

Everyone was in their own thoughts, worried about Mama.

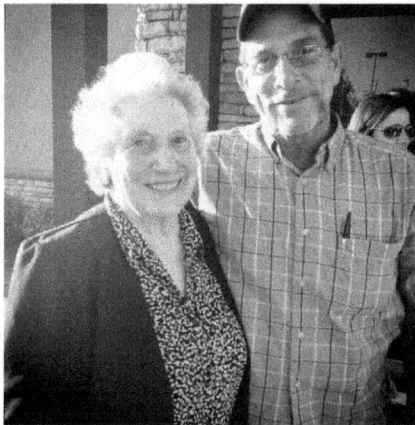

Mama and my brother, Paul

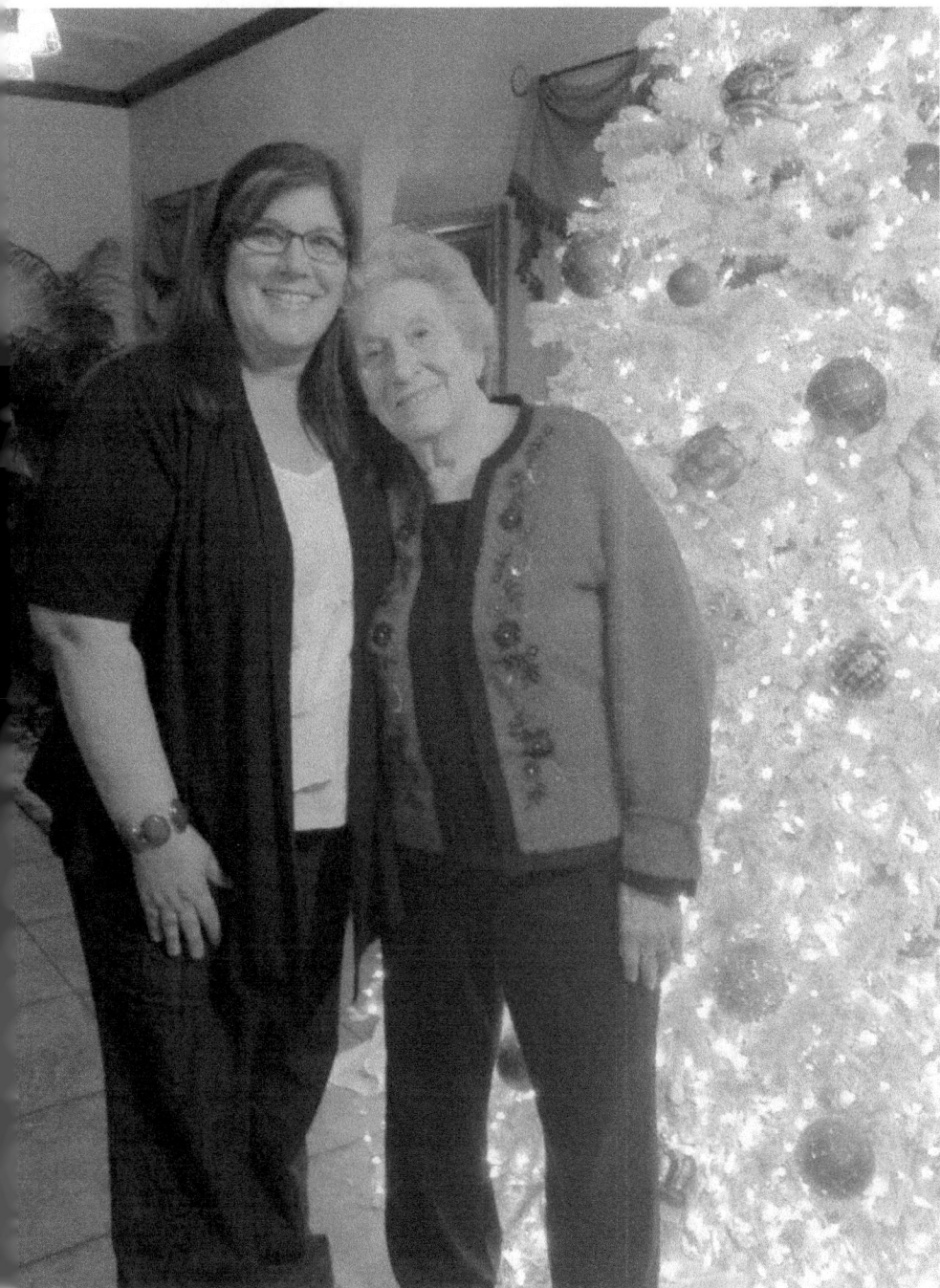

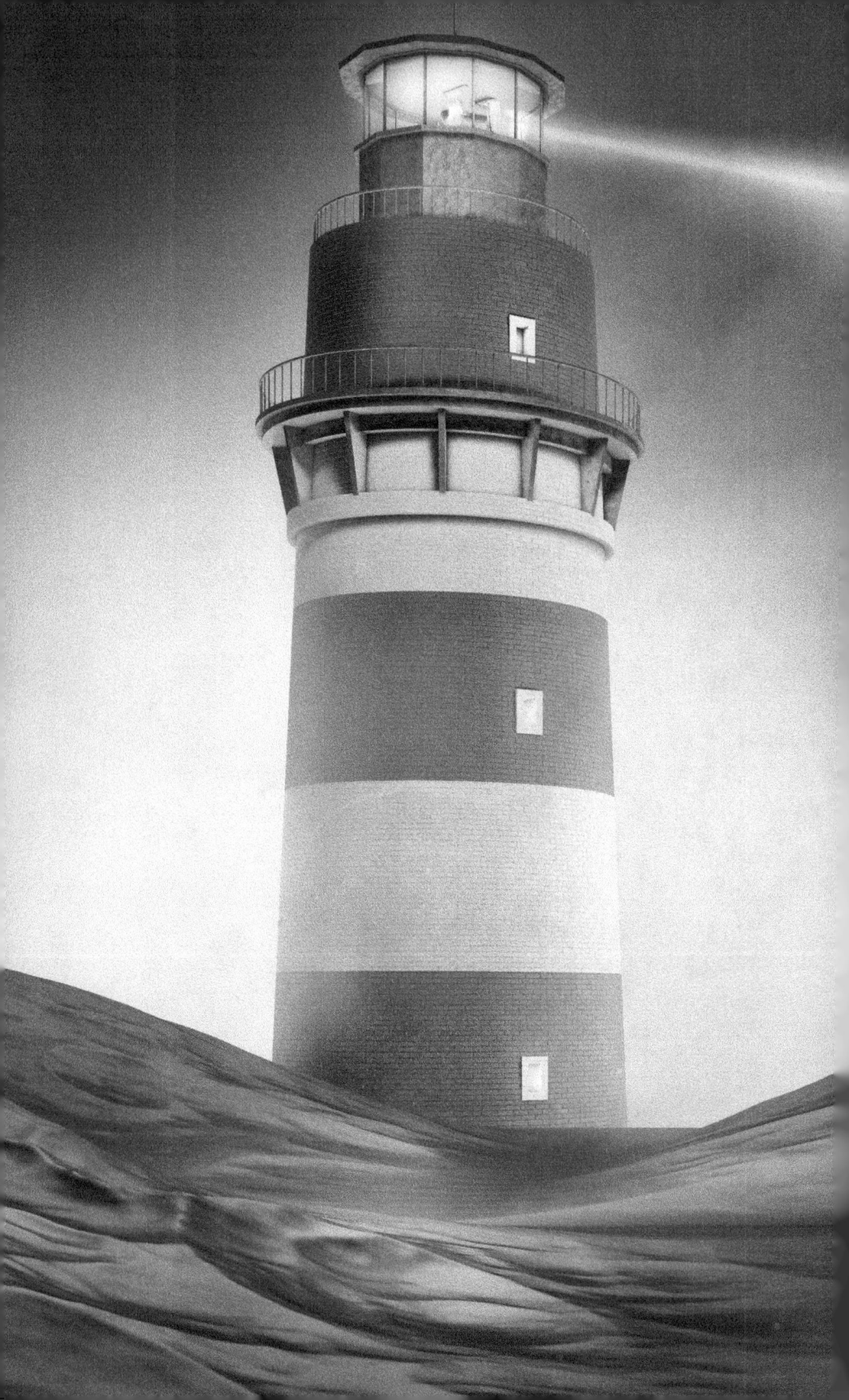

# CHAPTER 3

# SEARCH AND RESCUE

Soon after the holidays, I received a phone call from Mama's neighbors. They were dear friends and were very concerned about her. It seems one night as the wife was getting a glass of water, she spotted my mother through her window, tending to her flower beds. Here's the shocker! It was 3 a.m.! *Lord, what is going on?* I was thankful to have another set of eyes on that mother of mine.

---

We should never underestimate the value of caring neighbors, especially when they live next to an elderly parent.

---

Between the Christmas fiasco and the 'gardening by the light of the moon' episode, my migraine-inducing concern for her future weighed heavy on my heart. Mama's independent streak and spontaneity led her to drive alone for hours. She loved to revisit her old stomping grounds from her single days. Mama never told anyone where she was going, prompting me to head out on search and rescue missions after hours of radio silence. Sometimes, she was unaccounted for most of the day. I drove to her beauty shop, her sister's home, friends' homes, church, the big box store, etc. No one had seen or heard from her. This happened more times than I care to recount. When I finally found her back home, she told of her travels and how she knocked on the doors of houses or apartments she had lived in before she married.

My concern was that in 60-plus years, these neighborhoods had deteriorated substantially and were no longer safe for anyone, much less an elderly woman on her own.

After several "Where's Waldo" escapades or, in my case, "Where's Norma Jean," I devised new adventures while still allowing sweet Mama to enjoy a car ride. As we rode through town, we turned up the music. She loved to "play the drums" on the glove box, while simultaneously tapping the window with the back of her ring. It added a different tone to the mix. She loved oldies, country, soul, harmonies, zydeco, and anything with a good beat. The two songs she loved most brought a smile to my face. They were "Beat It" by Michael Jackson and "Tequila Makes Her Clothes Fall Off" by Joe Nichols. She loved those songs and acted like a 16-year-old on a Friday night, cruising downtown with the music up and the windows down. To make it a perfect day for her, I drove to Dairy Queen and ordered each of us a Blizzard. She was plum giddy. She held the cup in one hand, the long, red spoon hanging out the side of her mouth, and beat the glove box with the free hand. The more I took her out on these drives, the less she went out alone. My idea worked beautifully and unbeknownst to me, I had just passed my first test as a caregiver. The first with hundreds more to come.

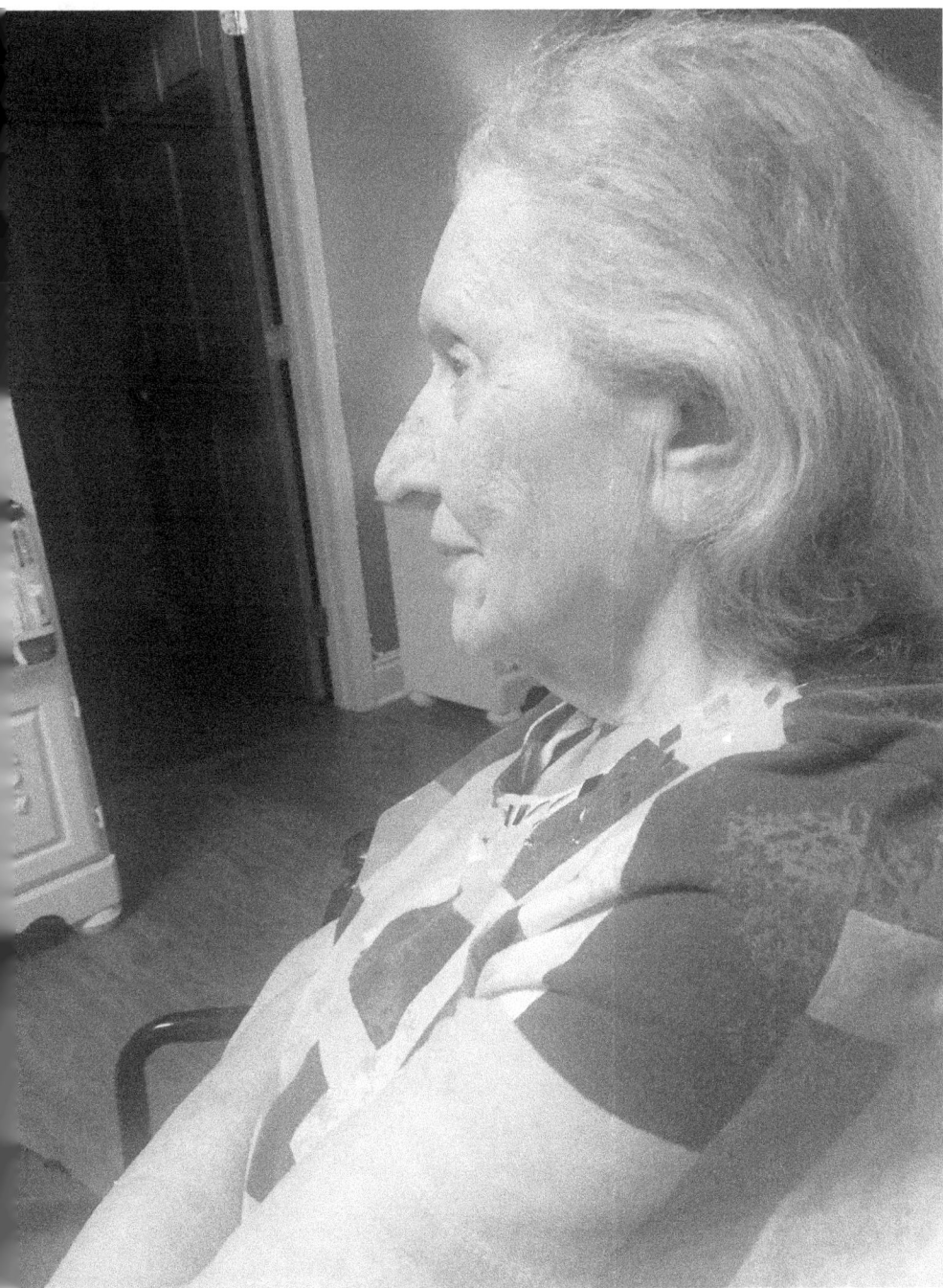

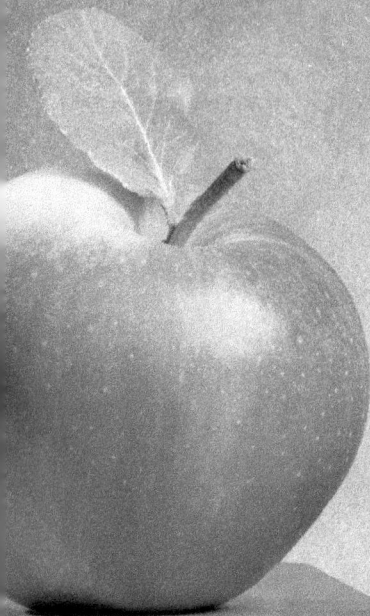

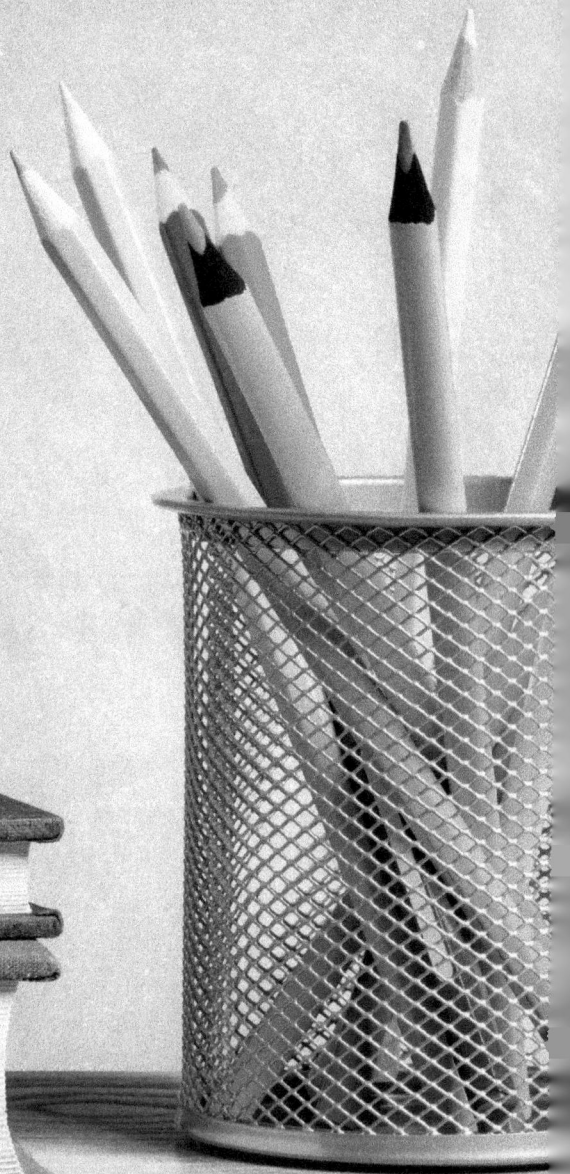

# CHAPTER 4
# SCHOOL IS IN SESSION

A FEW MONTHS passed with more symptoms surfacing, so I brought Mama to a geriatric doctor. He performed an "Alzheimer's" test on her. The doctor quizzed her on her name, birthday, the current president, today's date, etc. Next, he questioned her on what war occurred during her teenage years (WWII). She thought long and hard and retorted with her keen sense of humor, "I don't know what war was going on, but I had a good time at the USO with my sister." The more questions he threw at her in rapid-fire succession, the more frustrated she got. Mama's lips were pursed. Her scowled face was evidence this had gone too far. Next, we were moved down the hall into another office. There they tested her math skills.

*Side note: I've already told my family I would fail a math test every time. It is not an indicator of brain disease for me.*

Although Mama was a brilliant student and always remained sharp until these last few years, she could not respond correctly to the questions, not even the simple ones.

"Count to 100 backward by 10."

"Draw hands on the clock."

*Oh, wait. Did you say draw?*

She loved this one. I could tell by the sarcastic look she threw my way. She wanted to be an artist early in her marriage and even sent drawings to an art school. She scribbled flowers, grass, and a tree on the paper. The poor clock never acquired any hands. Mama was exasperated and mentally worn out. The doctor wanted to prescribe a medication called Aricept (also known as Donepezil) that could hopefully help her memory, but unfortunately, not cure the disease. The doctor hoped to prevent memory loss any further, but we declined. I had never heard of this medication, and this required more research. My to-do list continued to grow longer with each passing day.

⊰⊱

During this phase of Mama's progression, I had one son graduating from college and getting married later that summer; my second son was graduating from high school and preparing for college; my two daughters were also in school and very involved in church and sports. I worked full-time at a Christian school and also owned a successful photography business. My husband worked shift work plus overtime. I had a full plate already, but I needed a large platter for the multitude of responsibilities heading my way.

Without any previous knowledge of dementia, Alzheimer's, or assisted living, I slowly began to dip my toe into those waters. The learning curve was off the charts. Ready or not, here we go!

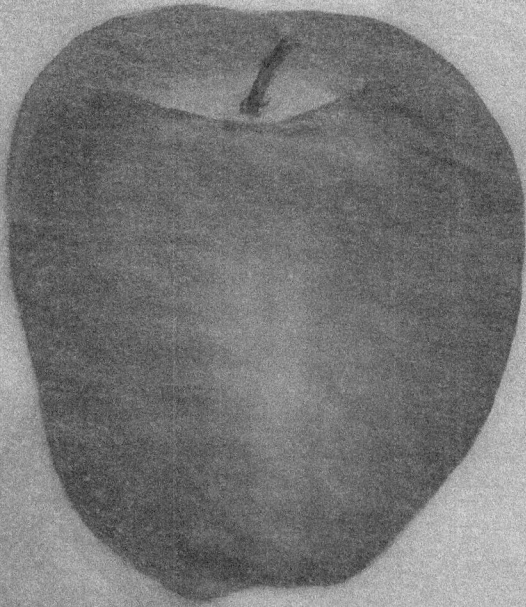

# CHAPTER 5
# A HELLION'S HEART

SWEET MAMA HAD a serious meltdown while at my house recently. She came over crying her heart out, worried if the "looney bin" was in the near future because of her memory loss. She was scared and said people told her all the time, either directly or indirectly, they knew she had lost her memory. *Why say something like that to her face?* She was a wreck. It broke my heart to see her this way. I've never heard Mama be so transparent with her thoughts and feelings. She was depressed and had been since the catastrophic storm, but this was different, more intense, dark. Here's a bizarre example. She heard on a TV show sunshine was terrible for you, so she locked herself in the house (not literally) but was going insane being cooped up inside. That's when she appeared at my house. I saw her rational thinking waning. She said the kids (my five siblings) don't come home because they don't have their Mama anymore. When I questioned her further, she said, "I am not the same. They know it, and I know it. They don't like it." I, of course, assured her that wasn't the case. Sadly, for the first time, she used the terms Alzheimer's and dementia when she referred to herself. This made me wonder how often fear and anxiety overtook her while she was home alone for hours on end. The sudden realization this may not be just a slight bump in the road had just become quite clear.

I attempted to take Mama to her family practitioner, but she refused to see him for this memory problem. I explained we needed to get a prescription from the doctor for Aricept; she insisted she wanted to see someone else, a specialist in this area. I decided to look into getting Mama some post-traumatic counseling (she actually had requested this in the fall). I felt we both could benefit from some professional help. Little did I know, how many more years we would travel through this foreign land and how difficult the navigation proved to be for both of us.

I took Mama to get her annual diagnostic tests ordered by her internist, including an MRI at the hospital. During the procedure, she experienced heart palpitations and a terrible headache. After the MRI, they took her to the ER for an EKG. The EKG was normal, but Mama's enzymes were elevated, a possible indication of a heart attack. The results of the MRI showed reduced flow in the blood vessels in the back of the neck. They wanted to biopsy the large flesh-colored mole on her left temple. Upon the completion of the tests, we walked down the hallway, and suddenly Mama clutched her chest and said she felt pain. Mama had never had any heart condition before this moment.

The doctors admitted her to the hospital for several days and they diagnosed her with bundle branch block. Two of her three arteries were more than 50% blocked.

I promise you I have never witnessed my mother be so confused and out of sorts as she was during her hospital stay. As I dealt with the child-like shenanigans Mama displayed, I was robbed of the ability to fully comprehend her new diagnosis. I do recall thinking, *Geez, both parents with heart problems. The scoreboard was not looking good team.* She ignored my request to get in a gown; but on day three, I succeeded and took a victory lap around the battleground. Mama did not want to take a shower. "I'll take one when I get home," she retorted while baring her teeth. When a kitchen staffer delivered a meal Mama angrily dismissed this innocent bystander from her presence. Mama summoned the nurse by screaming, demanding immediate action, instead of simply pushing the call button. When admitted through the emergency room, the protocol requires inserting an IV. She tried in vain to rip the tape off, justifying her actions with every tug of the tape. Her outbursts were quite embarrassing and absolutely exhausting. I felt the need to pull my long hair over my reddened face and just disappear.

I had never witnessed Mama behave in this manner. Imagine three days in a 12 x 14 hospital room with an unwilling, incorrigible, nearly 80-year-old displaying the worst rants I had ever seen. If the nurse's station had a "Naughty List," Norma Jean would have made the top of that list! Mama tried multiple times to "break out of jail." A nurse explained to her if she left without being discharged, insurance would not pay the hospital bill. Knowing that Mama was financially savvy, I took for granted she might comply. Strike one! "You don't know what you're talking about!" She was hotter than a firecracker. The nurse, staring into the eyes of a fearless lunchroom bully (played by my mother), quickly exited the room in disbelief. This battle was above her pay grade.

The nurses recruited two of Mama's male physicians for backup and they came in to reiterate what the nurses had already explained to her. Knowing how frugal Mama was, I was certain this two-man tag team had the expertise to give her an attitude adjustment.

Strike 2! No, it exacerbated the problem. Everyone on the fourth floor heard about her tirade. Much to our surprise and relief, the following day, she was released to go home. I assume the staff raised the white flag, but my concern for her mental health only deepened.

We saw the doctor for a check-up after her hospital stay and he reassured Mama everything looked promising. She found a sense of peace with the news and readied herself for the next major test. Mama went in for a nuclear stress test and the results were normal. Mama said she was going back to living her everyday life. She had such peace of mind and was in good spirits.

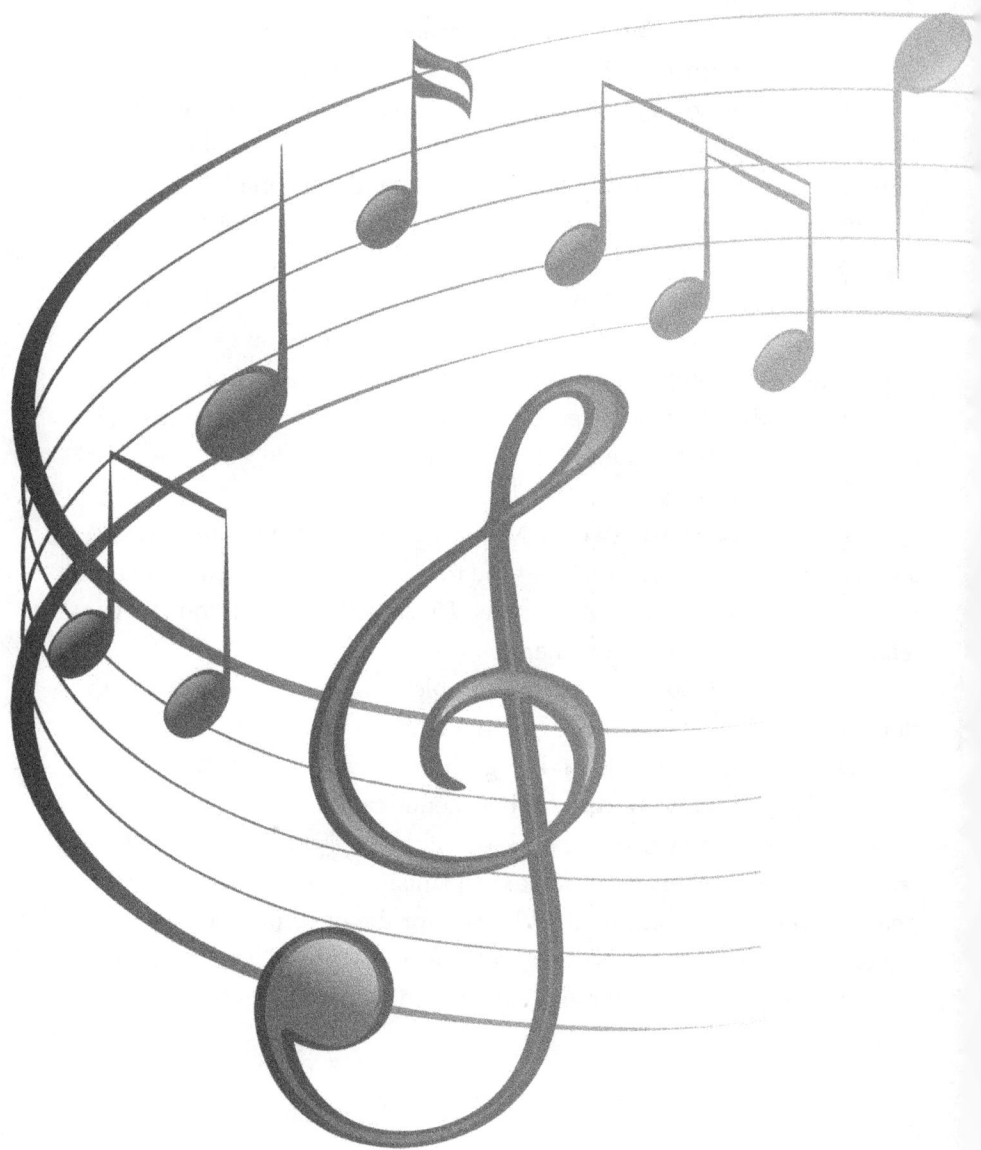

## CHAPTER 6
# DANCING GENES

Mama, her three sisters, my oldest sister, my cousin, and I all visited my Uncle Harris in the VA (Veteran's Association) nursing home. He also had Alzheimer's. The facility invited a Cajun band to perform that day, so we hit the dance floor. Mama's family grew up listening to the music on the radio and dancing in their living room. We continued that tradition as children when our aunts and uncles circled around us on Sunday afternoons. They played some of their favorite music like Zydeco and Cajun tunes while they tossed coins on the floor to encourage all the children to participate.

I sat with my uncle during a break from dancing and noticed the progression of his disease since the time he had briefly lived with my mother. He was funny, flirty, but trying in vain to put the pieces of the family puzzle together in his mind. It wasn't until I told him my dad was Billy that his eyes lit up and a smirk crossed his lips.

---

I am amazed at what triggers memories in this population. It might be children, music, a voice, a story, a color, an aroma, or food. There is no rhyme or reason.

---

Uncle Harris and I watched with delight his sisters two-stepping on the dance floor. It was an afternoon full of memories for me of a time when Mama embraced life wholeheartedly.

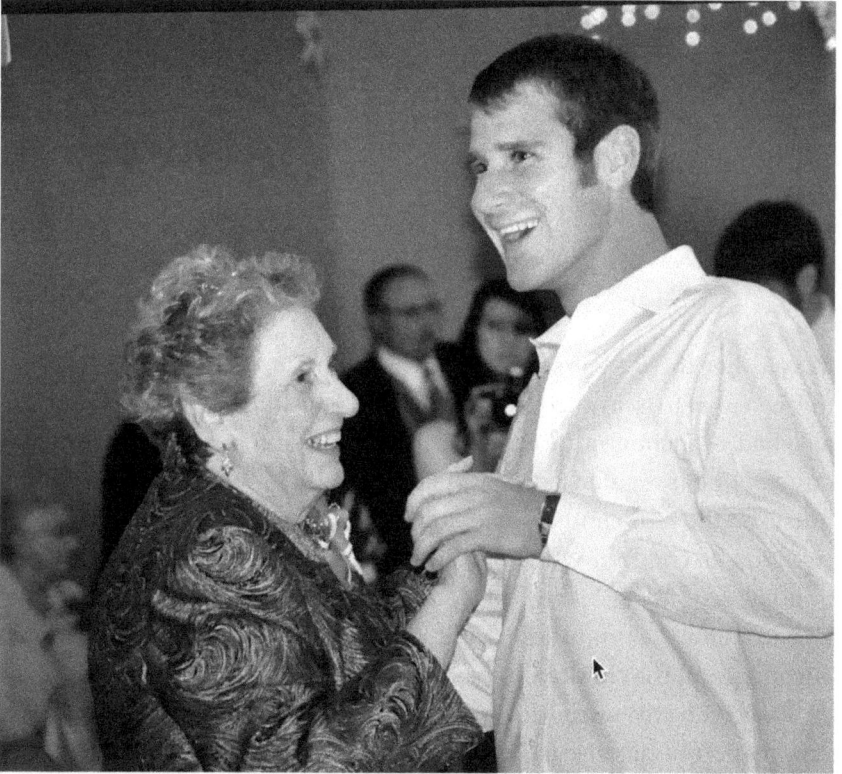

Mama with her grandson, Brett

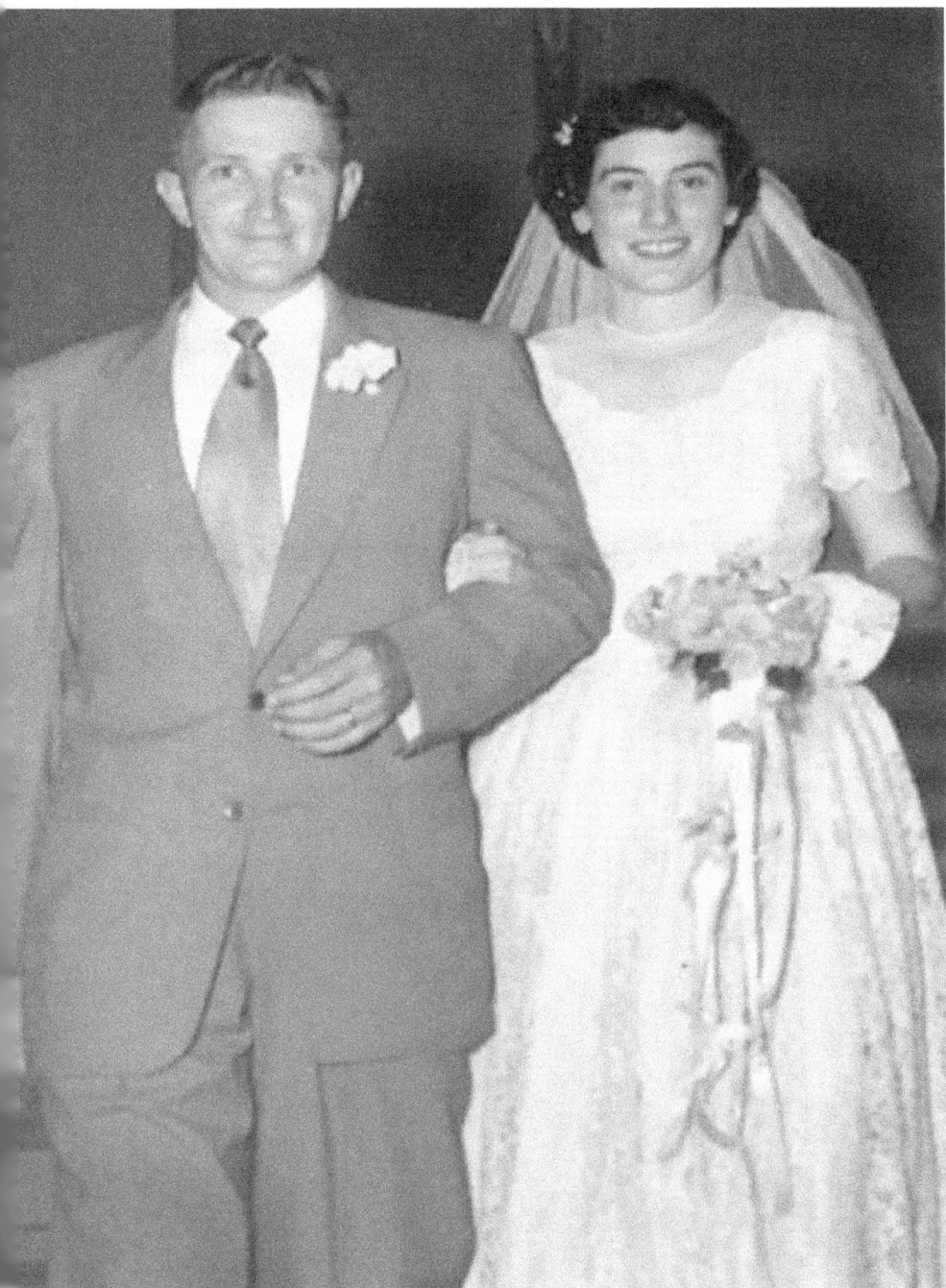

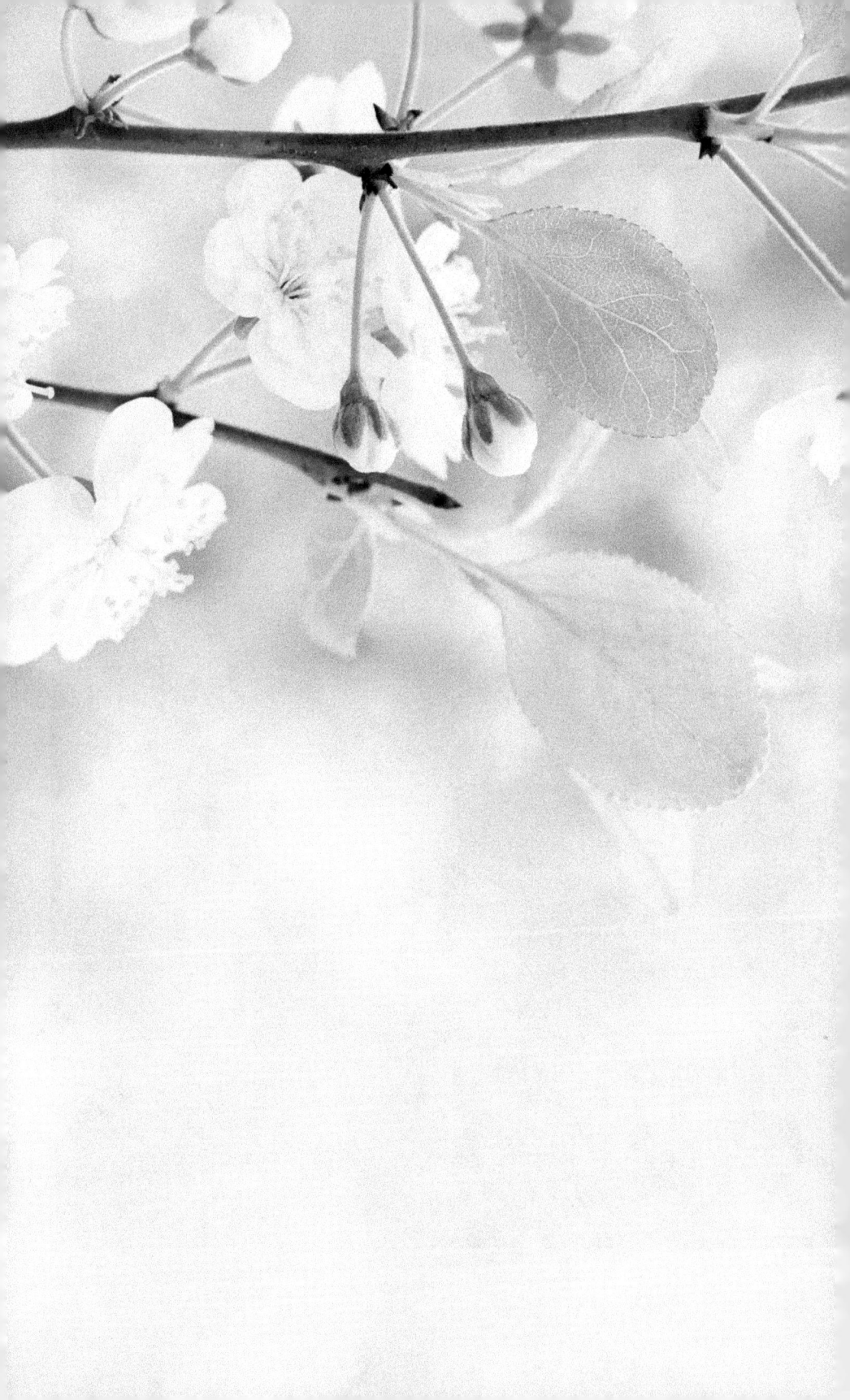

# CHAPTER 7
# HANDING OVER THE REINS

ON MY ROUTINE three-minute drive to Mama's house, I retrieved mail from her mailbox before I ventured inside to visit her. I noted a bright, yellow sticker slapped across the front of an envelope. Yep! I knew it wasn't going to be good. I teasingly hoped for that coveted title of the Publisher's Clearing House winner, but no, it was not to be. Instead, it screamed from the neon label, "Insufficient Funds."

An oversight dealing with anything financial ordinarily never happened, but after the recent insufficient funds letter, I became aware I needed to play a more active role in Mama's finances. I knew Mama was expecting a check for nearly $1,000 but she had not mentioned receiving it. I phoned the company sending it, and they verified the office had mailed the check two weeks earlier. The next time Mama came to my house, I told her she needed to confirm the delivery. She was flustered and didn't know anything about said check. She planned to look through her records when she arrived home; everything was fine if I didn't hear from her.

She was back at my house less than ten minutes after leaving with her checkbook in her hand. Mama couldn't find the deposit listed in her checkbook register (used to record financial transactions of deposits or checks). She asked me to look, and I quickly realized all deposits were unaccounted for, every last one of them! She seemed mortified. I called the bank to check their records, and found out Mama had deposited the funds. We were very relieved. I told Mama if she ever wanted me to take over her bills, I was happy to help her. Without hesitation she said, "Here, have at it!" I told her I didn't want to take away her independence, and she said, "Oh, I'm so over that!" We went to her bank and put my name on the account. I transferred all her bills to my address and began paying them. To quote Cathy, my sister, "Mama should only receive birthday cards in the mail." Mama's shoulders relaxed slightly as though I had lifted a heavy burden. She had wanted to ask for my assistance for a while but didn't want it to be an imposition.

Mama was extremely confused with mail and didn't understand the distinction between junk mail and regular mail. She got flustered easily. Her bills came directly to my address, but she didn't remember they did. She had three more past-due accounts because she forgot to give me the quarterly bill. We quickly took care of all of those issues.

Both of my parents were ultra-organized and meticulous in their record-keeping. For example, when we sold Mama's house, we found a black, tin box that held all the canceled checks back to at least 1960. It was interesting to learn what my parents paid for a car, vacations, or furniture still in use today. These documents were historically and sentimentally valuable to me, and I have been unable to part with the box's contents. The meticulous part of my mother's mind was slipping away. A little tin box contained the evidence and reminders of the woman she was before the hurricane.

⌦⌫

After being promoted to my mother's personal Accounts Payable department, I talked to Mama about her next move: assisted living. I wondered if she had heard friends speak of such a facility in our home-town. She responded, "Yes." Mama wanted to ensure they had activities and not just lounge around watching TV. A sedentary lifestyle was unthinkable for this mother of mine.

I made Mama aware she had the freedom and funds to indulge in anything her heart desired, be it a necessity or luxury. (I was secretly hoping to replace her broken couch.) Her response caught me off guard. "Oh, by the way, I know what I want to buy. I want to get the newspaper." Her simplicity and contentment never ceased to amaze me. It is truly the simple things in life that brought her joy.

I mentioned to Mama the possibility of my family moving to her home, and she said she didn't want me to be apart from my family. I responded, "Oh no, Mama, I mean all of us." She lowered her chin and said in a disappointed tone, "Ohhh." Yeah, let that one sink in. Mama grabbed her purse after an hour, and while we walked to the car, she said, "You know what you need to look for? One of those houses with the thingy." I said, "Mother-in-law houses?" "Yeah! I like that idea." With that off her chest, she drove away.

About an hour later, she called me to say she wanted to delve deeper into what we had discussed. I needed to return her call since I was busy at the time. When she picked up the receiver, she said without hesitation, "Hey, about the assisted living place in town. I wanted to ensure you knew I wasn't ready to move until after Christmas!!!" I said, "Oh no, Mama. I am talking years down the road when you can't care for yourself anymore." She reiterated, "I wanted you to know I planned to stay here until after the holidays," which was only three weeks away.

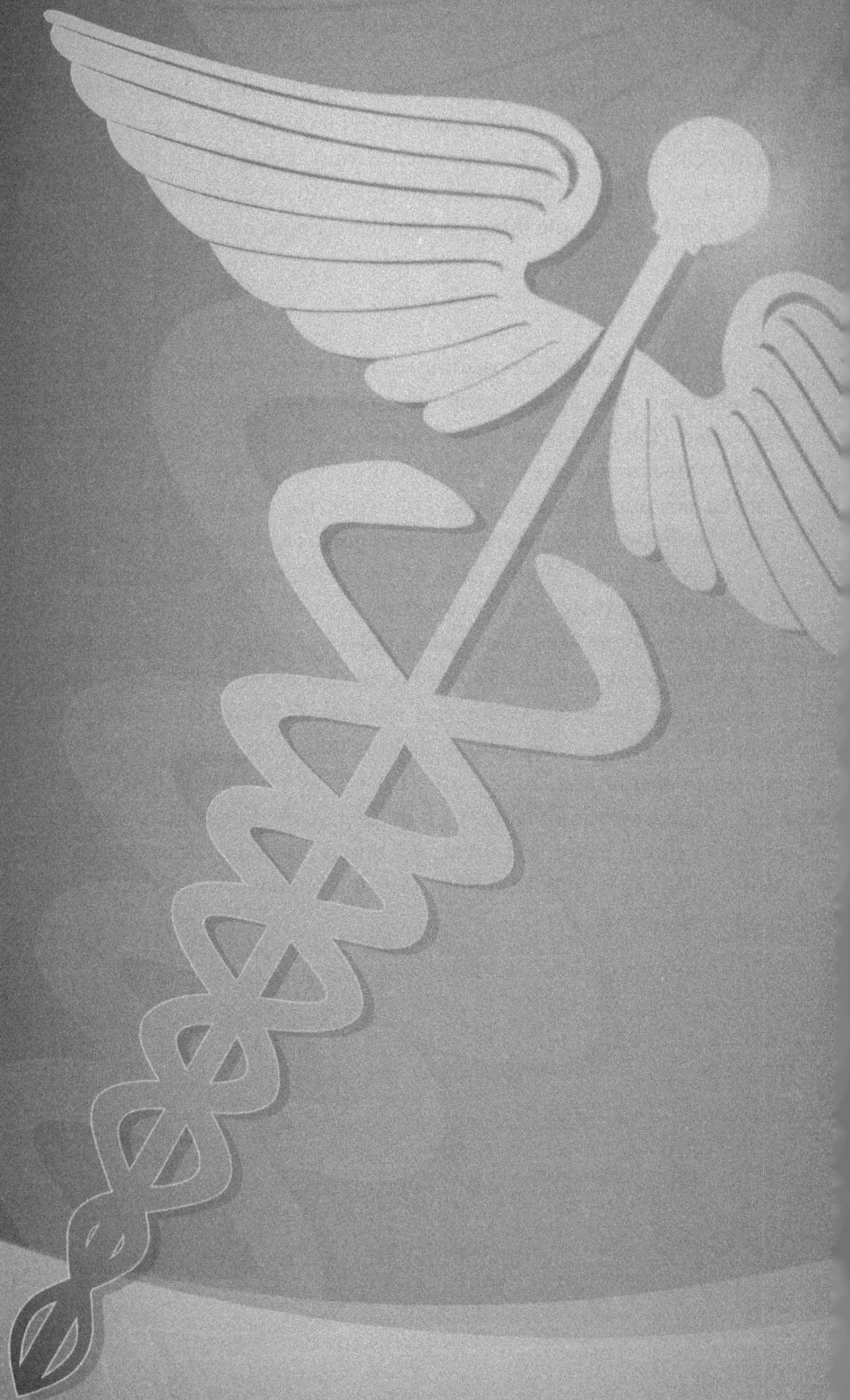

# CHAPTER 8
# IMPERATIVE TESTS

THE INSURANCE AGENCY phoned my mother and needed her to have a physical before they renewed her automobile policy. Mama dropped the forms off at her family practitioner's office, and a few days later, she went in to see her doctor. Immediately after the appointment, she drove to my house, clearly in shock. The doctor had completed the physical, but had taken it upon himself to call the geriatric doctor we saw last December. The geriatric doctor was questioned as to why he prescribed Aricept to Mama in the first place. Neither doctor was aware Mama had not even begun taking Aricept.

The geriatric doctor reported to the family doctor she could no longer drive alone. She needed to have a licensed driver accompany her. The family doctor wrote that quote on the insurance form. I was upset because the geriatric doctor had only met Mama once, and that was last year. I felt her family doctor was putting too much stock into what this man said.

I called Mama's doctor to see why he even called the geriatric doctor. Not getting to speak to him on the phone, I made an appointment with him to discuss Mama in person and at length. Meanwhile, Mama was slightly aggravated, depressed, and in denial; you get the picture?

I met privately with Mama's doctor, and he asked if the other doctor had ordered any testing to determine if Mama had Alzheimer's. *Why hadn't he asked the doctor himself, I wondered?* I told him about the card games and math and history questions that were part of the testing. He abruptly interrupted me and said, "NO! I mean MRIs of the brain!" There had been no mention of an MRI from the geriatric doctor. Oddly enough, he had, however, requested a biopsy of her brain, but I refused. Mama's family doctor was miffed at the other doctor because, and I quote,

---

**"You cannot diagnose someone with Alzheimer's unless you have an MRI of the brain. Secondly, you shouldn't prescribe Aricept if unsure of the patient's diagnosis.**

---

He said Mama may have three or four other problems that can be determined with an MRI. One he mentioned was normal pressure hydrocephalus or NPH. It's a treatable cause of dementia which is rare but possible, given her lack of balance. It's typically diagnosed with a CAT scan of the brain, but an MRI might be helpful. I asked if another geriatric doctor was in town, and he said, "No." *What were we supposed to do now?*

Long story short, Mama was never supposed to go to the doctor with the insurance form. It was for HER to fill out. Ugh! The agent said we didn't need a letter from the doctor.

Sure enough, Mama's family practitioner signed off on it at the bottom of the form, where it says DRIVER'S SIGNATURE *(Hello!!)*

I acquired a new form, filled it out, Mama signed it, and off it went. Mama was relieved. A month of stress for nothing!

⦿⦿⦿

I decided to start from ground zero and take Mama to see a neurologist and have a brain MRI done. I was constantly telling Mama this might bite us in the butt. She might have advanced Alzheimer's and not be allowed to drive anymore, or she might have something worse and still not be permitted to drive. Hopefully, it is something the proper medication might help. Whatever IT is in her brain, it has progressed in the last year, especially during the past six months.

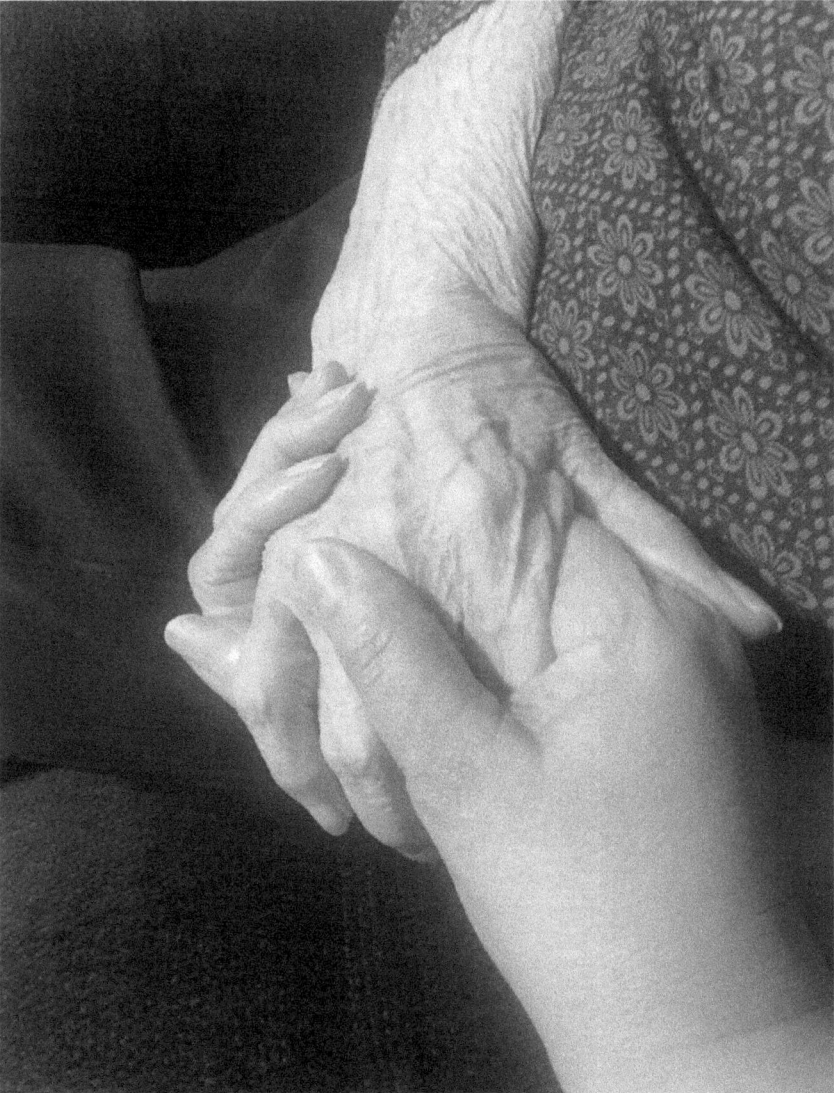

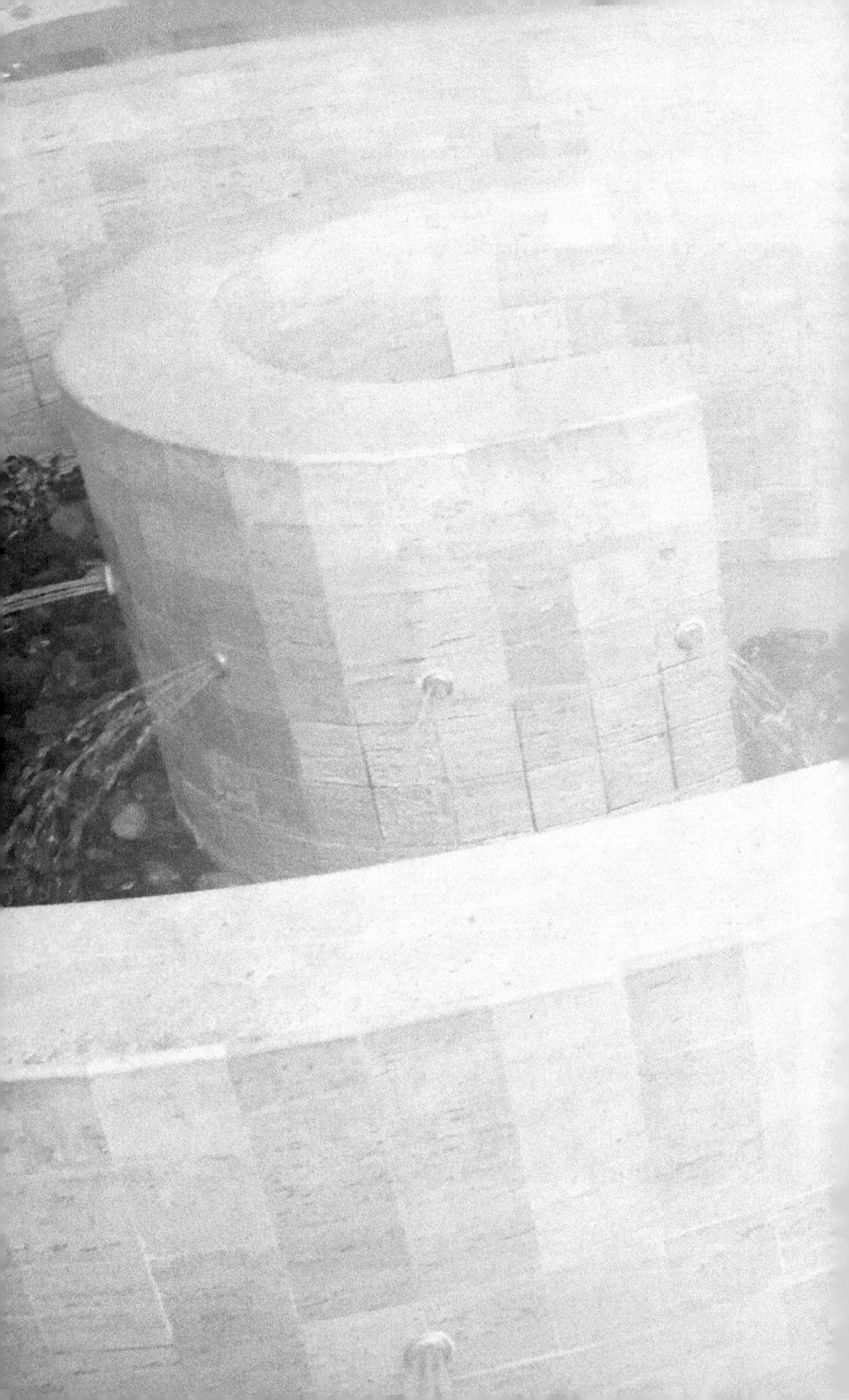

# CHAPTER 9
# THE MEDICAL MERRY-GO-ROUND

THE MRI TECHNICIANS had a difficult time keeping Mama still on the table for the test. If you have not had an MRI, it is imperative you stay completely still, and they prefer you don't talk. Mama didn't understand the rules; imagine wrangling cats. Oh, my goodness, she was a force to be reckoned with. I remember us both crying on the way home while we held hands. I called Mama's new neurologist Friday to see if they had test results.The hullabaloo was worth it; we got noteworthy results from the MRI. The nurse said they did get the MRI results, but were still waiting on lab tests to return.

The brain MRI #1 showed Mama had experienced seven TIA's (mini-strokes) and had vascular dementia. The doctor explained Mama did not presently have Alzheimer's; however, vascular dementia eventually turns into Alzheimer's. Her actions and her memory loss were clear indicators of the changes. He encouraged her to begin Aricept to prevent further memory loss and because I had researched the drug after the geriatric doctor mentioned it, I agreed.

My mother was thrilled because all she heard was what she wanted to hear-no Alzheimer's! She was jumping up and down and even kissed the doctor on the cheek.

Even though she was diagnosed with TIA's, she was happy she was not diagnosed with the "A" word.

After the diagnosis, Mama was doing better emotionally. At her request, we went to the local gym to sign up for a membership. We worked the machines and Mama was like a kid in a candy store. What a sight. She loved using the equipment. Thrilled and eager to go three times a week, it was great to see Mama happier. Mama informed me she wanted to start traveling again, wanted her teeth whitened, and to remove some moles. Talk about a new lease on life.

<hr />

It turns out Mama was a master at disguising her newfound shortcomings. Early Alzheimer's is not always obvious to outsiders and because it dealt with her brain, I knew we needed to be 100% sure what exactly Mama had going on in that little noggin' of hers. I did visit with a second neurologist that had been recommended. He was rude and unsympathetic. He was harsh and rough with Mama, demanding she sit still, asking why she wasn't answering his questions, and many more derogatory comments. This doctor ordered me to, "Be quiet or leave the room." You may be wondering what prompted him to say such a thing. Well, when Mama was posed with a question and wasn't able to answer, after a moment of awkward silence, I answered it for her; after all, weren't we there to find the root of her problem? We left the appointment early. No one should ever be treated in that manner; I even refused to pay the bill.

I brought Mama to a third neurologist. The first two neurologists had completely different ideas and I felt I needed another doctor to agree with one of them, something, anything.

He started evaluating Mama as soon as he came into the room by paying attention to her language skills while she and I talked and as he conversed with her. He told her that based on the one hour's worth of quizzes and paperwork she filled out and her ability to converse with him, he was pretty confident she may not have Alzheimer's. He said normally people who *definitely* have Alzheimer's have much lower conversational skills. He tended to agree with Mama her memory loss was due to the trauma of the hurricane. He even told her that was very insightful of her.

He began a touching test while her eyes were closed. He touched her lightly on the cheek, knee, or shoulder, and she had to say left knee, right shoulder, and so on. Sometimes, the doctor touched her in two places at the same time. After the third time, she stopped saying where he touched her, got frustrated, and just pointed to it. He said she showed fatigue, an early sign of Alzheimer's.

The doctor had her smile really big, and the right side of her mouth was more drawn. He pointed this out to me. He surmised that could mean she had suffered a mini-stroke (TIA) at some point, which had previously been confirmed.

He performed strength tests and her right side was significantly weaker than her left. She did not realize there was a difference. This weakness occurred in both the arm and the hand.

The doctor performed reflex tests, and when he got to her feet, she didn't feel warmth or cold on one foot, while on the other foot, she only felt vibrations in her toe. He said this might be a peripheral nervous system issue.

Mama told the doctor about the mole in her temple area and the pain she felt below it. He said it might be temporal arteritis, which is an inflammatory auto-immune disease of large blood vessels.

He checked Mama's balance. Sitting down, she was fine. When she stood and closed her eyes, she immediately swayed back and to the right. He repeated the test several times. Also, to check her balance, she sat down, closed her eyes, held her arms straight out, and counted to ten. Her left arm went five inches below her right arm. Again, he repeated the test. I asked him about her ability to drive. He said that based on what he saw in her paperwork and exam, he saw no reason why she couldn't continue driving.

The doctor advised staying on Aricept, emphasizing if a patient discontinued the medication, their memory may never be as good, even with just a brief six-week interruption. He said Mama might have a B-12 deficiency because of the foot issue. Shots, not pills, remedy that. He is also testing to see if she produces a protein against herself.

He suggested a nerve conduction test (because of the results of her foot test.)

Mama worded responses cleverly on the verb and cognitive tests and could pass more tests than she should basically because she started joking around with the doctor. Her humor was a powerful deterrent to the real issue at hand. She was a people person and loved to joke around. Simply irresistible. Mama fooled many people with the way she worded her questions and responses during conversations. It was a wonderful, hilarious gift. She was quite the entertainer.

This neurologist told Mama her humor was the highest form of intelligence, and he said he could tell she was an intelligent lady. He shared with us the tricky thing about intelligent people is they can fool you until the condition is bad. He told Mama she may have been brilliant and he may be missing Alzheimer's because he doesn't have a baseline of intellect to go on. You can imagine how great that made Mama feel.

He wanted to do an EMG, a test that measures muscle response or electrical activity in response to a nerve's stimulation of the muscle. We did a brain MRI #2 today. It will show if she had additional strokes and also if she has Alzheimer's.

What a day! My head is spinning. We left at 7:30 and returned home at 2:30. Exhausted puppies but happy. Mama was delighted with this doctor. It was a different experience from the geriatric doctor and the other two neurologists. We stayed in the exam room with him for over an hour, and it wasn't fluff. He was constantly monitoring her.

We received results on brain MRI #2. It appears on the MRI she had at least eight mini-strokes now. One more since the last test. It does not show she has Alzheimer's. Her liver, thyroid, SED rate, and blood vessels are normal. The doctor feels her memory problems are from mini-strokes and post-traumatic stress from the hurricane. He instructed Mama to stay on Aricept, start taking aspirin daily, and SHE CAN DRIVE.

Needless to say, Mama was elated! I had brought some pom poms to work on in the waiting room for my girls to use when they were cheerleading. They happened to match Mama's green and navy outfit.

When we exited the building, she grabbed the pom poms from me and started cheering. She was adorable.

Mama had a neurology appointment with a fourth doctor. I know it sounds absurd, but this was my Mama and the issue was her brain. This disease had long-term effects and I wanted to be well prepared for what we were looking at in the future.

I don't know if this latest doctor was the sharpest tool in the box. He asked Mama several times what she wanted from him. The doctor ordered me not to talk until spoken to. I wanted to scream, "She has four new symptoms, IDIOT." Things have changed since we saw the last doctor. He began doing a basic diagnostic test, including reflexes, walking, eyes, ears, and balance. Then he told her to have the following tests:

- EEG of the brain
- VNG – a test for dizziness. VNG determines if you have a disorder in the vestibular system (the balance structures in your inner ear) or the part of the brain that controls balance.
- DRIVING TEST - Here's what the idiot said to me in front of Mama. "I don't want to be on the defendant's stand when she **kills** eight people because I said she was okay to drive!" Mama was livid!!!
- BABY ASPIRIN - at least 2 or 3 times a week. He didn't care it gave her bloody noses. He retorted, "Take the damn thing, or you'll have a heart attack or stroke!"
- SLEEP STUDY – He surmised Mama's temple headaches were tension headaches, more than likely, and she was probably a tooth grinder at night. Poor Mama rubbed her head the entire conversation.
- NEUROPSYCH TEST takes three days, several hours a day. He suspected she could have dementia or pseudo-dementia, depression that looked like dementia. This testing shows precisely what memory problems she was experiencing. Dementia, depression, may be the beginning of Alzheimer's, or other problems. Unlike MRI scans, which show the brain's structure, neuro-psych testing examines how well the brain

works when it performs certain functions (for example, remembering). Impairment in many of these functions may exist because of brain abnormalities that cannot be detected on CT or MRI scans.

- BLOOD WORK
- DERMATOLOGY - lastly see the doctor to get the mole removed and send it off to the lab.

Mama was very depressed, as was I, so I stayed with her for a while when I brought her home. I called the driving test site in Lafayette to see what the tests entailed, but they were closed.

I went back to my house and Mama called me an hour later. She said to forget everything the doctor said. She refused all of the tests especially the driving test. She felt like driving in a large, bustling, unfamiliar city (Lafayette) was a prescription for failure. I honestly got turned around there myself.

Anyway, what a day! The doctor didn't think the temple pain and vision loss were connected. He couldn't tell me what caused her burning, tingling sensation. Mama whispered to me in the office, "IT" happened again." So there!

After the appointment, suffice it to say we felt as though Doctor #3 was the winner. The other three were not ever going to be recommended by me to anyone.

There were more frequent signs of memory issues and changes in her behavior, so I revisited some hard conversations with Mama about her living alone. I offered to let her come live with my family because we had two extra bedrooms. She frequented our home every afternoon and was very fond of my husband. With three of my four children still living at home, she thoroughly enjoyed engaging with them. She even took well to our furry friends. However, she quickly shut down my offer with this response: "I've lived alone for thirty years. I'm not about to live in a house with children." Well, alrighty then. I asked if she wanted to live with her sister. "No!" I brought up the new, popular assisted living facility in town again, and she raised her eyebrows, with a slight twinkle in her blue-grey eyes, she showed some genuine interest. Out of nowhere, she blurted out a confession: she and her sister had already gone on a facility tour. Okay, now we were getting somewhere. I was relieved it had been a positive experience.

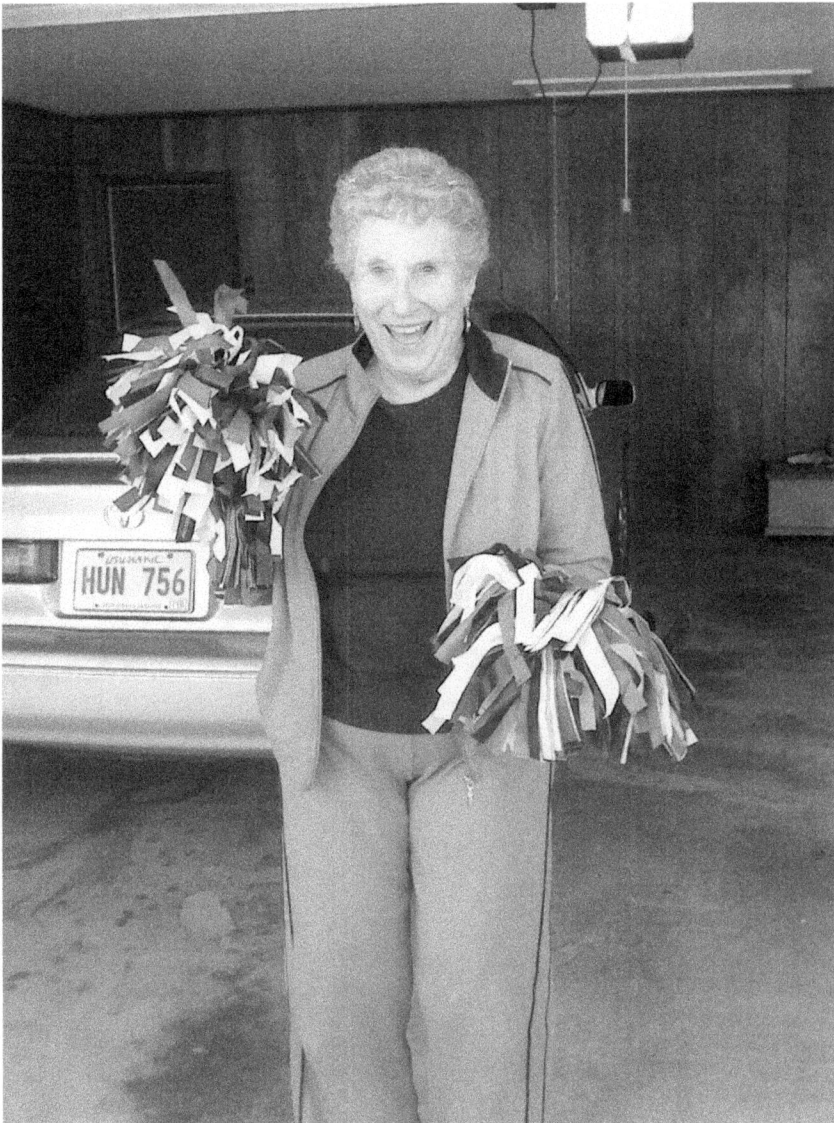

Meet my fun-loving mother.

# CHAPTER 10
# TEMPLE TESTING

MAMA and I went to see the family practitioner to get a referral to biopsy the mole on her temple. The doctor started from the beginning with his own examination and was not sure he agreed with the diagnosis of temporal arteritis (where the arteries, particularly those at the side of the head, the temples, become inflamed). Today, Mama also had terrible pain in the back of her head. Mama cried because her temple and the back of her head were hurting a great deal. She's one tough cookie and rarely cries with pain. Mama never even had headaches. She repeatedly asked me to get him to x-ray her brain—poor thing.

The family practitioner needed to make sure he treated the right problem, therefore, he ordered an MRI #3, as well as an MRA with contrast. The doctor felt she needed both tests, as the MRI creates images of the inside of the body, while the MRA zeroes in on the blood vessels. He also ordered a SED rate test to check for any inflammatory markers in the body. These blood test results eventually revealed temporal arteritis.

The doctor expressed his disagreement with the other doctors' findings regarding the warm and tingling sensations she had, emphasizing they were not indicative of a stroke. He had other patients who described the same exact phenomenon.

He said it could be TIA's or perhaps low blood pressure, low blood sugar, or tension. I told her doctor Mama had "an event" Friday night, and it only affected the arm and the leg. Armed with my additional information, his inclination began to lean heavily towards the possibility of a stroke. Mama was relieved someone was finally helping us and seemed to be on the ball. She burst out crying again.

⌐⋘◯⋙¬

During these months of testing, I tried to keep my photography business afloat but came to the realization, that I no longer was able to stretch myself that thin. I canceled all future photography bookings to concentrate on Mama. I finished all orders and temporarily closed the office. I made myself readily available, should Mama's health warrant my presence.

I quickly found myself regularly bringing Mama to her doctors' appointments: neurologist, podiatrist, dentist, ophthalmologist, internist, family doctor, physical therapist, and more. Oh, my goodness! Mama's favorite doctor was her ophthalmologist. When she had to lean into the equipment and place her chin on the bar, she waited until he rolled his chair closer and then either stuck out her tongue, blew him a kiss, or said, "Hey, good-looking!" She cracked me up every time. Cue the doc's blushing cheeks.

After the examination, he found the vision in her left eye was better, but her right eye was much worse. Even with the new glasses she received six months ago, she could only read the line under the big letter E on the wall chart. Her doctor made an appointment at Baylor in Houston with a neuro-ophthalmologist. Mama was eager to go because she did not want to lose her sight and license to drive.

⌐⋘◯⋙¬

I brought Mama to the hospital to sign release forms to get the film of her first MRI. When I arrived at her house, she was cutting the grass and turned off the mower when she spotted my car. It started thundering, so we walked inside. In casual conversation, Norma Jean proceeded to tell me her heart hurt all the time. She thought we were headed to see a cardiologist in Houston. I have no idea what brain cell that came out of but it was the beginning of many more discrepancies she shared in casual conversation.

I chose not to pursue the heart issue because nothing showed up on the EKG in the hospital when she wore the monitor. I haven't heard her speak of her head hurting in several days. I believe the aspirin a day has helped.

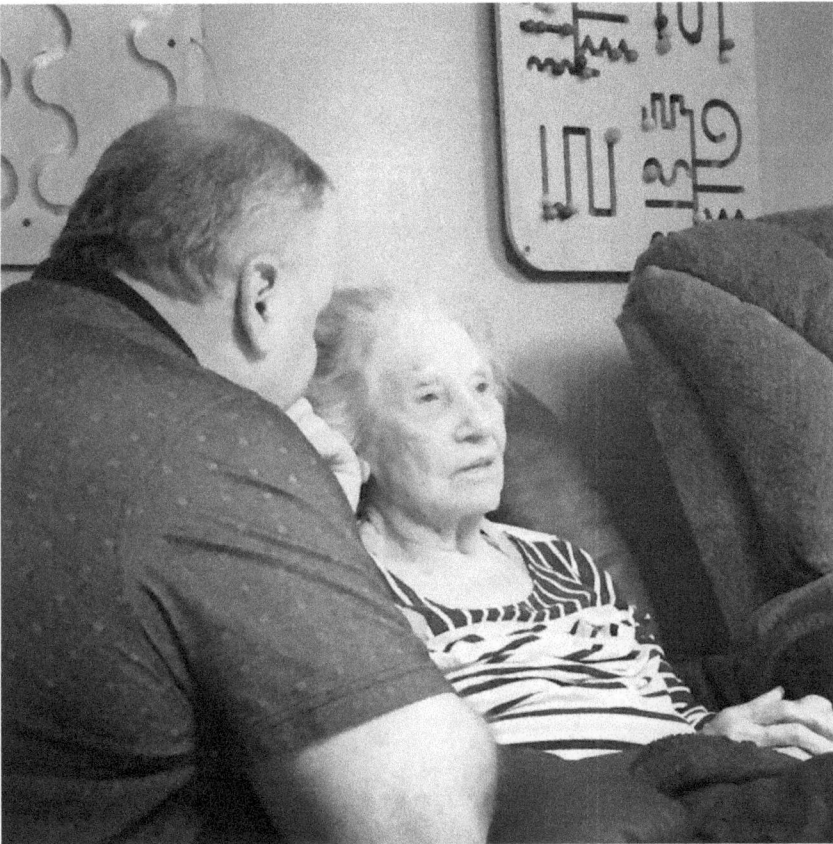

My husband loved Mama so well.

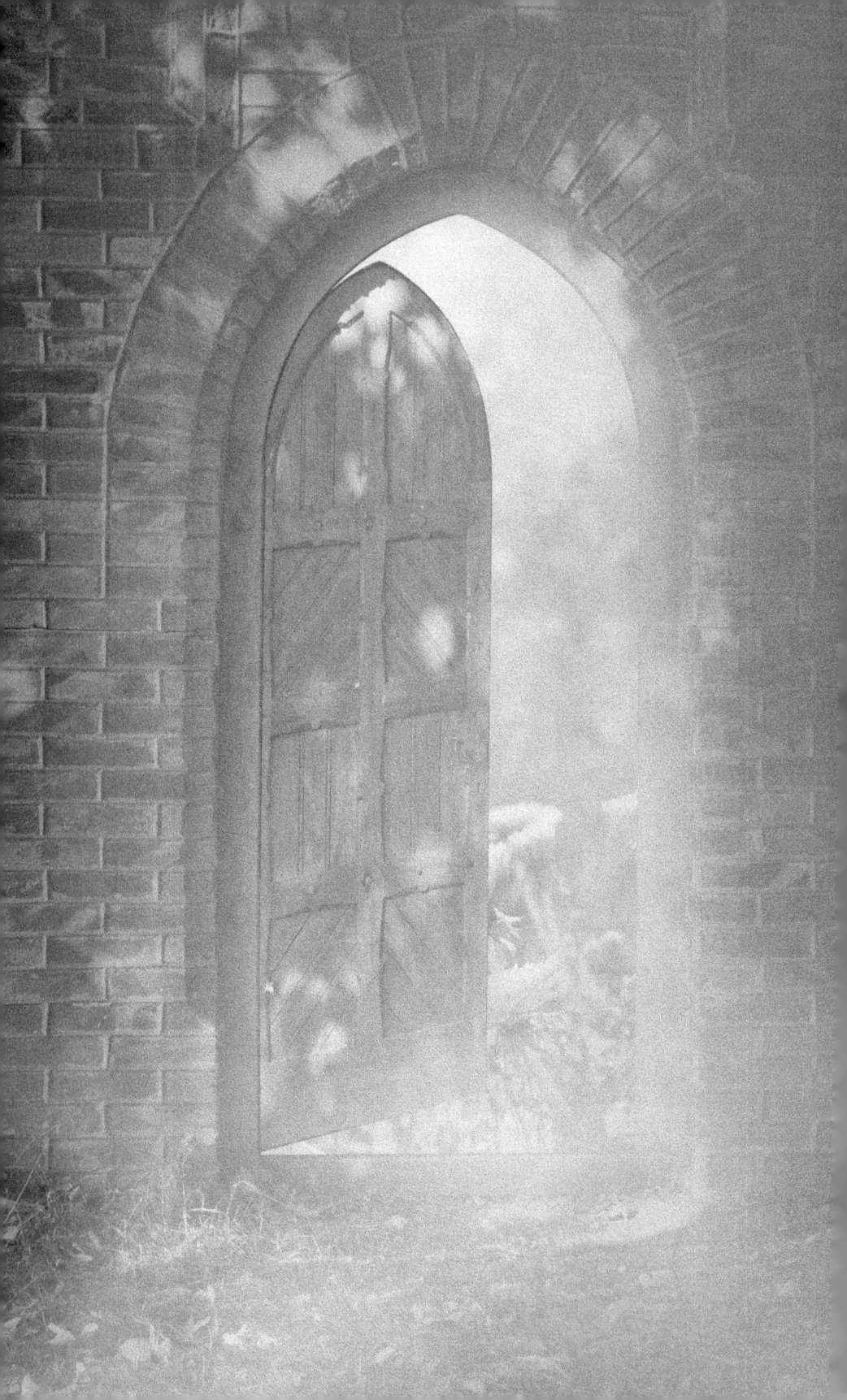

# CHAPTER 11

# PIVOTAL POINT

I RECEIVED a phone call from Mama, and she did not sound well. She was short of breath and sounded desperate. All she said was she needed me and James to come over NOW! Being the first call of this kind, we headed over immediately.

We entered her home and began calling out her name. We found her in the guest bathroom. She was pale and sweating profusely. She held a plunger in her right hand, and a myriad of towels were found in the tub, on the vanity, and all over the floor. She had chosen to use the guest bathroom, flushed, and water began coming up the drain in the bathtub. She retrieved a pitcher to collect the water and transfer the water to the toilet.

When she flushed the toilet, the water magically reappeared in the bathtub. It was an endless cycle, but it was all she knew to do. Just about the time the water went down in one place, it reappeared in the other—poor precious Mama. James jumped in and took over. He discovered the main sewage line outside had gotten plugged due to the roots of a nearby oak tree.

I took Mama to the living room, wiped her face, and brought her some cool washcloths for her face and neck. She confessed she had been fighting this monstrosity for hours.

Even now, the thought of her battling it alone makes me weep. She was a powerhouse and never a quitter. Never!

Once James had called a plumber, he joined us in the living room. Unbeknownst to us, this was the pivotal moment when Mama told us, in no uncertain terms, she was DONE with home maintenance and wanted to move into assisted living now! God works in mysterious ways, friends. I never believed the transition would occur under these circumstances. We stayed with her for a few hours, got her to rest, washed her towels, and cleaned the bathroom. When she woke from her nap, she wanted to sign up for an apartment at the assisted living facility. When Norma Jean made up her mind, well, it was done. No turning back.

Later that afternoon, the three of us drove over to the assisted living facility and met with the director. We took a tour of the facility and around every corner Mama seemed surprised and pleased, as if she had never seen the place before. Mama was very happy, and adamant she was ready to leave an independent, homeowner lifestyle.

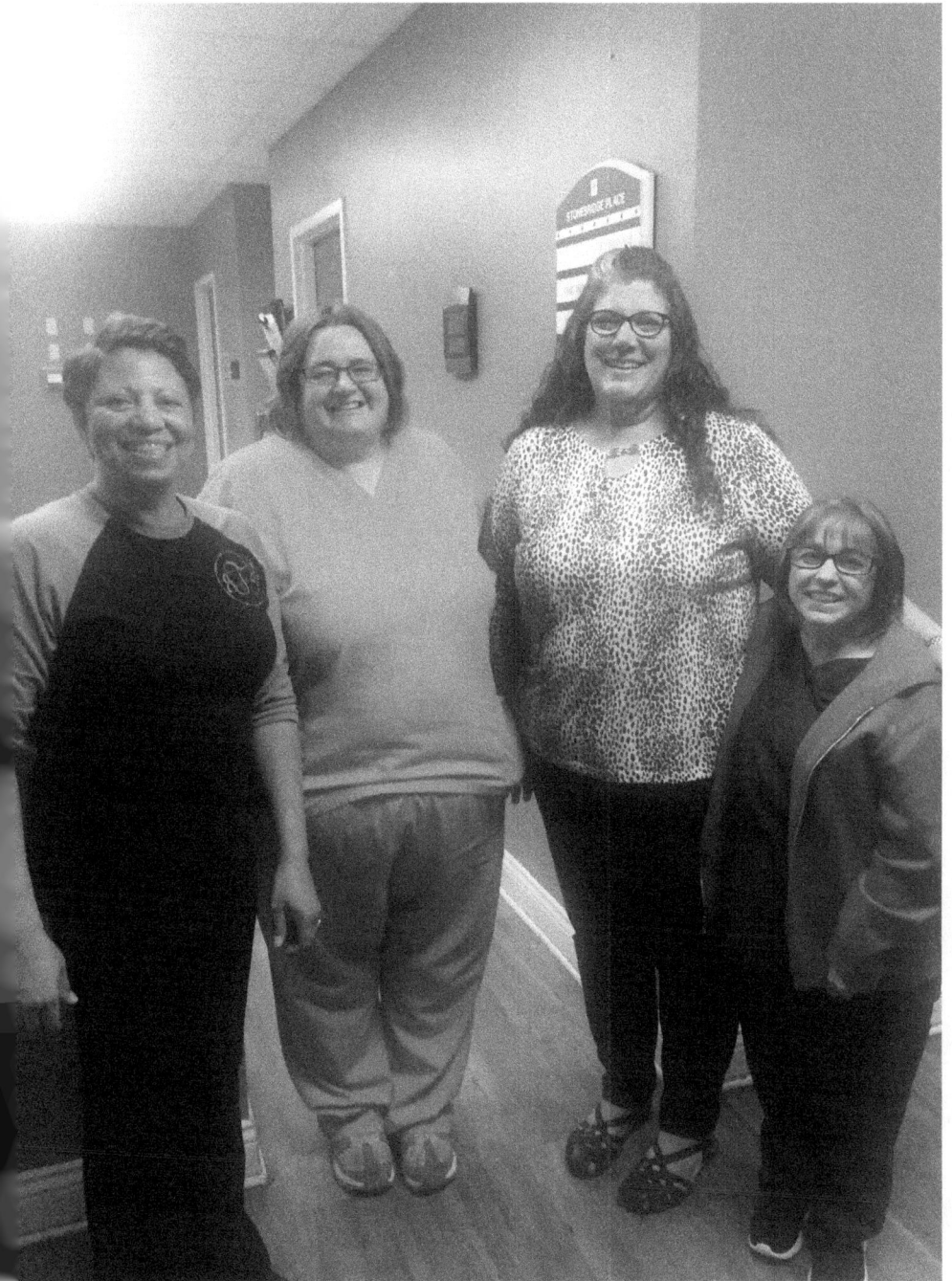

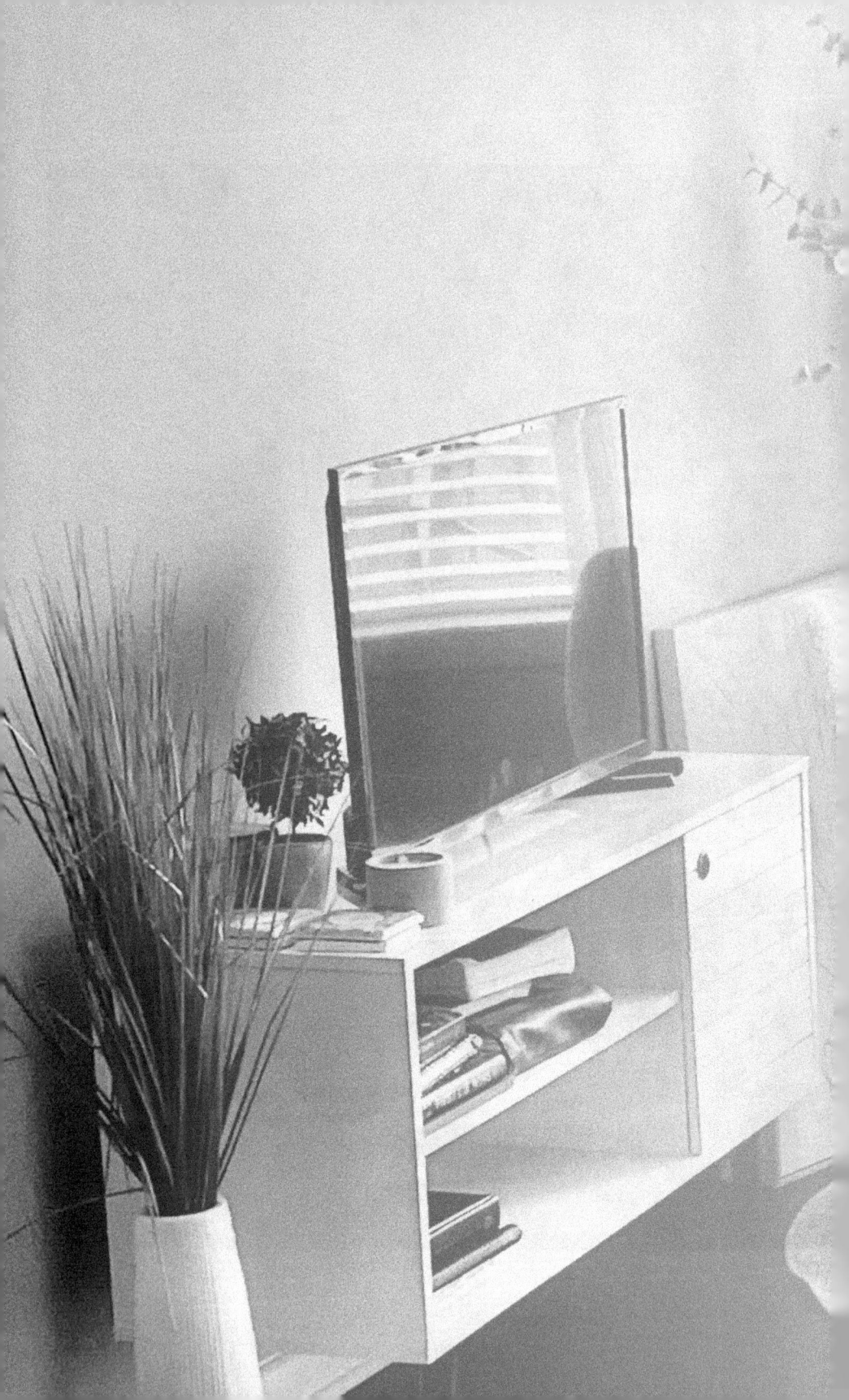

# CHAPTER 12
# NEW BEGINNINGS

CATHY, my sister, and Hannah, her daughter, were in town to assist us with moving Mama into Assisted Living. We brought them to tour the assisted living place and see Mama's new apartment. Mama was excited about the exercise room we passed as we walked in the front doors. She expressed her plan to put the equipment to good use.

As we walked through the back doors toward the gazebo, Mama was elated with the flower gardens and the gazebo awaiting her. Throughout the tour, Mama seemed delighted and was pleased to meet other residents as we strolled down the halls. Seeing some old friends thrilled her to no end. She was upbeat throughout the entire process. My sister said, "I don't know if she fully realizes how much her life will change." In hindsight, I was blindsided by how much this move, this disease, also changed my life.

I stayed with Mama all day since it was move-in day. At nearly 81 years old and with increasing memory issues, I was confident she appreciated some familiar company. I went with her to the dining room and met the ladies at her table and the kitchen staff. The staff attempted to match residents at each table based on their common bonds and personalities. After enjoying lunch, she returned to her new room, lay on her couch, and napped. After she awoke, I suggested we go downstairs to the cute ice cream/coffee shop.

Near the coffee shop was a beautiful sitting area around a fireplace. Decorated with ornate furniture, the setting consisted of two love seats and two plush chairs on either side of the fireplace. Mama perched herself in the chair to the right of the fireplace, which remained HER chair for five years. With a bird's eye view of the front door, the office, and the stairs, Mama loved sitting there because she saw almost everything going on. It didn't hurt she could be first in line for the meals since the dining room doors were within two feet of her chair.

This fireside chair was where she began meeting some of the staff as they stopped and introduced themselves. I loved they took the time to sit down and speak with her. Mama enjoyed all the attention. Two men, in particular, made fast friends with Mama. Ricky was the maintenance man and spoke French with her. Even with dementia, she was still fluent in her native French language. Ricky was quite the cut-up, as was my mother. This friendship lasted for a decade. He and Mama were always close, and I was confident he genuinely cared for her.

The other gentleman, Wesley, was the bus driver, assistant maintenance worker, and grounds keeper. He was quieter, but he and Mama bonded quickly. Not only did they share the same birthday, but she respected him immensely for his work ethic. They shared stories of their families, their love of gardening, and the latest happenings at "The Big House," which is the name we gave the assisted living facility. Mama moved into her apartment in August, and her first birthday in her new home was in November. Wesley could have taken that day off, but he chose to work to share their special birthday together. He continued to do that every year until she died (ten years later). *Who does that? Especially for someone with dementia who won't even remember your gesture?*

Wesley did, and I loved him all the more for it. Over the years, Wesley and I grew very close. He watched over Mama without being asked. I don't know if she was like a mother to him or a sister, but he doted on her every chance he got. Words cannot adequately express my gratitude to him.

**Take notice of all the special people caring for your loved one. You'll notice some go out of their way to bring a smile, or engage in conversation with them. Show them your appreciation.**

These two men, Ricky and Wesley, randomly let me know, they had checked on Mama, just to make sure she was adjusting well. For the first two or three months after Mama moved, I spent all day every weekday with her. I wanted to help her get acclimated to her new environment, and I was interested in meeting other residents, just like I enjoyed meeting her neighbors when she bought her new home.

I needed to keep abreast of any behavioral changes in Mama since this was a significant life-changing event.

**My time with Mama was also an excellent opportunity to build rapport with the staff.**

Overall, Mama seemed happy, but as I noticed how other residents set up their apartments, I made suggestions to Mama, hoping it might make her even more pleased with her new lifestyle. One such proposal was to leave her door open when she was in her apartment so others could drop by to visit her. She absolutely refused to try it. I walked with her down the hallways and pointed out those who used this methodology, but it totally turned her off. To this day, I don't know why.

Another suggestion was to sit in the different areas they offered to residents, i.e., the front porch outside or the large sitting areas midway down the hallways. Nope! She loved her fireside chair. Other residents stopped by and visited with her, so she found her own way to connect with people. Very slowly, she began to make new friends.

I attended daily Mass with Mama at her church and brought her back for the weekend Mass on Saturday afternoon, followed by dinner at her favorite restaurant. Some weeks my family joined us. It all depended on what kind of mood she was in that day. Every other Friday, I brought her to the same hairdresser she had used for nearly 40 years.

Numerous funny stories took place within those four walls. I saw first-hand what a character my mother was and enjoyed every minute of it.

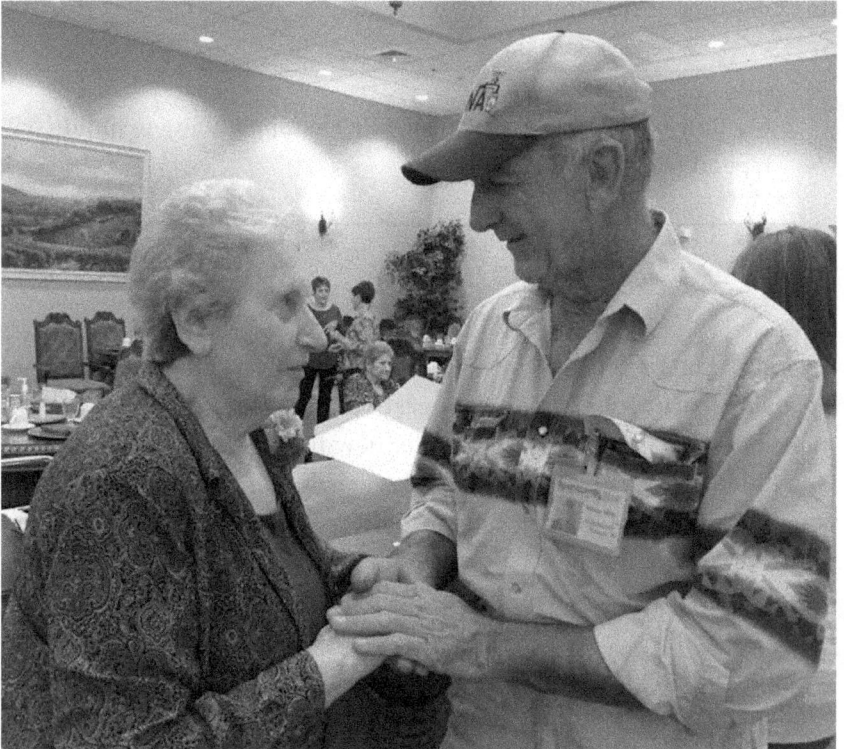

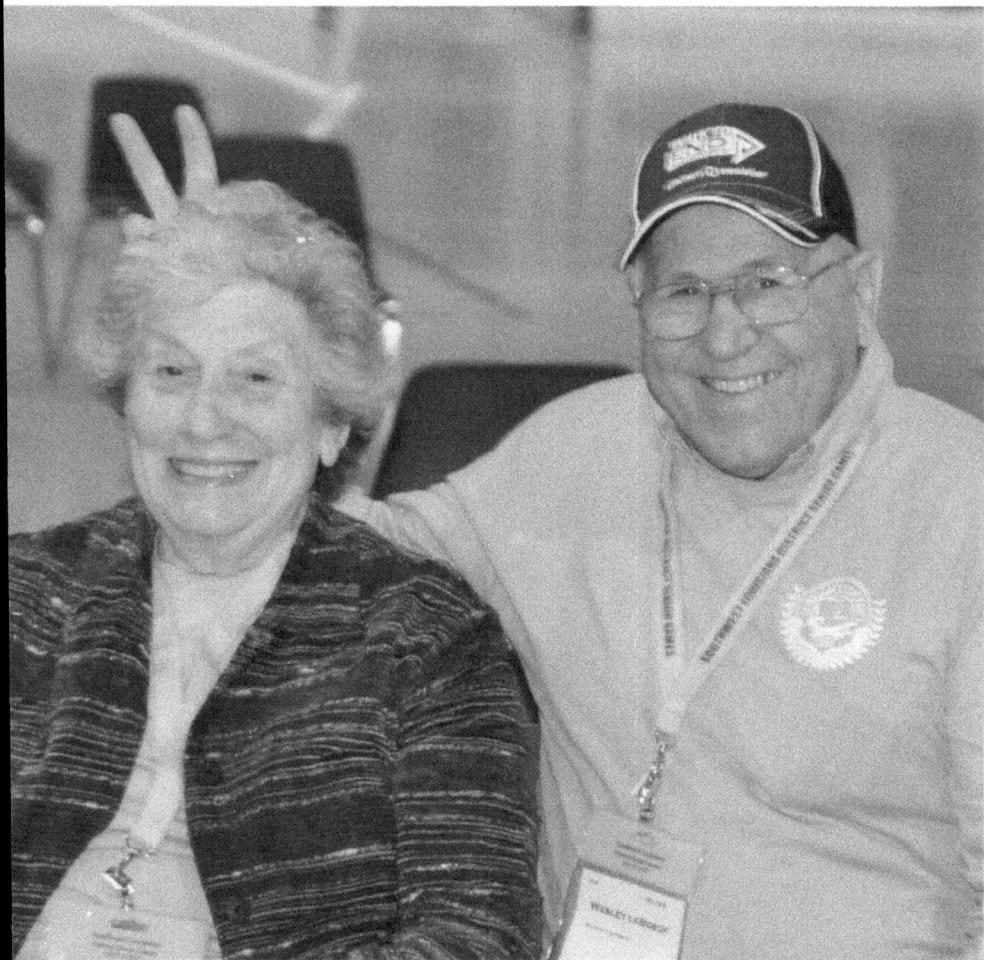

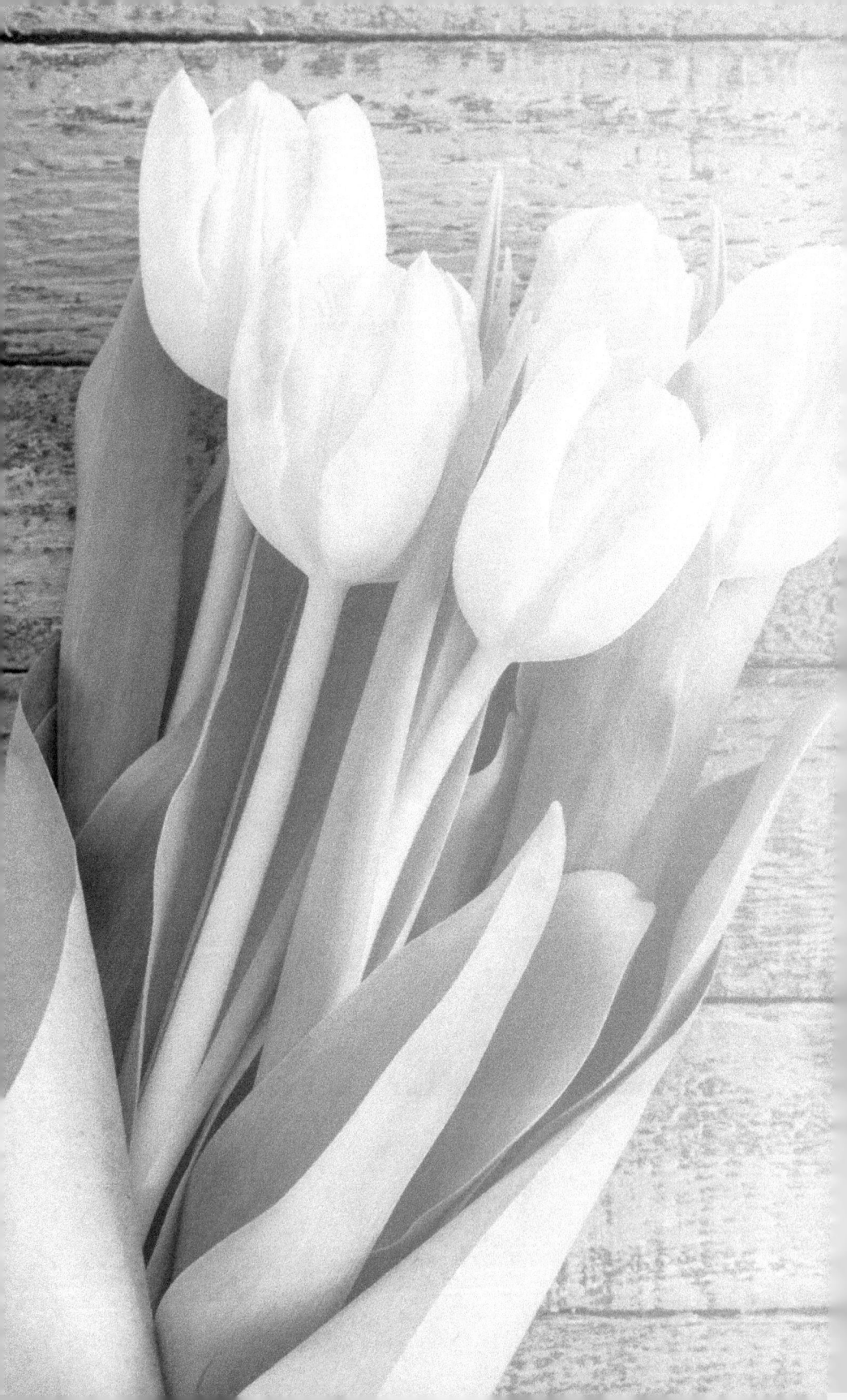

# CHAPTER 13
# PLOT TWISTS

AFTER MAMA MOVED into the Big House her overall status was good. She seemed to not be in any pain, i.e., hip, temple area, chest, etc. Not killing herself with yard work eased some of the pain. She seemed happy. However, after I returned home from a conference, I called her and she had been by her old house to "play" in the yard. She said she thought she wanted to go home. She missed her yard. I reminded her of the sewer issues and the loneliness. I also reminded her how much better she felt physically. I asked if anything was wrong at the assisted living facility, and she said, "No, I just miss my yard." I called one of my aunts, and she said Mama was unhappy and didn't want to tell me because she felt like we put her in the Big House.

With this new information, I called the facility's director and told her what Mama was thinking (about moving home), and she was shocked. She said Mama participated in everything, laughed, and cut up. Mama had numerous friends and never missed a meal. She asked if we had sold her house, and I said, "No." The director said, "That's the problem. It's unfinished business. She remains drawn to it as long as it's there." She planned to pull Mama into helping with the yard work at the facility. They had just begun to plant winter plants. I knew they didn't want to lose a good resident like Mama, and Mama was safer there with others keeping watch.

<hr/>

Mama's memory began to decline quickly. This is just one example and the first time it had ever happened. One morning, she called me about an answering machine issue. We discussed this in detail over the 20-minute conversation. She needed to go to the restroom, so we said our goodbyes. She called right back and started the same conversation as if we had never spoken. The time difference was less than five minutes. This was the first of its kind. There are more stories about her memory, but suffice it to say, it was worsening.

<hr/>

Lately, instead of introducing my daughters by their names or me, for that matter, she simply said, "This is my daughter and her girls." No names. Then she nudged me and said, "Tell them." The first time stung but, I can't lie, it continued to hurt every time it happened. She knew our names, but on the spot, she couldn't recall them.

<hr/>

Mama missed a luncheon with her siblings. Her sister called her around 11:00 and invited her to come over, and Mama gladly accepted the invitation. By noon, she had yet to arrive at the gathering. I called the facility, and Mama was eating in the dining room. She never made it to her sister's house. She totally forgot about the invitation. I drove over to visit Mama and asked her if she had seen her siblings. She said, "Yes, they came over to my place. The facility had a Siblings Day, and they all came." I said sarcastically, "Really?" I asked the secretary if they had a Siblings Day, and she said, "No, but her siblings did visit her." Similar incidents happened all the time, a prime example of her quick thinking to cover up overlooking some detail or conversation. I was thankful someone else helped me watch over her.

During one afternoon visit, Mama informed me she wanted to sell the house after the holidays. *GASP!* She was holding out hope that everyone would arrange their schedules to be home for Christmas; I informed my siblings if everyone came, we could pack up the house. I thought it was funny; the only thing Mama requested from the house since she moved seven or eight weeks before was her iron and ironing board and her croquet set. I thought that was pretty impressive.

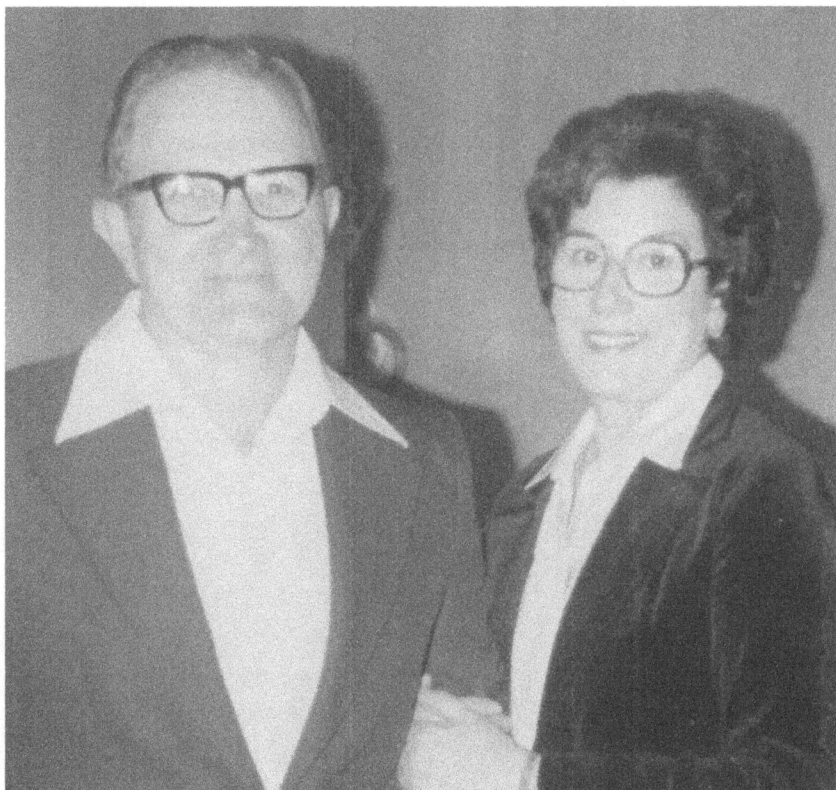

My parents on an anniversary date

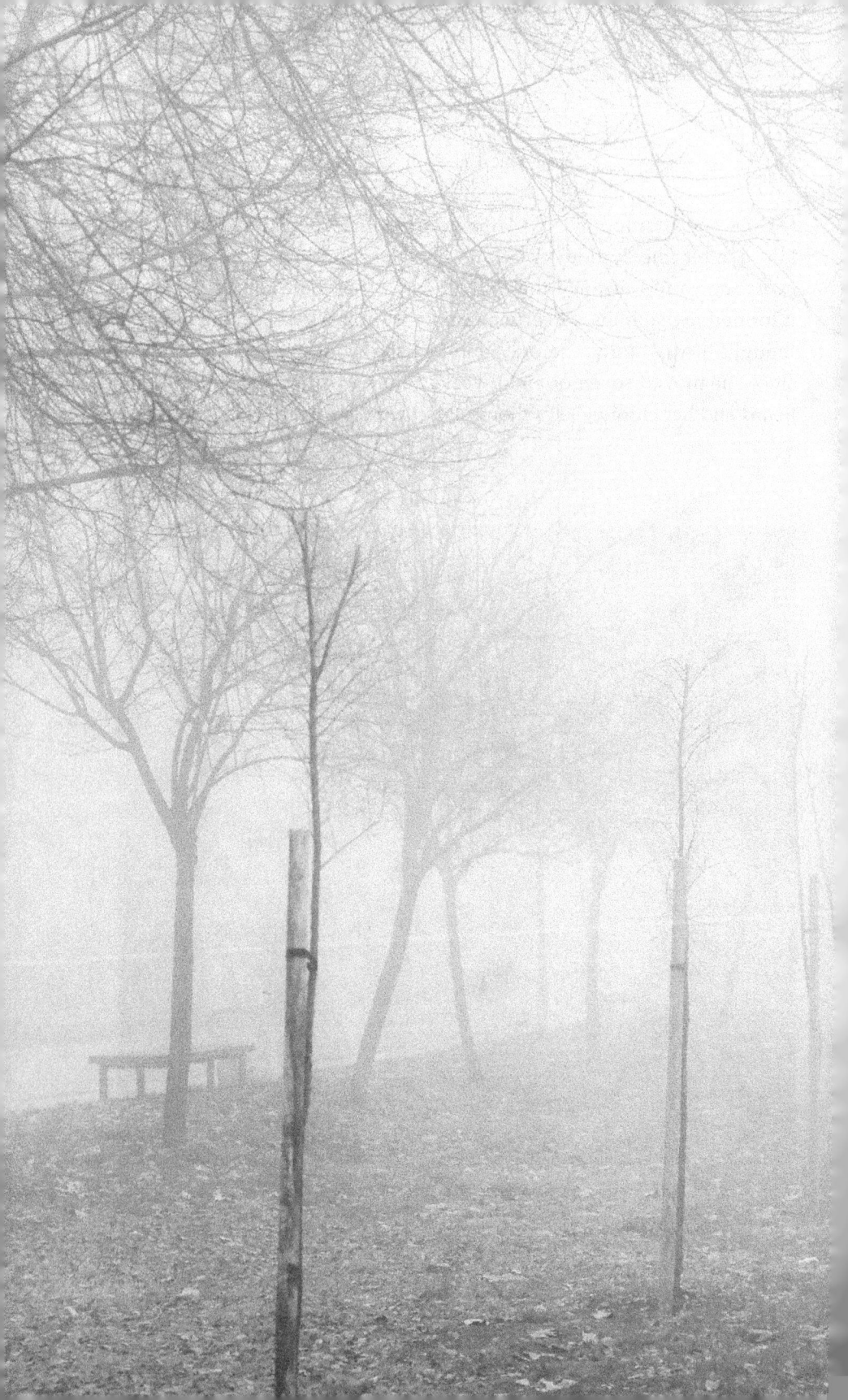

# CHAPTER 14

# ROADBLOCK

MAMA HAD NEVER BEEN TOLD DEFINITIVELY by doctors she couldn't drive, even having had numerous TIAs, so she brought her car to the Big House. I was not overjoyed about this. Thoughts ensued about how horrific it might be if she were ever responsible for maiming or, worse, killing someone. I couldn't bear to live with myself. In my attempt to wean her from her driving habit, I often took her for a drive to get her out of the Big House on my visits. She enjoyed our time together.

***

Mama's friend, Shirley, visited from Texas, and they went for a drive with Mama behind the wheel. Since Shirley was from out of state, Mama planned to show her the town.

Later that afternoon, Shirley reported to my brother Mama had been lost for over 30 minutes and unable to find anything that looked familiar. The experience frightened both ladies. Ralph talked to Mama about not driving anymore. I later discussed with Mama she should stop driving due to her eyesight. Oh, don't even think she fell for that line. I told Norma Jean, with colder weather upon us, we needed to store her car in the garage; I mean, out of sight, out of mind, right? I had spoken to my sister and her husband, and they were interested in buying the car for one of their daughters. The car stayed in the garage for a short time before Mama began to ask more frequently for it.

I decided to call her doctor and let him deliver the bad news and in essence, be the 'bad guy'. I told the nurse on the phone what the purpose of the appointment was so everyone was in on the game plan. We arrived, waited briefly, then were brought back to the room. The family doctor entered the room and began an examination of Mama and asked her rote questions. When he finished the exam, he wished us well and opened the door.

*What? Did he not get the memo?* I walked out to the waiting room, sat Mama down, and told her I needed to pay the bill. When I reached the secretary, I reminded her of the "game plan," and she told the doctor immediately. He signaled me to bring Mom back to him.

Same song, second verse. We walked into the room, Mama hopped up on the examination table, and the doctor came in. He went over her list of medications. He asked her if she was on Aricept. I answered yes after she had turned to me for help. He informed her anyone on Aricept should not be driving. He also said he was sorry but she was not allowed to drive anymore. Oh, Norma Jean played it cool. Despite the exchange of all the expected niceties and well wishes, when we got inside my car, she cussed him from here to eternity. Wow, was she ever mad! "Who does he think he is anyway? Nobody's gonna tell me not to drive!" The cuss words flew out of her mouth like I never heard before. I was thankful Mama took this out on the doctor, not me.

---

**A valuable lesson I learned that day. Let the professionals take the hit instead of you (the family member). You need to be their ally and constant, reliable loved one.**

---

When I took Mama for a drive, I was struck by her fascination with two things: the trees and the 18-wheelers. She never failed to comment on them, and I admit, it was quite remarkable considering her diminished eyesight. To maintain my sanity, I devised a game for myself. Each time she made a comment or asked a question about these objects, I challenged myself to provide a unique response. Not only did it serve as a coping mechanism to prevent me from losing my ever-loving mind, but it also became an educational exercise, expanding my vocabulary along the way.

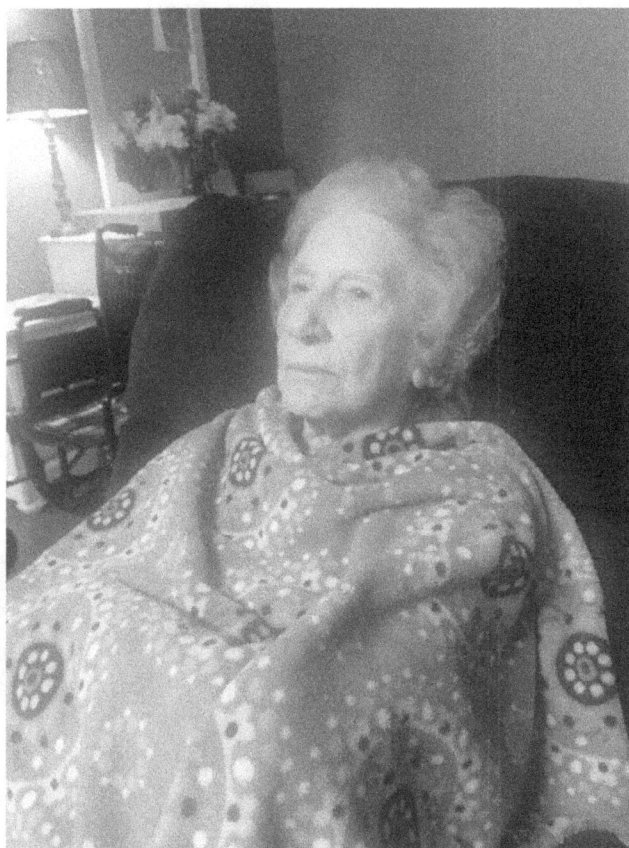

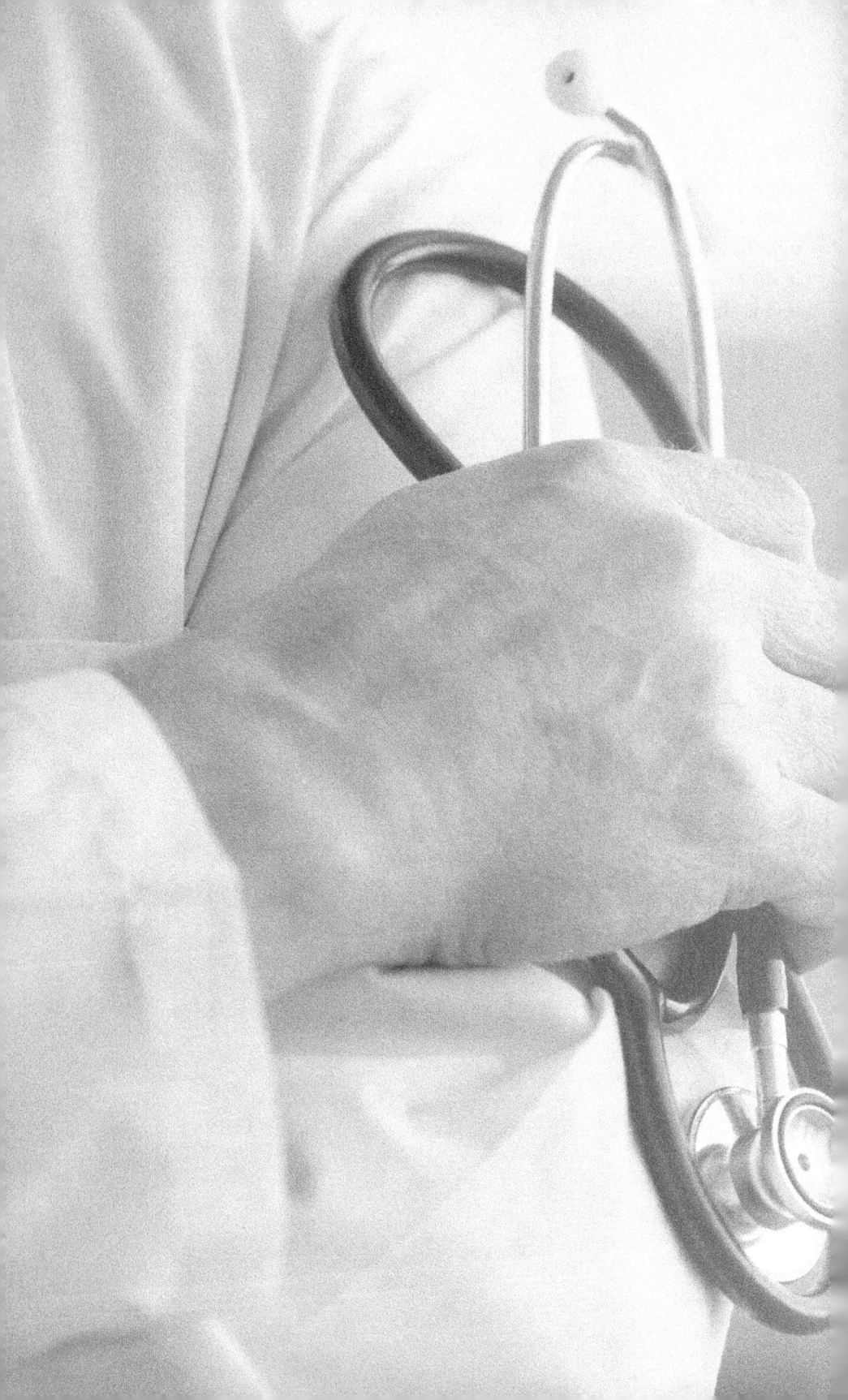

# CHAPTER 15

# ANATOMY LESSONS

IN THE WORLD OF CAREGIVING, survival is the name of the game – you do whatever it takes to endure.

Mama's hip had been hurting for weeks. She quit attending morning Mass and preferred to stay home and on a heating pad. She went to the orthopedic doctor and they ordered X-rays. The doctor believed it was degenerative spondylolisthesis. They sent her for an MRI. Mama said her leg "faded" as she walked; It would catch then give out on her. She was in extreme pain. In addition to the heating pad, she used anti-inflammatories and Darvocet, yet, her hip still bothered her and caused her to lose sleep. Her pain radiated down to her calf on the left side.

I reached out to a family friend in the field and was told her diagnosis wasn't good. Mama's problem usually required either surgery to completely fix it or physical therapy. It required being hospitalized for a few days.

With this news, I spoke in depth with an orthopedic surgeon's assistant with years of experience, and he said the surgery was horrible. A person Mama's age might likely never recover. I believed our best option was epidural injections several times a year.

The assistant gave me the name of a reputable doctor in town who gives injections. I was concerned about how much worse her memory might be if Mama were to be put under anesthesia for surgery. We brought Mama her mother's walker and wheelchair to use as needed. She was thrilled to have them.

Mama and I had an appointment with the pain management doctor. He said Mama's arthritis is severe and squeezing the nerve. He wants to do a medial branch block on this nerve. He said he uses anesthesia on the nerve which only lasts for two hours. He then repeats the procedure except with different anesthesia (all local). The second anesthesia lasts for four hours. If both of these relieved the pain, he knew he had the right nerve and source of pain. He would then cauterize the nerve. As a result, the pain is likely to be alleviated for almost a year.

I sent the information to my family friend I had spoken with previously and he reported back the plan from the pain management doctor was a good one. He obviously knew what he was doing because he was following the correct protocol. By using the pain management doctor's plan, he was not changing any of the architecture/anatomy, so the injections were worth a try, and if they didn't work, no harm, no foul.

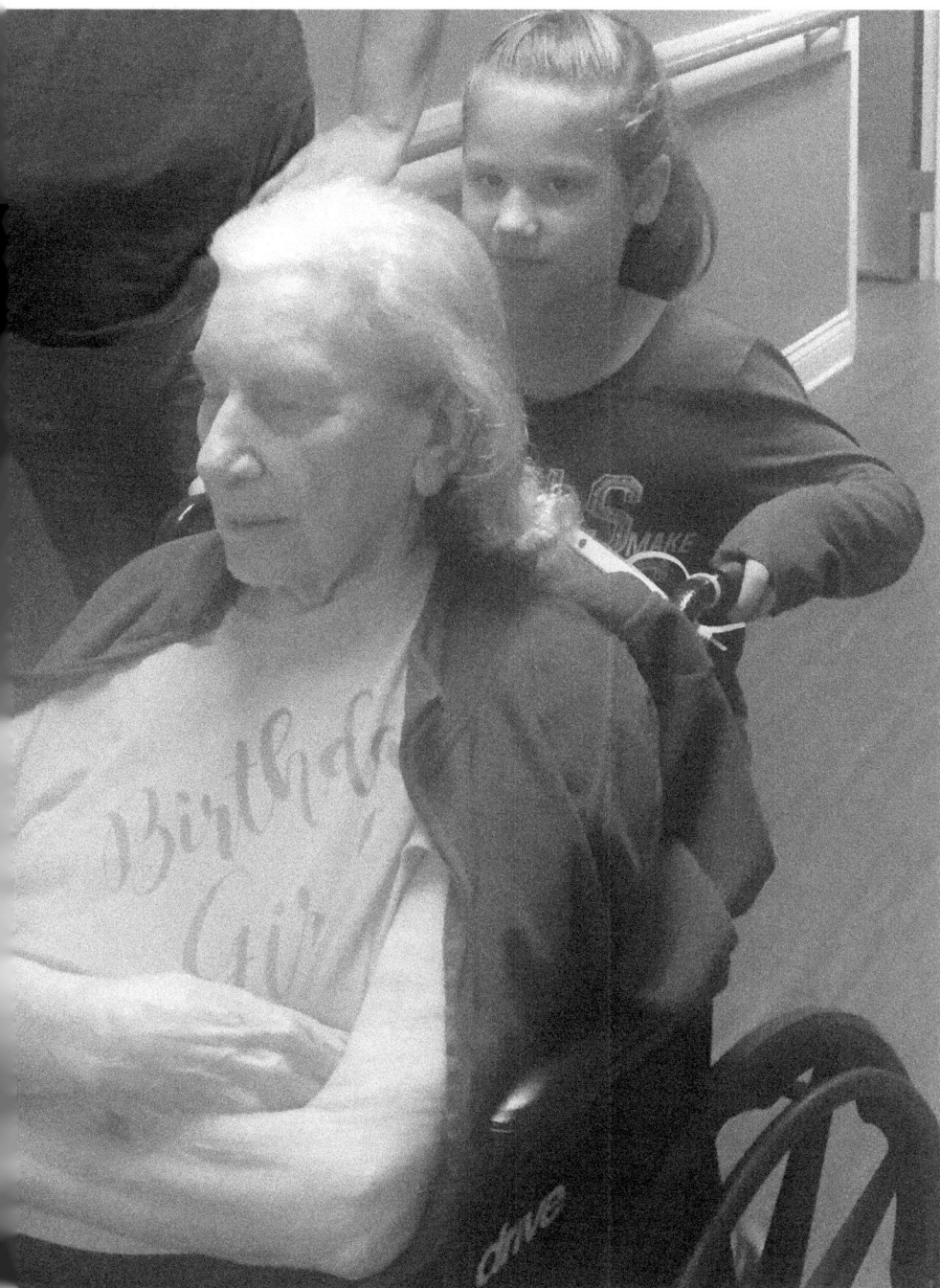

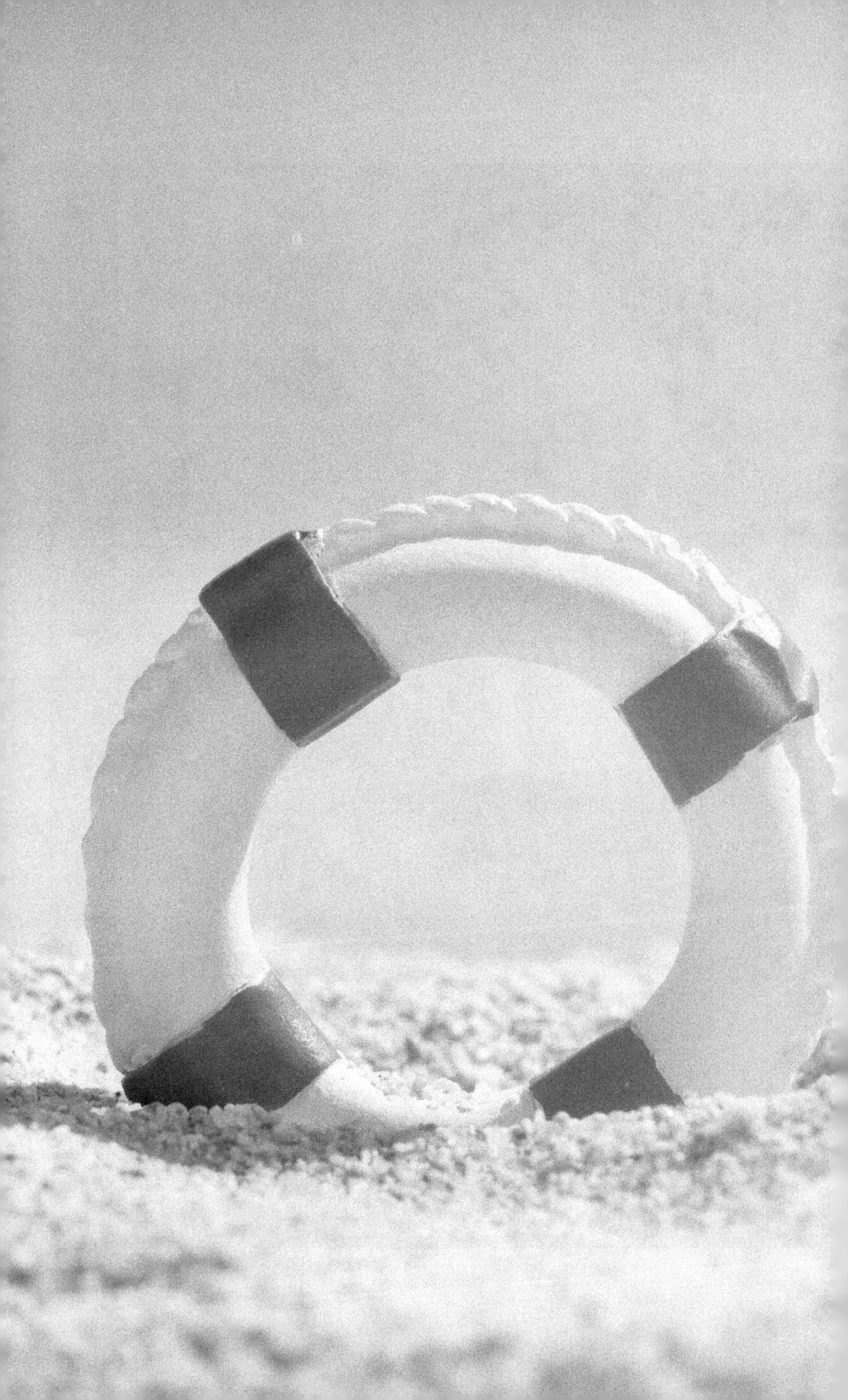

## CHAPTER 16

# REINFORCEMENTS FORTHWITH

THE BIG HOUSE puts on an extravagant, very popular Halloween festival every year. It was opened to the public and welcomed over 500 attendees. I personally did not participate in Halloween; however, knowing how much Mama loved children and missed her own grand-children, this was an excellent opportunity for Mama to interact with hundreds of little ones. The residents were encouraged to hand out the candy as the children went down the hallways and stopped at each open door. Other residents were gathered in large sitting areas. We purchased ten large bags of candy, and she only had half of one bag left over at the conclusion of the festivities. Although Mama was temporarily in a wheelchair due to her hip and back pain, she was ecstatic about all the candy and the children. I have wonderful pictures of her through the years of this annual event.

I placed her outside on the front porch because she was enthusiastic and an excellent ambassador for the Big House. It amazed me even the scariest of costumes didn't frighten her in the least. She pinched, hugged, and tickled the trick-or-treaters and laughed the entire time. My girls came with me and enjoyed seeing their Mamaw so animated.

In the following days, Mama was admitted to the hospital with severe pain that could not be controlled with over-the-counter medications. I had been at the hospital with her by myself for a very long week. Sharon, my sister-in-law, who lived four hours away, sent me a lengthy email offering to give me a much-needed break. In the email, she had some statements I feel all caregivers need to put in practice, although not always as easy as it sounds.

*In the future, you will have to tell us what you need – we don't need you going down in the process. We all have limits. If you don't care for yourself and your family, you cannot care for Norma Jean. You have a LIFE – a job, kids, etc. just like your brothers and sisters. You cannot carry this load by yourself.*

*He (my brother) cannot read your mind, and he will not make a move until you tell him. It's not that he doesn't care, but he doesn't think like that. He's thinking of emergency care, not ongoing help.*

She offered to bring a bed-sized heating pad, crossword puzzles, and a book. She even went so far as to bring a casserole for my family.

At the time Sharon wrote this letter, my husband was trying to be Mom and Dad on the home front, coach his daughter's games and work 12-hour shifts.

Mama was discharged from the hospital and had an MRI. We laid low at her apartment all weekend and eagerly waited for the MRI results and a treatment plan sometime the following week. It had been a long week for both of us.

<hr>

I called Suzy, my sister, to tell her how out of her mind Mama was recently. I wondered if Mama had another mini-stroke because she was very antsy, very hot, and not feeling well, but not sick. Shortly thereafter, her mind was a storm of confusion and chaos. It stayed that way for the remainder of the day. The following day she was perfectly fine.

Based on the MRI findings, home health was sent to the Big House for Mom to receive physical therapy. She needed to learn how to move properly when getting out of bed, etc., and they discussed putting a brace on her neck.

***

I'm thankful for my sisters, Suzy, Lydia, and Cathy, who were such good listeners today while I rambled. God knows who and what you need, just at the perfect time. I am blessed with family, friends, and even strangers who reach out at the ideal time to say something that may not seem profound at that particular moment, but in a few hours or days, or weeks, I could see God used them to prepare me for what was to come. He orchestrated those people to plant a seed of faith in me or speak a word of affirmation over me.

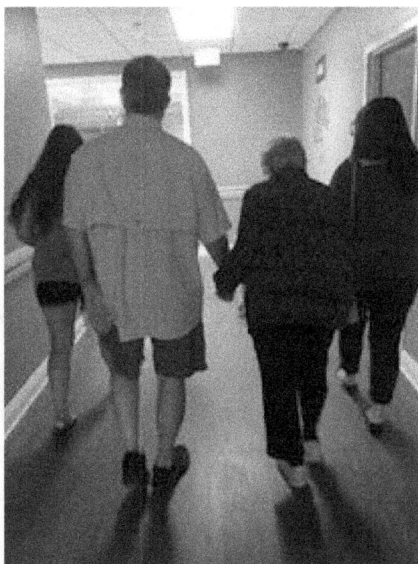

My tradition of taking photos of all the walks down the hallway

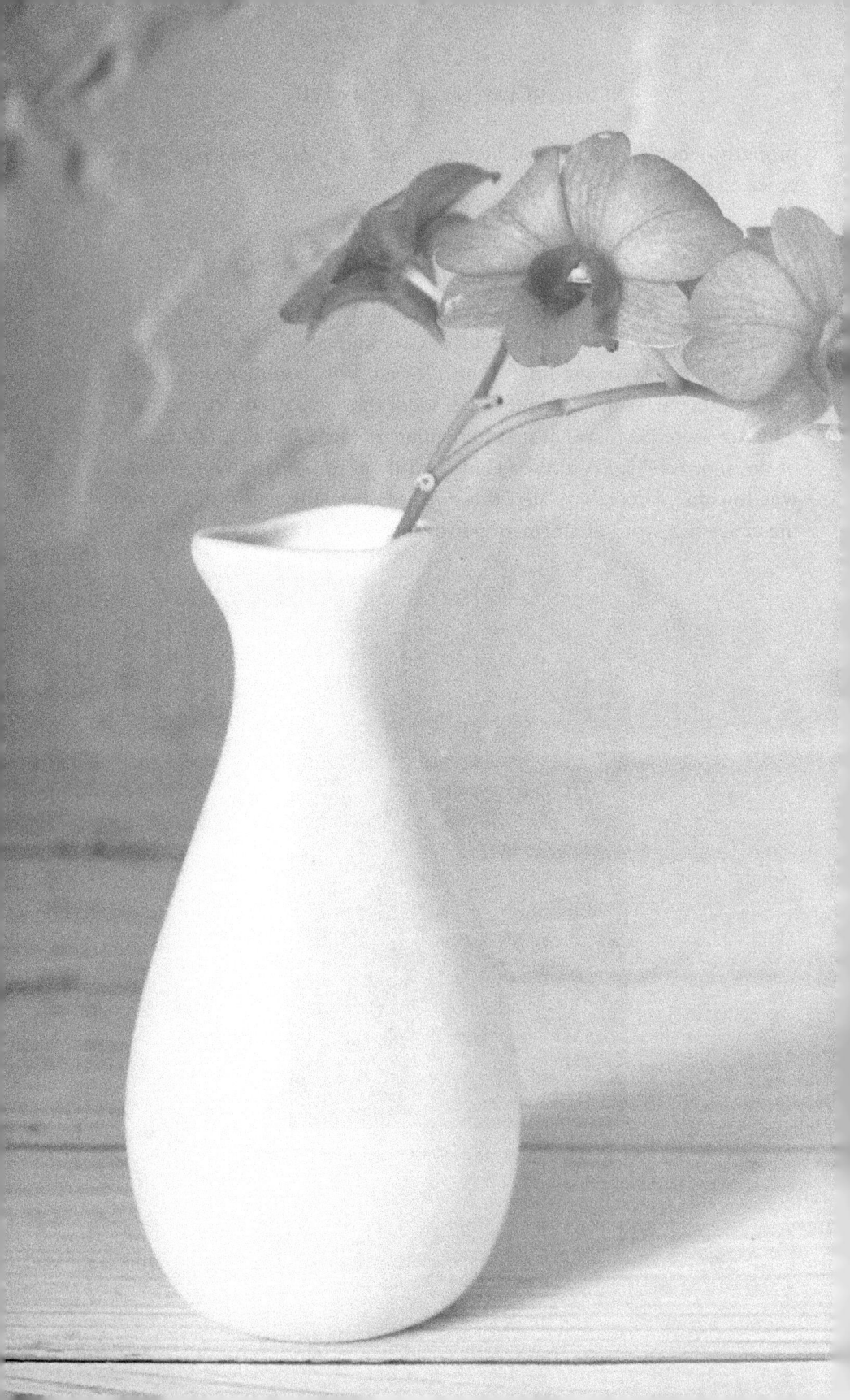

# CHAPTER 17
# EARLY ALZHEIMERS

I FOUND an outline on the three stages of Alzheimer's I picked up in one of the many doctor's offices we frequented. Doctors diagnosed Mama as having vascular dementia, but I believe all dementia leads to Alzheimer's at some point; at least, that is my understanding based on the neurologist's comments. I've included information on the stages in the **Resource** section.

Mama had been "maintaining" the same phase for a couple of months, and it was hard to manage, hard to watch, well, just plain hard. The most challenging aspect was I anticipated it becoming more difficult. I prayed and prayed for God to take her before it got too bad. I did not want to have to move her to "The Back," otherwise known as the Special Care unit or, worse, a nursing home. Even the thought of either of those situations made me sick to my stomach. I also didn't want her to suffer through any major illness.

In an attempt to get my siblings more involved with Mama's care, I sent them an email with some simple ideas:

*How can I help, you ask? Well, the best way is to call Mama, espe-cially in the evening. She starts calling me persistently around 5:00 p.m. and doesn't stop until 7ish. Take one night every week to call*

*Mama. This would help me and make her momentarily happy and pre-occupied. You can say the same thing – she won't remember. She asks about all of you every SINGLE DAY. I've given her your phone numbers several times, but she lost the paper. Please call her.*

*If you have time, those of you who are letter writers, please send a thank you note to Uncle Leonard and Aunt Bobbie. They have helped me tremendously. Aunt Bobbie tries to take Mama out at least once a week for an entire day. They usually return to Aunt Bobbie's house for lunch with Uncle Leonard. After lunch, they drive over to see Aunt Phoebe. Ethan and Jaci take Mama out to eat to give me a break, too. I feel she needs to get out of the facility for a change of scenery, but the director recently told me it could actually worsen her paranoia. This disease is relentless!*

---

My time was consumed with transporting Mama from one place to another...church, neurologists, podiatrists, dentists, internists, and family doctors. Add to that, the beauty shop and perhaps a trip to Dairy Barn. Don't forget the car rides we enjoyed. I had hoped someone might offer to help and take on a couple of the weekend drives or perhaps bring her to Mass. Thankfully, one kind gentleman from church offered to pick up Mama for Mass. Very few friends came by to visit her. One church friend shared with me how much she enjoyed visiting with Mama. She recently lost her husband and was working through a host of emotions. She knew her secrets were safe with Mama because of her dementia. Consequently, she found her time with Mama very therapeutic. I never thought of it from that angle, but she was right. It amazed me to watch family and friend's reactions to the changes in Mama. I knew she was different, and it was awkward, so I loved how her friend used it to her advantage while simultaneously providing some much-needed company for Mama.

Simple gestures have a powerful impact. It just takes your time and patience. Have a cup of coffee with her. Join her in the ice cream parlor.

Sit outside on the porch. I found myself thinking her world was shrinking with each passing day.

---

My sister-in-law came to my rescue again and stayed with Mama at her apartment while I attended a business conference. She reported after Mama's shower, she sat her in her recliner and Mama started sweating profusely – her hair was drenched and she was flushed. She wasn't confused but was having difficulty breathing.

Sharon concentrated on Mama's breathing and getting her to relax. After 30 minutes, it finally passed, and her temperature returned to normal.

---

In lieu of updating my brothers and sisters individually, when I felt the changes in Mom warranted an email, I gave precise details of recent events to keep them abreast of the medical and behavioral updates. My latest email was necessary to inform my five siblings how serious Mama's health had gotten. She had experienced numerous 'episodes' in 17 days. She experienced one every day for the previous three days. Home health was on speed dial! The 'episodes' or possible TIAs manifested themselves by sudden redness all over and appeared to be a severe sunburn or scalding, profuse sweating, and tingling or prickly feelings. The "event" usually lasted less than an hour, and pain was never involved. Afterward, she was agitated, and the episode definitely affected her memory. I did not bring her to the ER because they said she needed a stent because of the 70 percent blockage, previously diagnosed, but Mama did not want a stent. Secondly, she couldn't take aspirin anymore or blood thinners because they cause serious bleeding issues. Both Sharon and Suzy witnessed these symptoms.

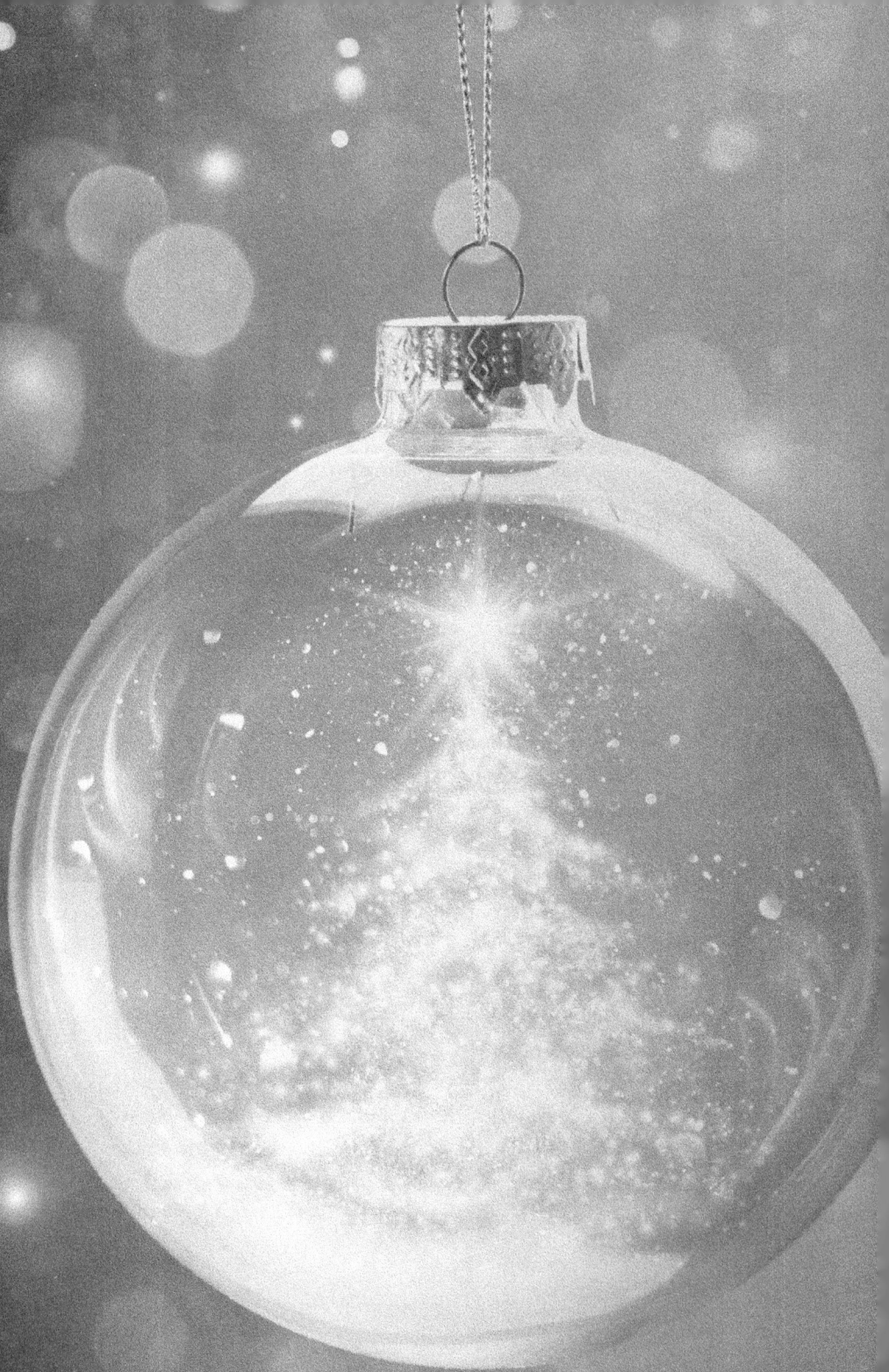

# CHAPTER 18
# A CIVIL CHRISTMAS

TODAY WAS A LONG-AWAITED DAY. All six of Mama's children came back home for Christmas, and now it was time to go through her belongings and get the house ready to go on the market. I'm proud to say we were very civil as we carefully divided Mama's belongings. Siblings expressed their wish list of the more prominent objects, i.e., a dining room table, bedroom suites, living room furniture, etc. After that was dispersed, we considered the grandchildren and collected items to give to them.

Regarding the smaller but still significant objects, we chose to go around the circle, and each sibling picked an object. We did this until everything was gone. It went smoothly, and the house was emptied. We would list the house at the first of the year per Mama's instructions.

After the holidays, we painted three walls in Mama's house, steam cleaned the carpets, deep cleaned the house, fixed the issues in the guest bathroom, fixed the rattling heater sound, and gave the living room furniture to Care Help. We planned to have the yard mulched and cleaned, and hopefully, Mama's house on the market by the weekend.

Mama was still on board with the sale of the home.

I suddenly realized with the expectant sale of the house and Mama already settled in her new apartment in assisted living, coupled with her steady decline, my life took a profound turn. From that point onward, I stepped into the role of Mama's primary caregiver for the remainder of her time on earth. There was no turning back from this point forward.

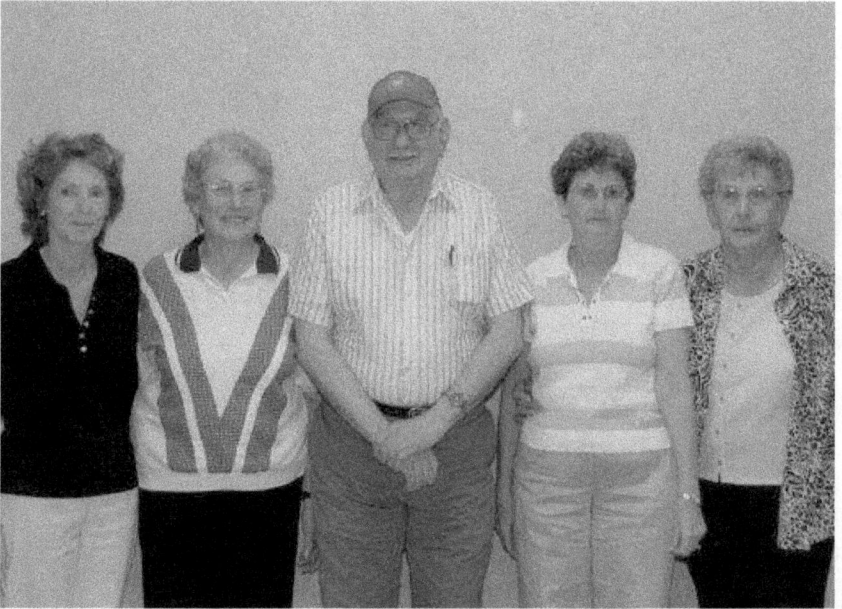

My Uncle Harris and Mama with her three sisters

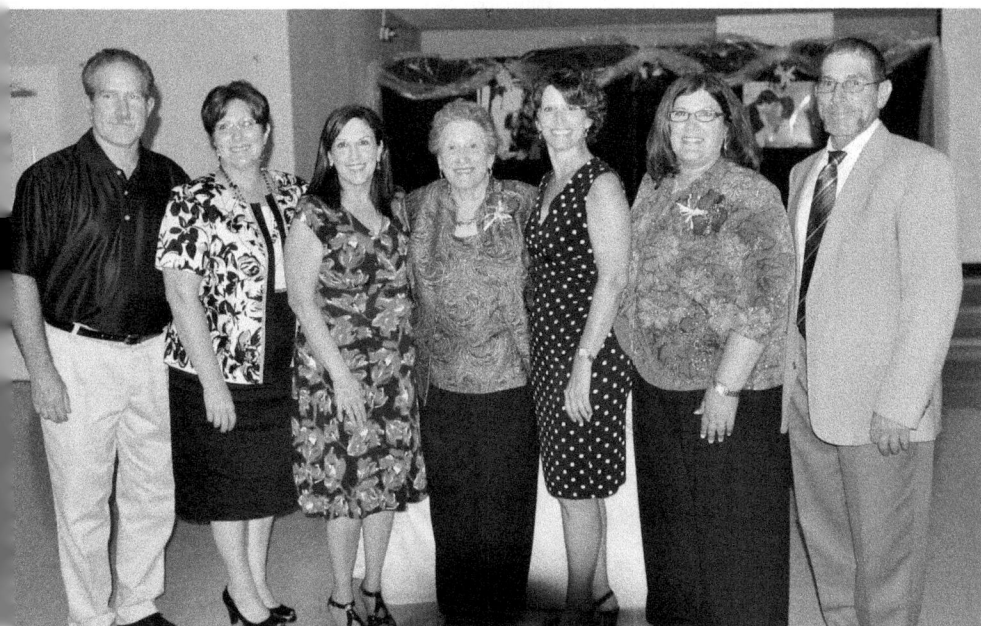

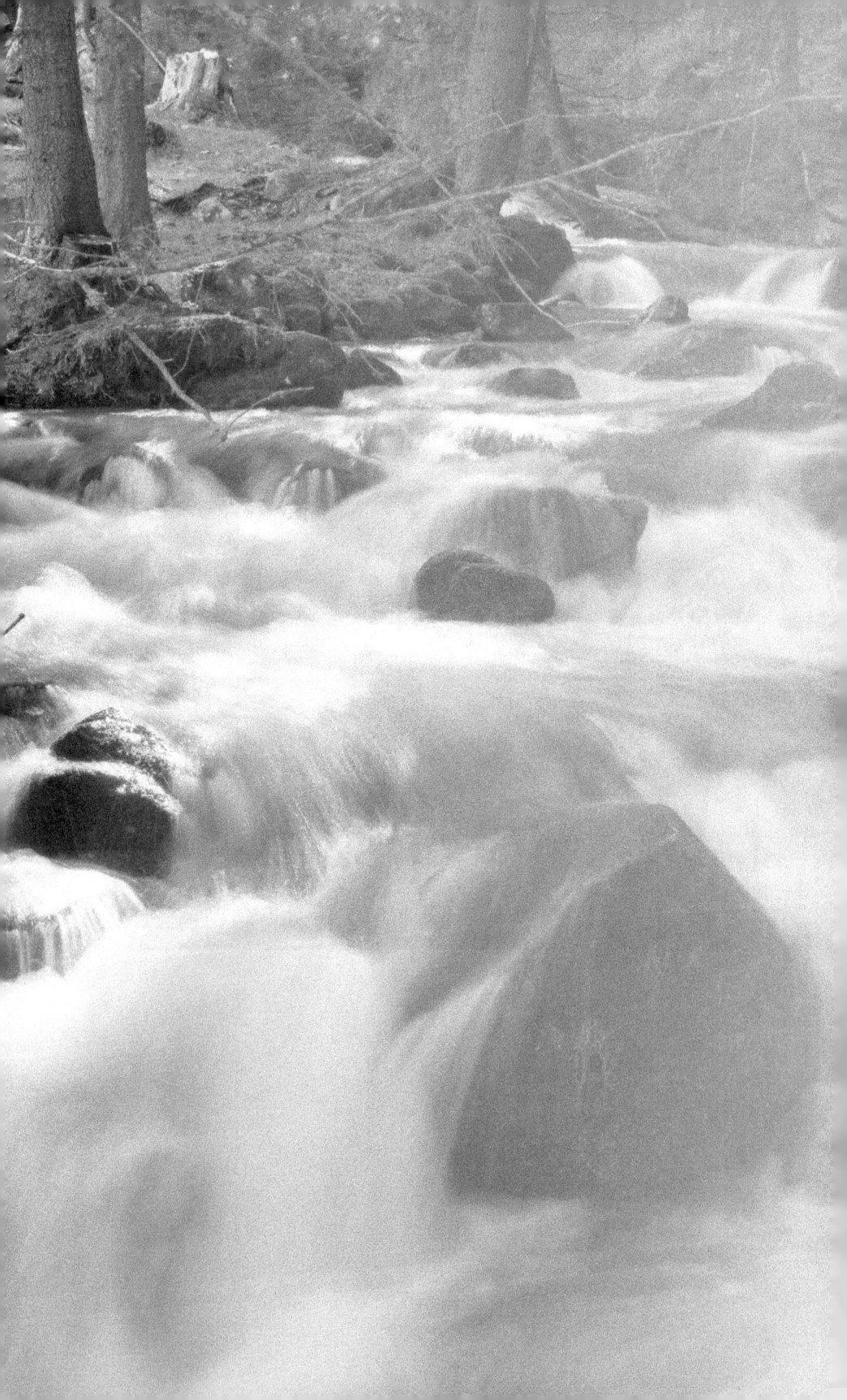

# CHAPTER 19
# EMBRACING THE UNEXPECTED

AFTER SEVERAL MONTHS HAD PASSED, Mama asked me for her car because, somehow, she remembered it being stored in her garage. This disease is so frustrating. She didn't remember my name and I saw her every day at length, continuously having to repeat my name, but somehow, some way, she remembered a car she hadn't driven or even seen in months. She had no memory of the doctor taking her car away. The complexities of her mind are truly remarkable, and a testament to our Creator and the intricate workings of the human brain.

---

On a recent visit to Mama's, I straightened her living area and I noticed some Social Security mail in her trash can. I took immediate action to change her mailing address with them to my home address. I thought I had transferred all her mail to my house, but I inadvertently over-looked this one since she received the check by direct deposit and rarely received any mail from them. Long story short, I was able to change the address with them; however, in order to do so, I had to become a Payee, which meant the checks were directly deposited in her account but made out to me for Mama.

I was required to complete a yearly report indicating how the funds were used. The representative said to list the cost of the assisted living apartment and that should suffice.

<hr>

When I found extra time on my hands, I went through the boxes and boxes of paperwork I inherited from Mama after clearing out her house in December. As I went through the cards she saved, I found a prayer card where Mama paid for a Mass to be offered for *herself*. The card stated she was scared she was losing her mind. To see her handwriting and to know how pained she must have been to pen those words -- what a heavy burden this was for her to bear. Oh, how I cried as I held the card to my chest.

Another poignant card I noticed was a beautiful, delicate card my father had given Mama on their 25th wedding anniversary. With his beautiful cursive handwriting, he signed it, "I can't wait until the next 25!" The reality was he only lived for another year. Twenty-six short years together. It grieved me to know they missed out on many memory-making events: more grandchildren, weddings, empty nest, retirement, and travel.

---

**This is a lesson for all of us. We don't know how much time we have with the ones we love, make every moment count!**

---

<hr>

Mama's house finally sold after ten months in a sluggish housing market. Hallelujah. I was overjoyed to have one less thing to contend with on my ever-growing list of responsibilities. I shared the news with Mama and she was happy. I was thankful there were no signs of remorse.

<hr>

**When a caregiver has an out-of-the-ordinary banner day, you celebrate your victories.**

Mom and I had a wonderful Friday morning consisting of morning Mass, coffee with her friends, and shopping for a new purse and a Mother's Day dress (a feat in and of itself). She was pleased with our purchases.

In order to give me a break, the following morning my sweet hubby woke up early after having worked a graveyard shift, and he brought Mama to her hairdresser and to the nail salon next door to get her all gussied up for Mother's Day. He is a rare breed. I love that man.

Well, fiddlesticks! I bought Mama a corsage to go with her new Mother's Day dress and planned to bring her to church followed by a nice meal with the family afterward. I arrived at her apartment and found her on her couch, in her pajamas and coughing.

She wasn't interested in doing anything. Instead of getting dolled up in her new dress, with hair and nails on point, and a beautiful corsage for extra flair, we ordered Chicken Della Casa from Joe's (our favorite Italian restaurant) and ate quietly in her room. I felt sad for her. On the other side of town, James had a wonderful morning with his mother. We were a house divided, both caring for our parents.

With Mama's aches and pains, especially in her knees, I decided we needed to opt out of daily Mass at church. Bless her heart, she couldn't stop herself from kneeling and paid the price soon after, every time. I brought her instead to the chapel service at the Big House. They did not have kneelers. Problem solved. She enjoyed the chapel and, as always, loved the hymns.

My son's wedding was approaching and after the rehearsal supper, I rushed Mama to the emergency room because she complained of chest pains. I couldn't take a chance she might have a heart attack during the wedding the following day. They didn't find a reason to admit her, so she was discharged and we laid low at her apartment. The next day at the wedding reception, Norma Jean was on the dance floor with all of her children and grandchildren dancing the night away. No one could have guessed we were in the hospital 24 hours earlier.

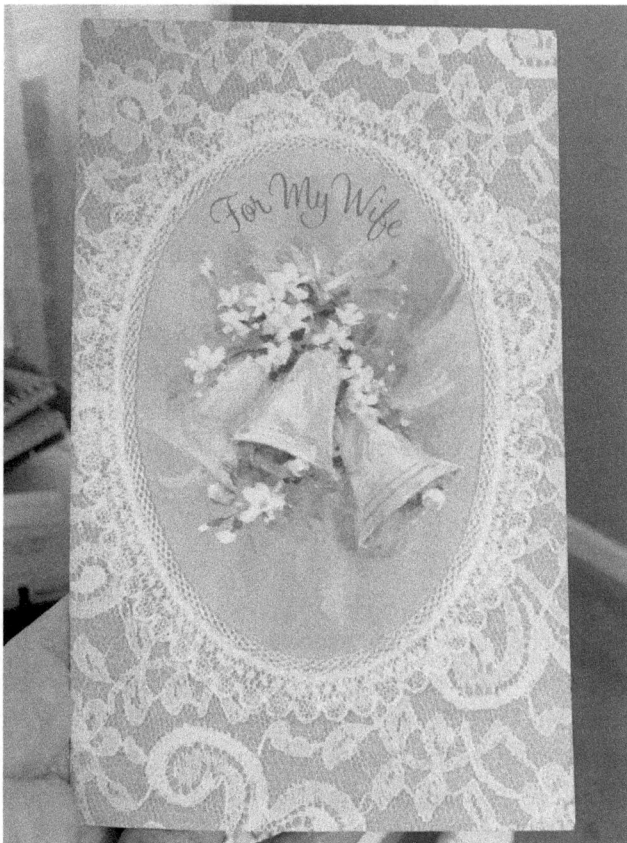

Happy Anniversary
(25)
With All My Love
Hope we have
25 more. Love you,
Bill

BINGO!

# CHAPTER 20

# LET THE GAMES BEGIN

I AM grateful for all the activities the Big House offered its residents. Mama participated in bingo, bean bag baseball, and painting classes, and anytime there was a band playing in the dining hall, you could find Norma Jean front and center. I tried to be there when she was participating in the activities because watching her in action on her good days was so very good for my heart. Her athleticism shone through every time. She didn't always know I was there because I wanted to see how she behaved and interacted with others. Some might call that spying.

Other times, I sat next to her and joined in the games or if she felt good, danced with her while the band played. My treasure chest of mental memories is bursting with precious times we spent together doing some of Mama's favorite activities.

I was delighted to hear Mama had picked up her paintbrush and was painting again. I thought it was gone for good, but Kelly, the activities director, provided art teachers to help the residents paint. Mama was not as good as she once was with her failing eyesight, but she enjoyed it. Chrissy, my daughter, visited her often and joined in on this type of project. My home office now houses several of these collaborative paintings.

I had a wonderful time with Mama at the Big House playing bean bag baseball with them. I was pretty good with this "sport," although nothing to write home about. But today, during my first practice run, I hit the 3-base hole. Mama was proud, and I heard the residents say, "She takes after her Mama." I played the best game ever. I hit two home runs and a triple. Oh yeah, and then there were those two outs. Oh well. It was great fun.

I headed to bed later than normal and checked my phone one last time and saw an email from a common first name. I clicked on the letter and saw it was from a relative.

Although we only see each other once every ten years, her huge, kind-hearted gesture for my mother had me blubbering like an idiot. I was speechless. I had tears on my pillowcase that night. The writer informed me she sent some puzzles made specifically for dementia patients for Mama and other residents to enjoy. What a unique gift.

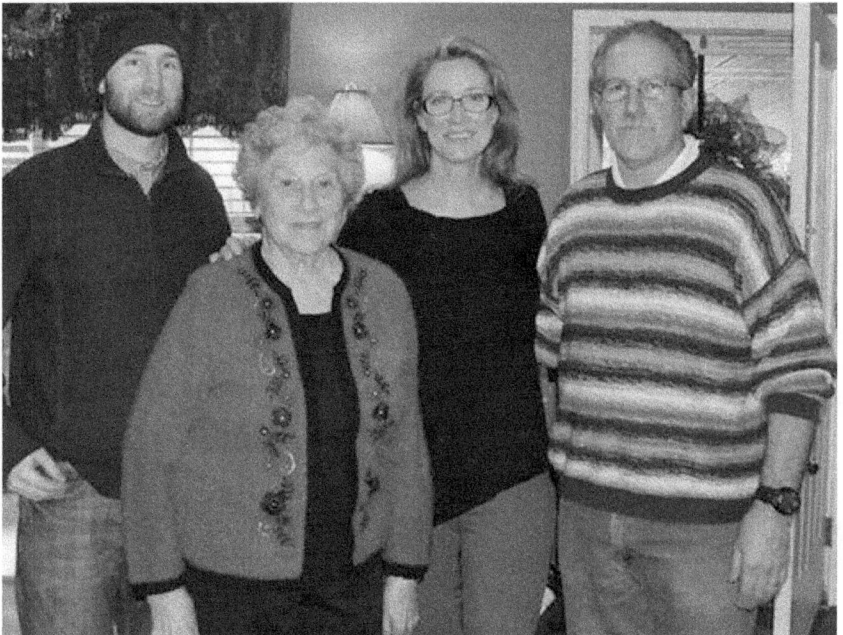

Ralph, Sharon, and Neal visiting Mama

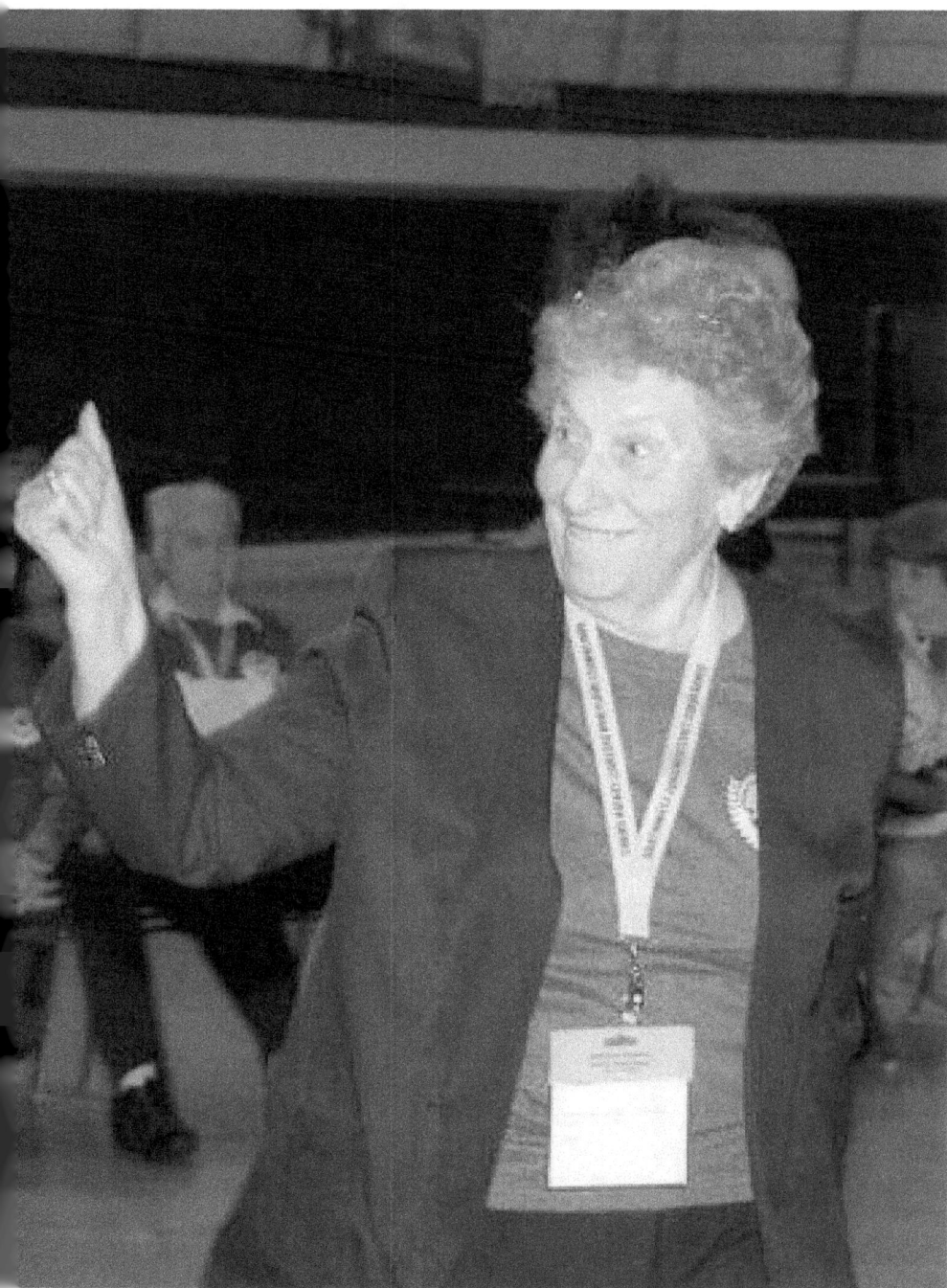

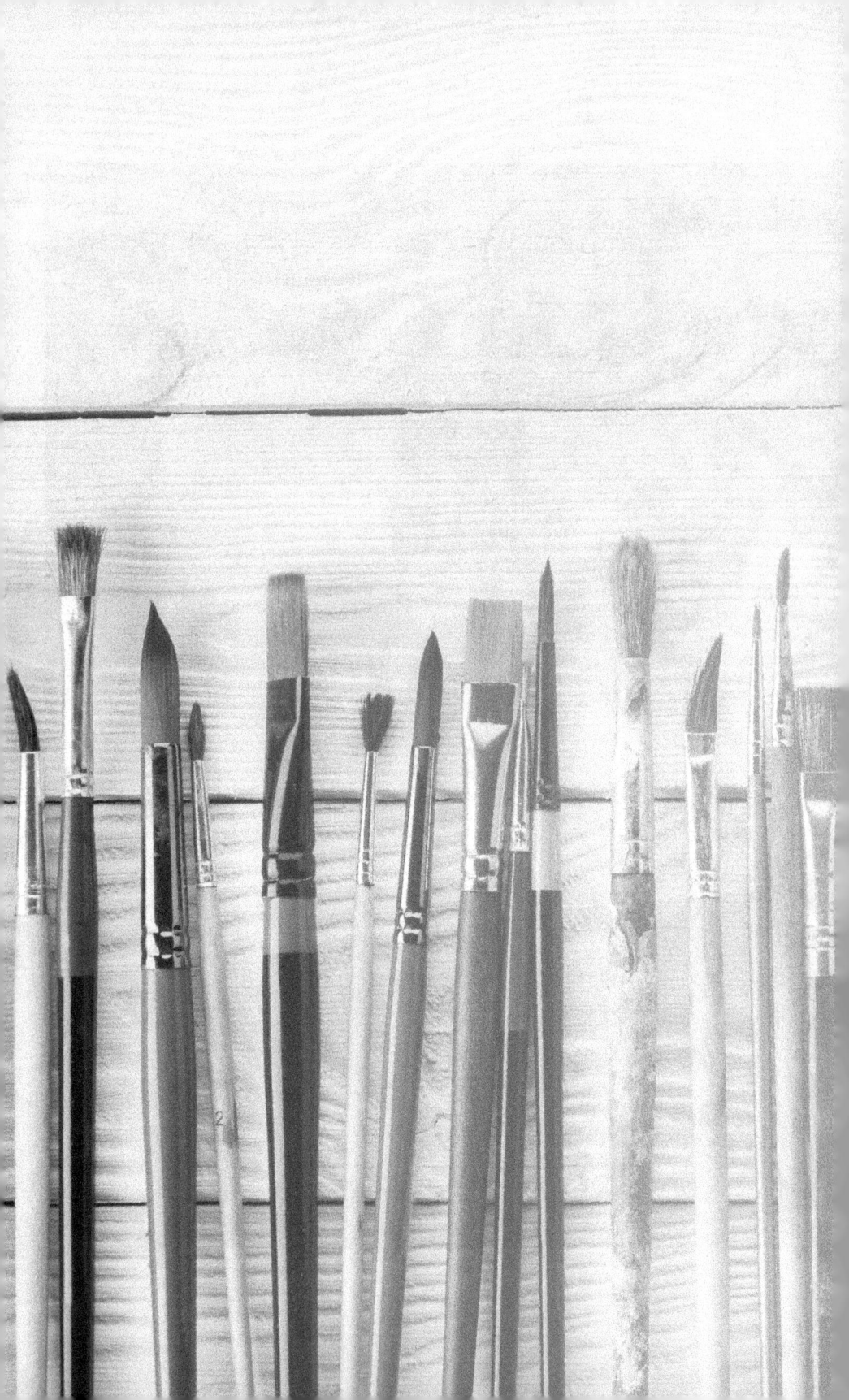

# CHAPTER 21

# MOTHER OF INVENTIONS

MAMA'S 83rd birthday had come and gone. It struck me as funny because last year, I didn't know if I had another year with her. I coveted each day with her. It was a gift. Thank you, God, for giving me (and my five siblings) the most amazing mother - full of laughter, intelligence, love, and honestly, the mother of inventions!!! I must tell you two of Mama's most remembered creations, so to speak.

Pompom bushes lined my mother's curved sidewalk when she lived on St. Joseph Street. Several of the bushes had died, their once vibrant green now a brown hue, prompting Mama's creative instincts to come to the rescue. Knowing she might not find a replacement the same exact size, she purchased green spray paint and sprayed the dead plants, miraculously bringing them back to life. They matched the original bushes perfectly and looked amazing. The neighbors were none the wiser.

Mama was the best at creating something beautiful out of nothing. Take her macrame sandals, for example. She was unable to find shoes to match her grandmother-of-the-bride dress, so you know what she did? She painted her off-white macrame sandals with nail polish, the color of the teal dress. It was an exact match, and she received compliments from everyone, including the bride, on the wedding day.

# CHAPTER 22
# A SUSPICIOUS MIND

MAMA'S HEALTH was changing again. Mama had begun to be paranoid above and beyond normal in the last six weeks. She believed (even during the day) that everyone had left the facility and left her there all alone in the Big House. She was on the verge of having a panic attack. She roamed the halls in the evening (what they call sundowning), and could not be convinced residents were in their apartments. She felt they were scheming behind her back and intentionally leaving her out of the group trips. This resulted in seven or eight phone calls to me a day. She didn't remember we recently talked and called again. I received three or four calls in a 30-minute time frame. I quit answering some of them because I knew what she was calling for – she was lonely and paranoid, but I was either cooking supper or at one of the girls' games. Unfortunately, I changed Mama's ringtone on my phone to Piano Riff. Every time I heard that ring, I dreaded answering it. My heart skipped a beat every time. I changed it to an upbeat tone because I realized I was sabotaging myself and my mood. Problem solved.

Mama's personality was unstable and ever-changing. Aunt Bobbie and I caught her sitting by the director's door, facing the window toward the circle driveway. She told us she was waiting to be picked up by someone. No names, no reason, no time frame. But no one was coming to get her. The two main people in her life stood right in front of her and she was fixated on looking outside believing in the scenario she had concocted in her mind. I witnessed her multiple times standing by the front door and reading the visitor's log to see where everyone had gone when there were six friends she could have joined on the front porch. I reached for Mama's hand and brought her outside to join the "front porch crew." Mama enjoyed the time with them.

---

**As a caregiver, if you watch, listen and learn, you will soon find the value of redirecting your loved one at appropriate times.**

---

Another time Aunt Bobbie walked into the Big House and found Mama near the front door, seated in a wheelchair, facing the elevator, and just staring into space. Aunt Bobbie asked Mama what she was doing, and she replied, "Waiting for someone to bring me to church." She was also found on occasion standing over the upstairs railing while she watched who entered and exited the building. Do you get the picture? She was obsessed.

Mama unplugged her TV and computer in her living room because she did not want anyone playing on them. She believed the employees and other residents came in her apartment when she wasn't there and used her electronics. I believe that was part of the reason she was stir-crazy. She had nothing to do in her room but sleep. Mama had loved playing computer card games and typing letters to her friends, children, and grandchildren. She created beautiful keepsake cards for special occasions. Again, another activity she could no longer enjoy. She didn't enjoy reading because she couldn't remember what she read on the previous page.

Mama had developed a very short temper and had alienated most of her friends in the Big House. This broke my heart more than anything because she had been a people person my entire life. I wished I could stop the progression of this disease. I didn't like the myriad of changes I saw in my Mama.

I liked to join in on bingo games with the residents and reconnect with some classmates' parents who were also residents at the Big House. However, Mama began to embarrass me during these games. If someone so much as whispered to another player (between the games), she snapped at them, slammed her hand down on the table, and told them to, "Shut up!" Their reactions said it all. So sad.

⁓⧼⧽⁓

I had a new situation on my hands, one an adult child never thought they would encounter, but I did, unfortunately. As the following scenario began to rear its ugly head, I remembered reading about this in the stages of Alzheimer's although I held out hope, Mama might bypass this one. Hygiene was its name, and it was no game!

Mama had begun fighting me to change her clothes. When I recruited the aides for reinforcement, she fought them, too. She adamantly opposed changing her clothes and consequently wore the same outfit three or four days in a row. When I asked her to change, she argued with me. Her voice was raised and she didn't hide the fact she was agitated with me.

---

**This was when I learned to apply a life lesson I used while raising my four children...pick your battles!**

---

More often than not, I redirected the situation by offering to take the items home to remove the dreadful stains. Thankfully, she finally succumbed to my request. I threw away most of those stained clothes because no amount of scrubbing removed the spots.

Aunt Bobbie and I noticed when we visited Mama, she never had

93

toilet paper in the bathroom when I knew good and well, I just brought her 12 rolls a few days before. She hid the toilet paper everywhere because of her suspicions. She didn't want the workers to steal the toilet paper. I engaged in an adult "Easter egg hunt" to find the hidden toilet paper, and replenished the bathroom stash until my next visit, when I discovered the "eggs" had all been hidden again. So frustrating!

It is natural for you to wonder what she used instead of toilet paper. Well, we wondered, too. Aunt Bobbie visited Mama one afternoon and mentioned to Mama she was out of toilet paper. Mama replied, "Oh, I'll just use a wash rag!" The mystery was solved. The story was out. I can't even imagine what she did for a BM. Sorry to get graphic, but caregiver to caregiver, I am trying to be honest here and prepare you. This was my life. This was my mother. She was unwell and becoming different with each passing day. Prepare yourself. Psyche yourself up.

I wondered if management knew how bad her hygiene situation was because I certainly didn't have the heart to tell them. Obviously, they were aware of the fact she wore the same outfits repeatedly, but I needed to find out if she even showered. She never smelled, so there's that. All of this was disheartening, and not like Mama. I hated this part of my journey. It made me sick to my stomach, not arguing with her, but knowing her disease had reached this level and in all likelihood, would inevitably worsen.

<hr />

When Mama exhibited serious signs of paranoia, I called the director and asked for an assessment of Mama. Without having to find her file, the director rattled off about eight items. Everything was correct. She didn't mention Mama's hygiene, and I didn't give that information out. I tried my hardest to keep Mama from "The Back." I didn't know if I would ever be strong enough to make that move.

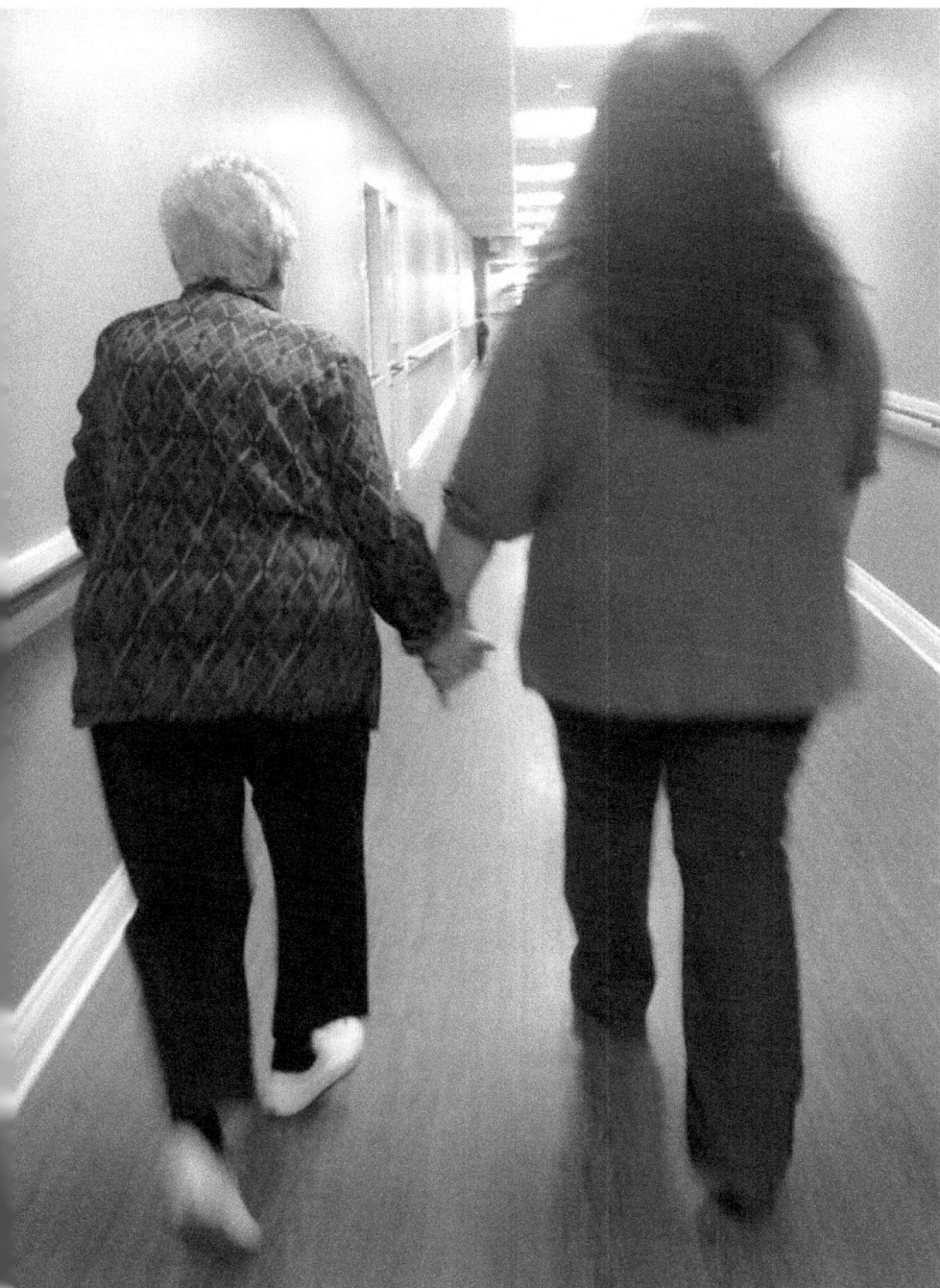

# CHAPTER 23
# BIT BY BIT

MAMA'S MEMORY was getting shorter and shorter if that was ever possible. I spoke with her about all the new great-grandchildren to join our family during the year, and she informed everybody she was going to become a great-grandmother soon. I said, "Mama, you already have eight great-grandchildren." She replied, "Really? Who are they?" Inser lump in my throat.

I became a grandmother to two beautiful girls, born only two months apart. I was over the moon in love with both of these little bundles. One was born locally and the other several hours away. I prayed they would grow up to be best friends and close cousins.

I was touched when my Aunt Bobbie came right away to the hospital to meet our new grandchild. She stood in the gap for my mother, without even being asked. It meant so much to me for her to be there with me.

The following day, my Mama was having a good day, and knowing how much she adored children, I thought I might bring her to the hospital to meet her new great- grandchild. I sat Mama in the rocking chair and placed the baby in her arms. Mama looked incredibly awkward holding the newborn. She had no idea how to hold the baby.

It was not coming back to her. I stayed right by her with my hanc on the newborn. This saddened me a great deal. *My mother, a mother to six, grandmother to 17, and great-grandmother to more than ten children could not remember how to hold a baby.* I laid the baby in a different position in her arms, and Mama still appeared uncomfortable. We took a picture of her but it was not a happy memory to me. Yet another realization of the most endearing pieces of Mama's mind were gone.

Another memorable event was when I had taken Mama out to eat with me and my girls. I dropped all three of them off at the front door of the restaurant and by the time they were situated in a booth, Mama was holding her chest and breathing hard. I chose not to pursue the issue because the doctors typically run countless tests which she hated and she had made it abundantly clear she had wanted to die for the past ten years, and we all knew her mantra, "I gotta die of something." So there. The queen had spoken.

Mama's bones began to hurt more often, and she got absolutely no exercise. Although the Big House did have an exercise room available, she got ticked off because someone had the audacity to adjust the height of the seat on the bike. She never went back. It showed, too. She was not nearly as mobile.

Mama recently had two urinary tract infections, and I learned something new. When someone has dementia and any infection, it could alter their personality. Isn't that interesting? I'm learning volumes about the elderly population, dementia, healthcare, and myself.

Mama's vision was completely gone in one eye, and it became more and more difficult for her to see. She was content staying in the Big House even when she hadn't been out for some time. This is also typical of the dastardly disease.

Mama's memory was rapidly waning. She couldn't remember how many children she had or where she had worked. Those were the two significant changes from the past month. I informed my siblings, that she won't remember when you come, but YOU will know you came and made a difference to her if only for a few moments. Bit by bit, pieces of my mother's memory, significant pieces, were being stripped away by this disease and I was left with a person I hardly recognized.

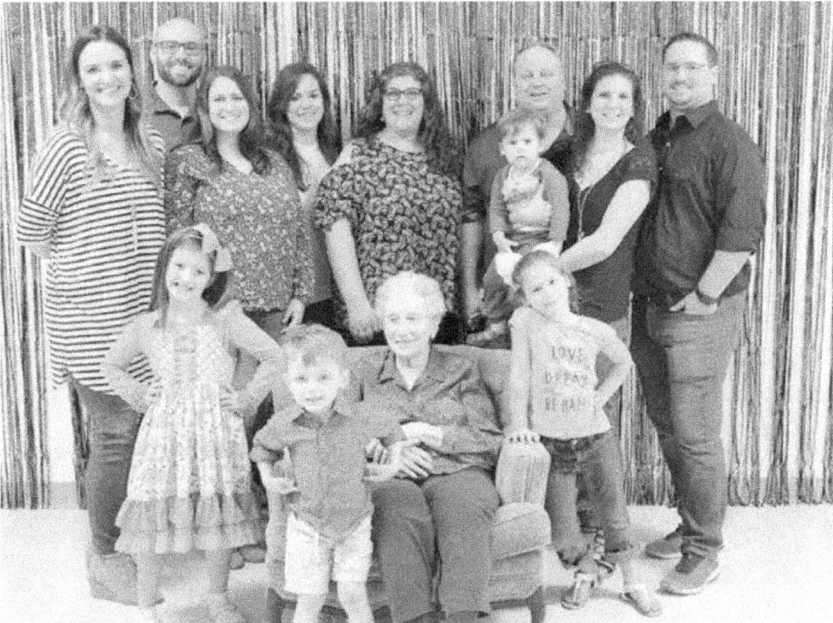

My family at Mama's 90th birthday party

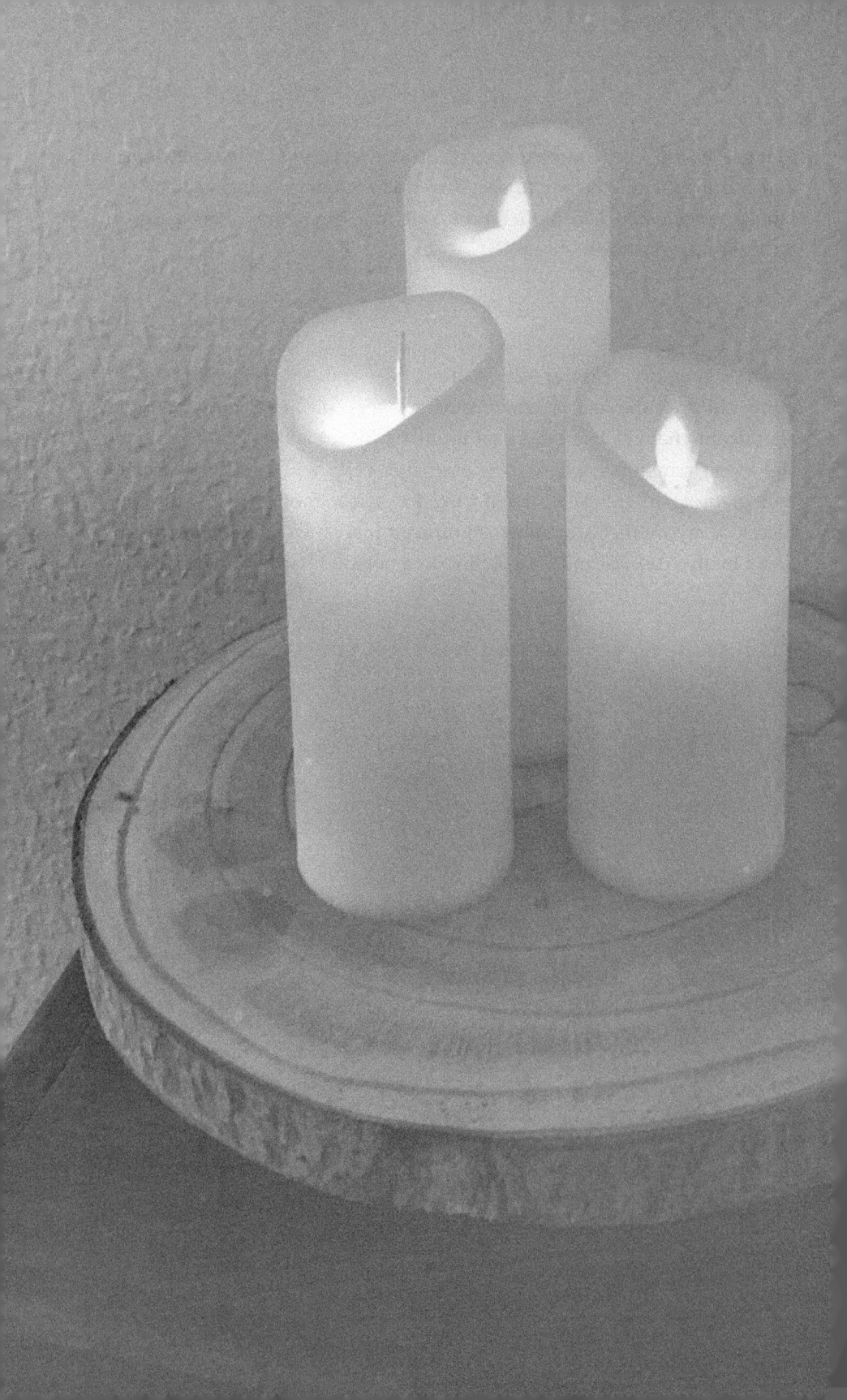

# CHAPTER 24

# SMOKE SIGNALS

GROWING UP, my father chewed on cigars, perfectly angled out of the side of his thin lips. He had previously been a smoker and at 39 suffered a massive heart attack; hence, the tobacco habit became unlit cigars until his premature death at age 50.

My mother was also a smoker, but I categorized her as a social smoker. The funny thing was I never once remembered her clothes or breath smelling of smoke. I don't recall our home having any unpleasant odors either. Mama gave up smoking every year for Lent, and she quit smoking a couple of years after Daddy died. She was in her mid-fifties around that time.

Fast forward to her life at the Big House. Smoking was not allowed inside; therefore, all the smokers gathered on the front porch in the rockers. Those smokers were a close-knit group and enjoyed each other's company. They were often seen sitting together at least a few times a day for a lengthy visit. They loved the opportunity to interact with all the visitors to the facility.

As I did every day, I drove to the Big House to visit my mother. I parked my car roughly 50 yards away from the front entrance. As I approached the porch, I instinctively and mischievously tapped into my investigative skills, eager to discern who was sitting on the patio. This particular day, I was stopped cold in my tracks.

I recognized the residents outside, even from a distance, but imagine my shock when I realized my mother was smoking a cigarette! *NORMA JEAN, what are you doing, woman?*

I hid behind a large, brick column and just watched in amazement. Some 30 years later, she smoked as if she had never quit. I cracked up. This was a true "candid camera" occasion. I was tickled she had regularly supplied me with never-ending comedic material during our journey together. It helped to keep me balanced when I was faced with difficult times. I wiped the smirk off my face and approached Mama. She didn't even attempt to hide the fact her old habit had resurfaced and, quite frankly, didn't act like anything was new under the sun.

That woman, what a character. As we sat on the porch and visited, my wheels were turning at warp speed. So many questions! *Where did she get the cigarette from? How long had this been going on?* I never brought up the subject with Mama. I wanted to see how this played out. I told the staff, and they were aware she was smoking. They wondered if she had smoked when she was younger. Norma Jean, my very own version of Lucille Ball.

Time went on, and I saw Mama smoking more often and wondered how in the world she acquired her cigarettes; then I saw it. *She was a moocher!* People enjoyed her company and offered her one, and she gladly accepted. I refused to buy her a pack because I didn't want to encourage her to smoke. I thought surely, at some point, her porch friends might grow weary of her mooching.

Months go by, and while Mama napped on her couch, I straightened up her bedroom. She had a French Provincial bed, two bedside tables, an entertainment center, and a dresser in her bedroom. I dusted the entertainment center and found one of her trademark, bright yellow kitchen cups behind an 8 x10 photo. *Why did she hide that cup?* Because it contained a cigarette and a lighter. *That turkey! Was she smoking inside her room?*

*Where did she get the lighter?* I thought it was VERY humorous it was positioned next to her beloved statue of the Virgin Mary. Oh, Norma Jean, in the untouched crevices of your mind, you were still a character.

I removed the cigarette and lighter and couldn't wait to share this discovery with my siblings. Mama never asked about the missing paraphernalia.

---

That was one huge advantage with Alzheimer's disease. I discreetly handled necessary matters without her knowledge. The disease diminished her frustration with me tremendously, because she forgot as quickly as it happened.

---

Less than a year later, I never saw Mama smoke again. I don't know if she lost her "supplier" or just grew tired of the habit or the company, but I will always love the memory of catching her red-handed.

Oh, and the yellow kitchen cup is now housed in my office. The contents? The winnings from one of her bingo games – a couple of dollars and some change. I couldn't bear to part with it. My recollection of this entire event brings an enormous smile to my face, even now.

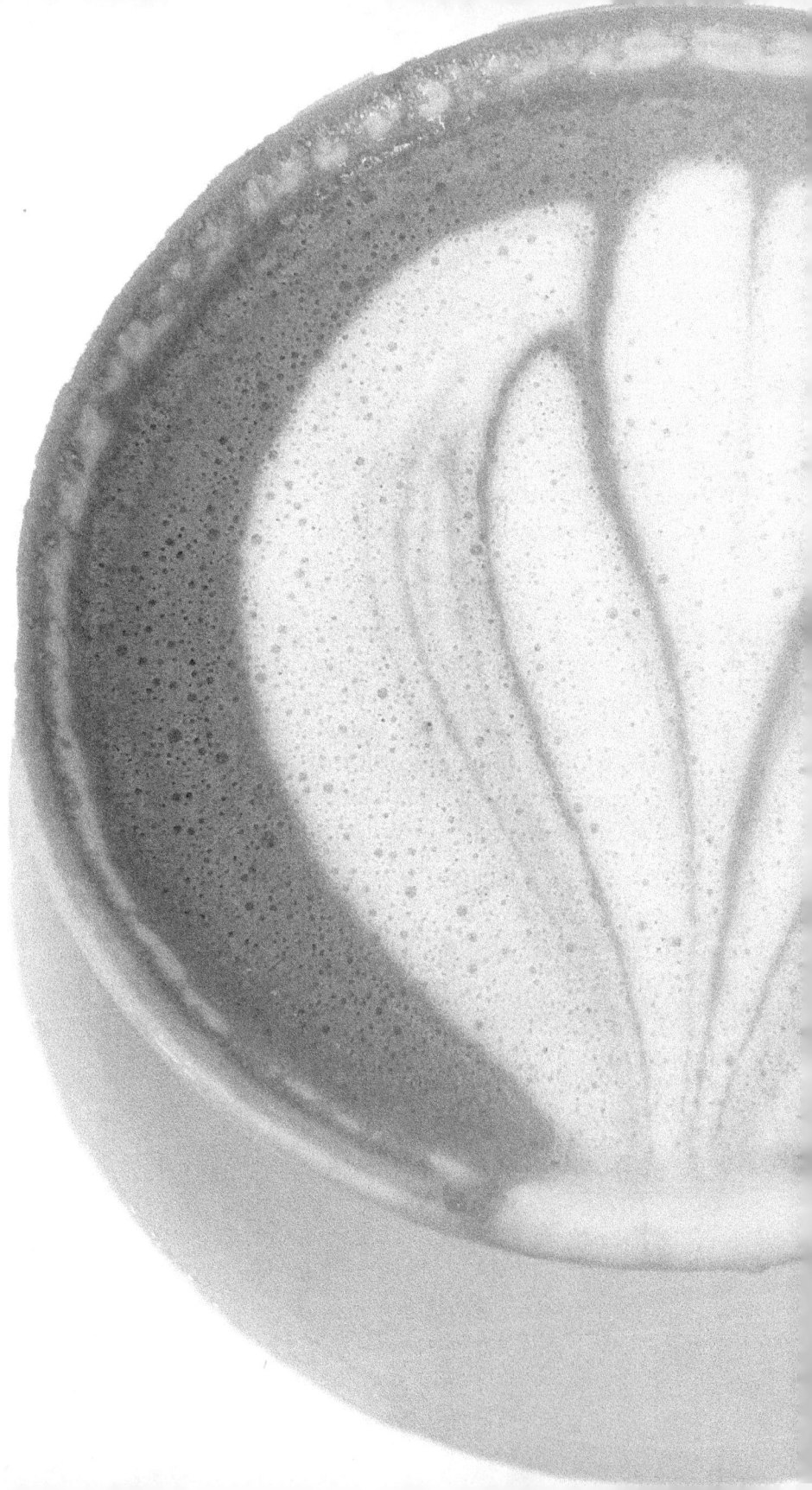

# CHAPTER 25
# SOCIAL GRACES

I FOUND as Mama's vision continued to decrease, she would not get quite as easily agitated in a well-lit room. In addition, she didn't like excessive noise. She reacted quickly with outbursts. Because of these new issues, the ability to locate a restaurant that met all my requirements and ensure Mama enjoyed the meal was difficult. Today I chose to bring Mama for a late lunch at Cracker Barrel to avoid the crowds. The young male host went to seat us at a table and, because Mama was happier in better lighting (I'm not kidding either), I asked if we could sit by the windows. Without hesitation, he moved us to a window seat and raised the blinds which provided plenty of light for Mama. He had no idea what one little gesture meant to us. Mama didn't complain the entire meal about "how dark" it was; it was one of the most enjoyable meals we had in a long time.

---

As Mama's Alzheimer's progressed, her eyesight diminished. She only saw slight shadows. She maneuvered down the hallways without assistance in the beginning. As time went on, however, I noticed other changes. I noted a significant change when I visited her one evening for supper. She was with three other residents at her regular table in the dining room.

After I pulled up a chair and settled in beside her, I saw her using her hands to eat. She touched the mashed potatoes and then, *with her hands*, put a dollop of them in her mouth. As she felt around the plate, she touched the carrots and, again, hand-fed herself. I was extremely embarrassed this precious mother of mine, who NEVER EVER in her *right* mind would have fed herself like a toddler, was doing this repeatedly and not thinking anything of it. Her tablemates were alarmed and appalled. Each day I tried to help Mama and coax her into using her utensils, but she always reverted to eating her meal with her hands. This new behavior was disheartening. Some women who sat at her table requested to be moved to another table because they were repulsed by her newfound table manners. One by one they left, leaving Mama to eat alone. I understood their motive, but Mama wondered where her friends went—yet another thing this disease took from my mother.

Mama seemed to be more awkward in public situations. She has said inappropriate things about people and to people. She hides tissue in her bra, pulls it out to blow her nose, and stuffs it back in her bra when finished. I've even had her offer that same tissue to some innocent bystander in need. I intercepted the pass!

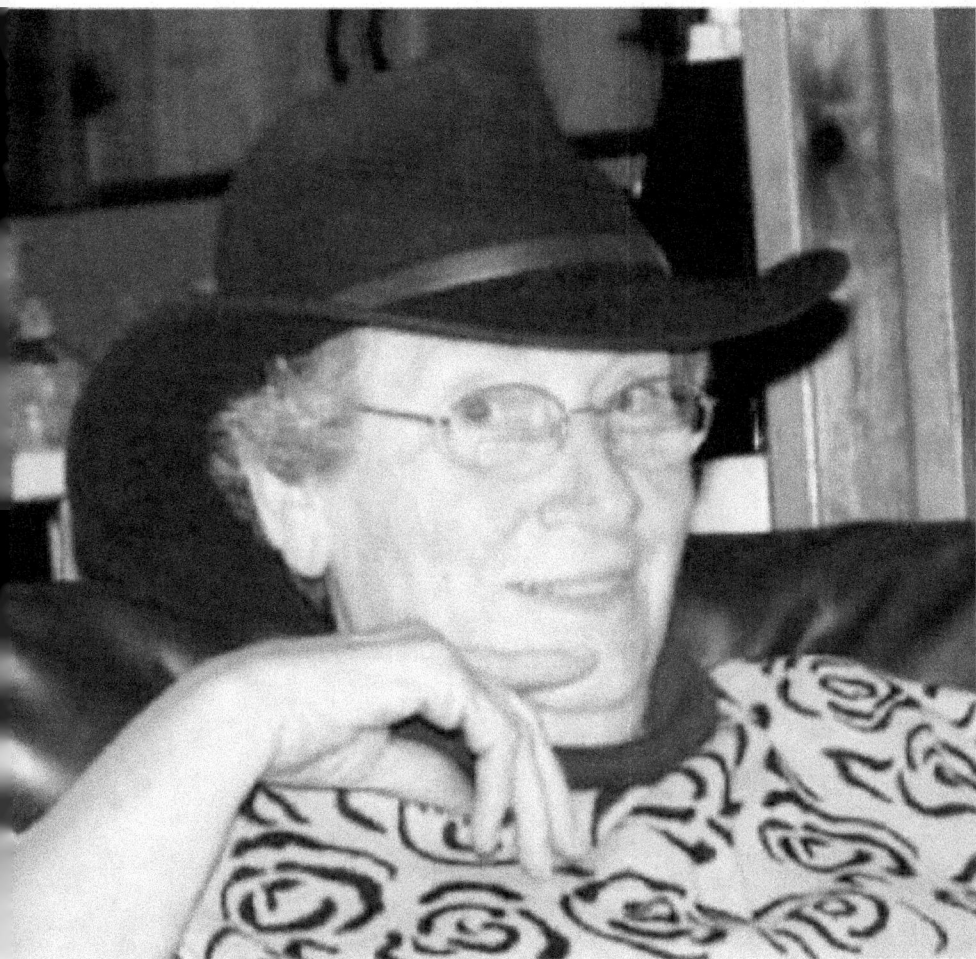

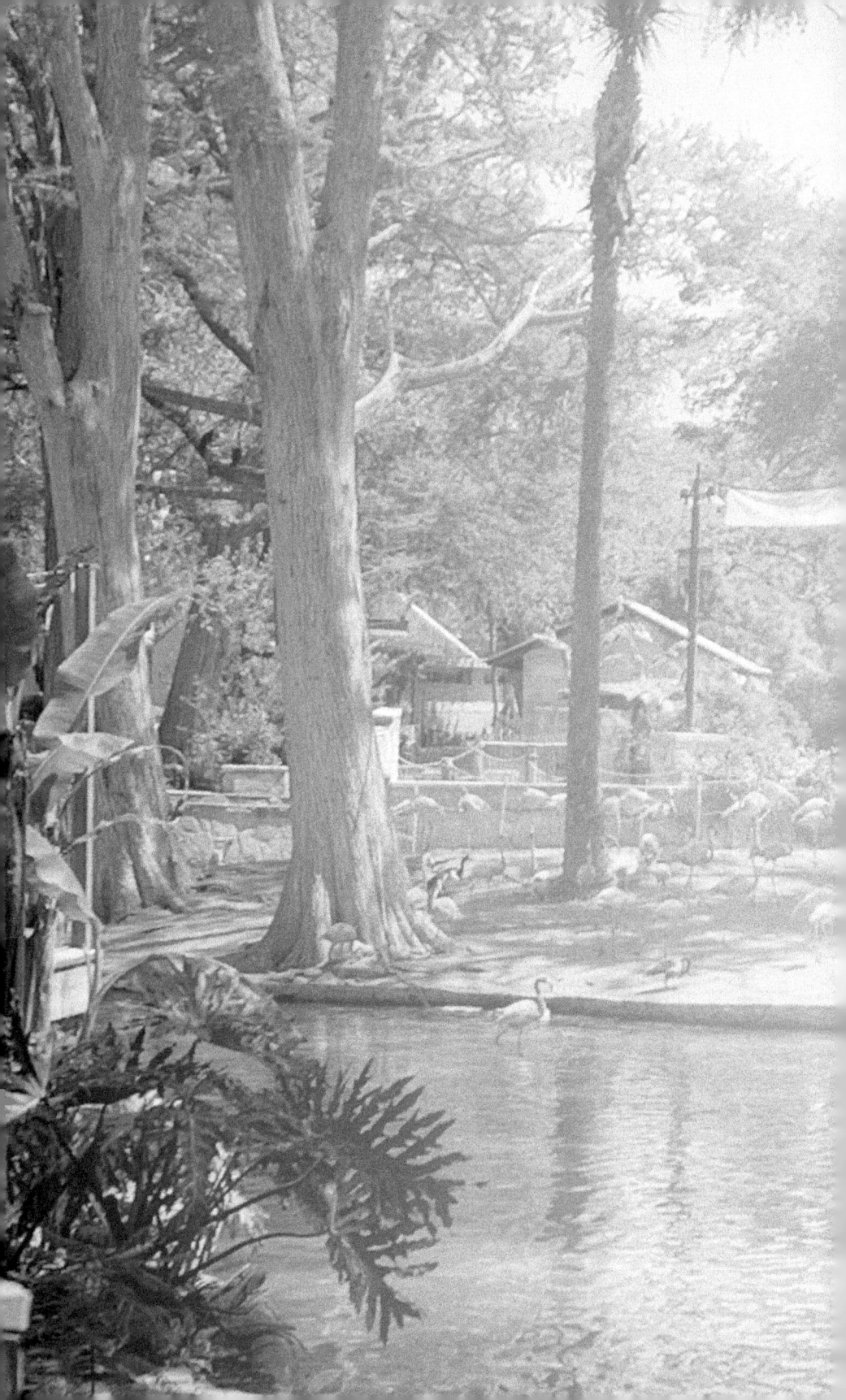

# CHAPTER 26

# NORMA JEAN COMEDY HOUR

MY SWEET MAMA had such an eventful day. We went to the salon for a manicure, and she kept saying funny things to the kind man helping her. He never made eye contact or smiled at her or acknowledged her antics. However, when we walked toward the door to leave, he followed us outside and asked me her age. I told him she was almost 86, and he lowered his head and shook it side to side in disbelief. He said, "I thought she was a lot younger." He walked off, seemingly very disappointed.

At our next stop we saw our dear, sweet, family friend, John, at his office. Mom and I were seated in the reception area waiting for him to return. Once I saw him walking toward the door, I told Mama to tell John, "Are we still on for Friday night good looking?" She rehearsed it several times, and I figured there was no way she was going to remember what to say. Lo and behold, John walked in the door, and Mama said her rehearsed lines verbatim and John was shocked! It was a memorable, hilarious moment for all. Later the same day, I received a picture of Mama playing with puppets provided by a church group visiting the Big House. Mama was having way too much fun cutting up with them. These were the good days, and I didn't take them for granted.

Mel (Mary Ellen's nickname) offered to give me a much-needed break and brought Mama to the beauty salon. Mel later relayed a story that an older lady in the stylist's chair waved to Mama, and Mama quickly turned to Mel and asked who the woman was looking at her. Mel mentioned she looked familiar but had no idea who she was. When the woman's hairstyling was finished, she jumped out of her chair and walked straight over to Mel and Mama. The woman greeted Mama in French and Mama seemed to respond properly in French. They carried on their conversation like they were old friends. When the woman left, Mel and Mama immediately looked at each other, shrugged their shoulders, and chuckled out loud. That's my Mama: *Fake it till you make it!* I'm delighted my children and grandchildren learned to enjoy the company of individuals who might not be fully themselves but are still incredibly lovable.

My daughters went to visit their Mamaw after school one day. Mama asked them about their grades. (I found it interesting how she quickly surmised since these were young ladies, they must be in school.) Chrissy asked Mama about HER grades. Mama asked, "Which ones?" Mary Ellen piped up and said, "Your awesomeness!" Mama quickly replied, "Oh, that's 100%." I am so thankful my girls did not shy away from their Mamaw.

They knew she had changed. She was different. But they looked past the change and had the knack of bringing out the comedian in her, and it was a beautiful thing to witness. Those three shared countless laughs. What lovely memories.

During our routine trip to the beauty salon, the male salon owner climbed on top of a ladder located right next to the door and cashier area. He tried in vain to repair the neon "OPEN" sign while Mama and

I stood near the register and paid the bill. Remember, we were positioned right beside the ladder with the gentleman on it. Something told me to look at Norma Jean. I turned around and glanced at Mama; she was staring up at the gentleman with a big, mischievous smile on her face and slowly raised her hand. The stylists and other clients all held their breath. We were certain Norma Jean would slap the poor ole guy on his rear! We waited and watched as she gave him a firm karate chop across the back of his knee! Everyone exhaled at once! It was hilarious. The whole salon, including the victim, was in stitches. Oh, how I love these moments with Mama.

<hr>

Another trip for Mama to the hair salon, followed by a trip to the nail salon was in order for the day. None of the technicians in the nail salon spoke English. When the employees were talking to one another, Mama, not one to be left out, chimed in with French dialogue with animated body language, and the room burst out in laughter. Mama was genuinely trying to teach these ladies French.

<hr>

Let me share a prime example of Norma Jean and her mischievousness. After getting her hair fixed at the salon, another hairdresser says, " Miss Norma, you are looking so good, to which my mother quickly replies, "You were looking at my backside when you said that, it must mean you like what you see!" I can't make this stuff up.

<hr>

It was time for another visit with the eye doctor. The nurse turned the light out while Mama's eyes dilated and Mama immediately said, "I look prettier in the dark, don't I?"

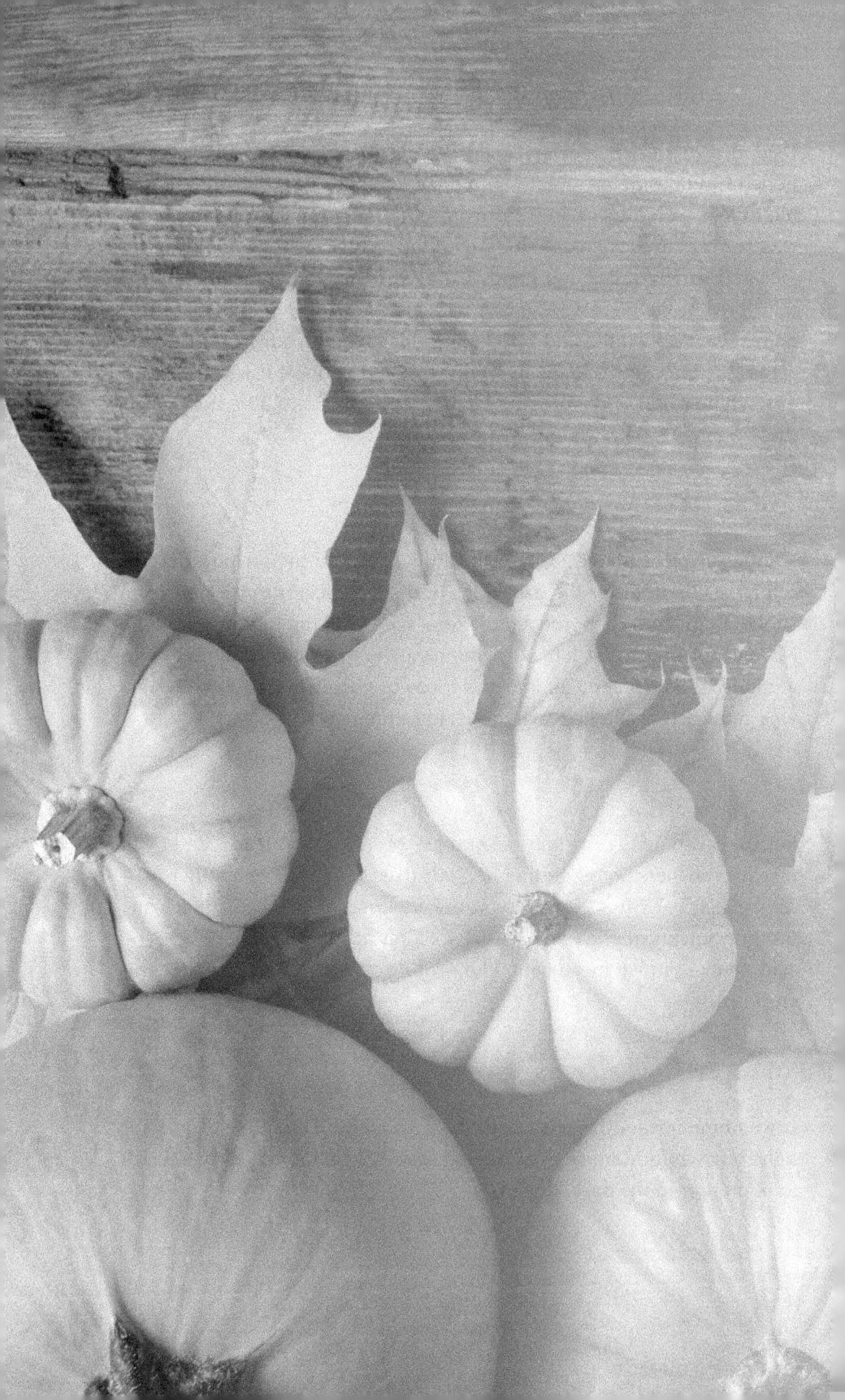

## CHAPTER 27

# MORE TRICKS THAN TREATS

THE ANNUAL HALLOWEEN festivities rolled around at the Big House, and although Mama became increasingly awkward in public, I chose to let her sit in her chair and hand out candy to all the children who passed through the facility. She enjoyed the children very much. I couldn't take this opportunity away from her. I sat right next to her while my daughters were on the other side of her chair.

Before the first child arrived, Mama started eating the candy in her bowl. She wasted no time enjoying this gift from the gods. The first family approached Mama, and the child moved close to her. Mama picked up a piece of candy from the bowl, unwrapped it, and popped it in HER own mouth. The child's face was pathetic. I couldn't help but laugh, though. I told Mama the candy was for the children, and she immediately removed the half-chewed morsel from her mouth, put it back in the wrapper, and dropped it in the child's bucket. *OH MY GOSH*. I was not expecting that at all. I apologized profusely to the child and her parents. I thought surely this was just a fluke. Unfortunately, I was wrong. She did the same thing when the next child came. The parents' faces told the story. They were mortified.

My laughter turned to sadness. I gave Mama a smaller bowl and let her eat the candy. My girls handed out the candy to the children. Mama never noticed the changing of the guard.

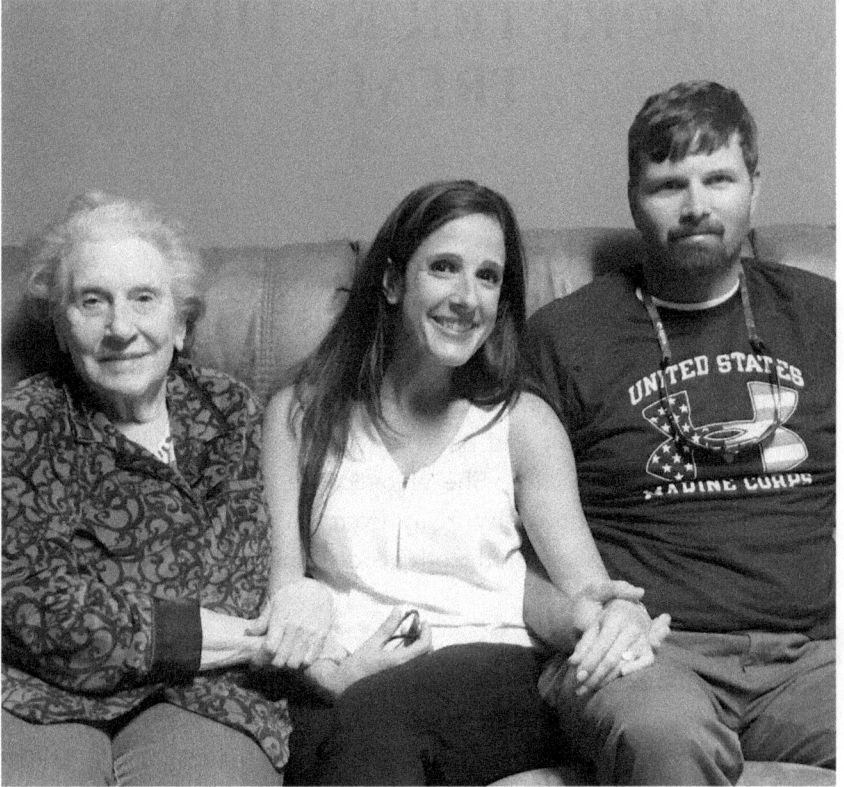

My Mama, her granddaughter, Katie and her husband, Jason

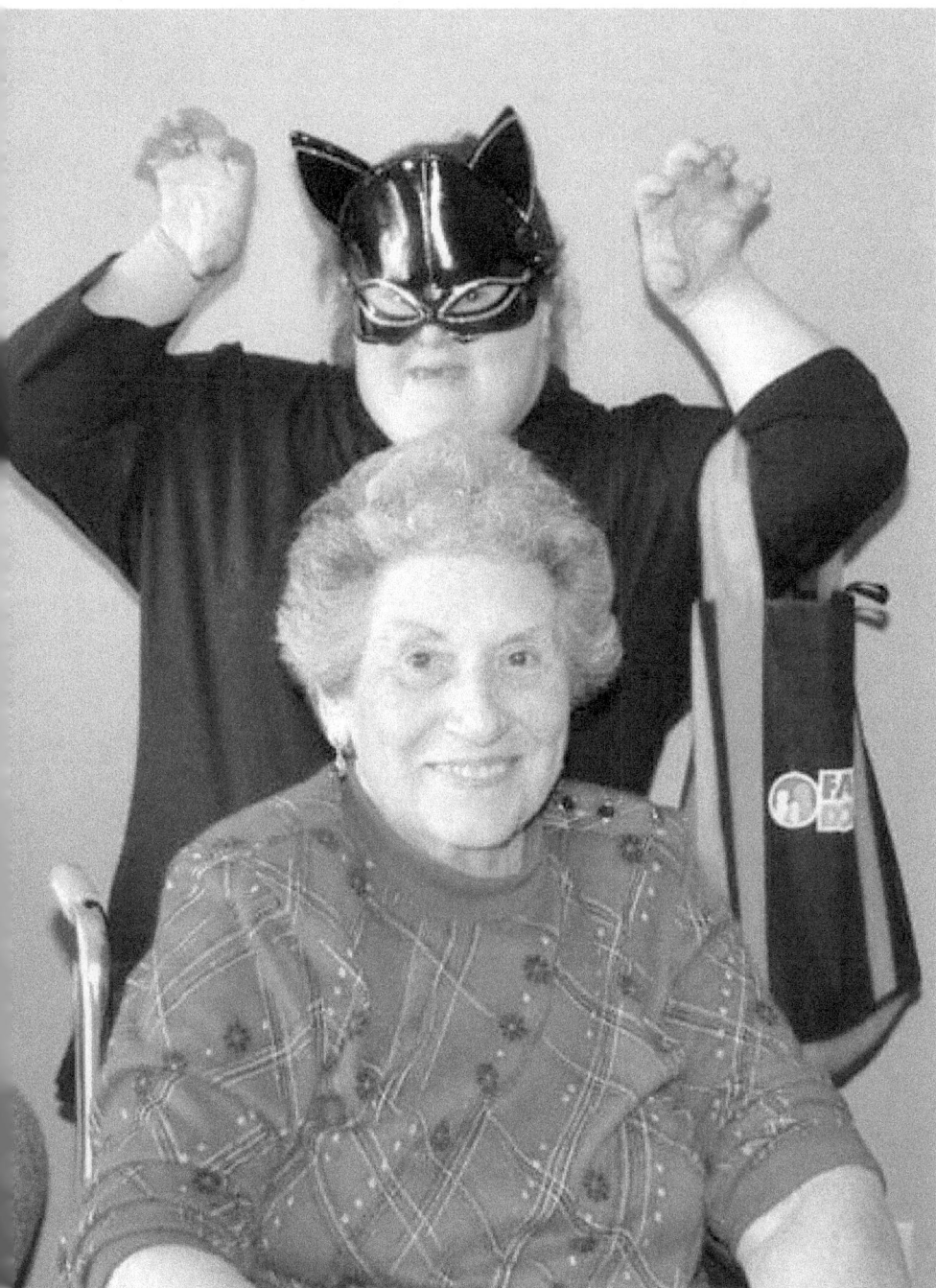

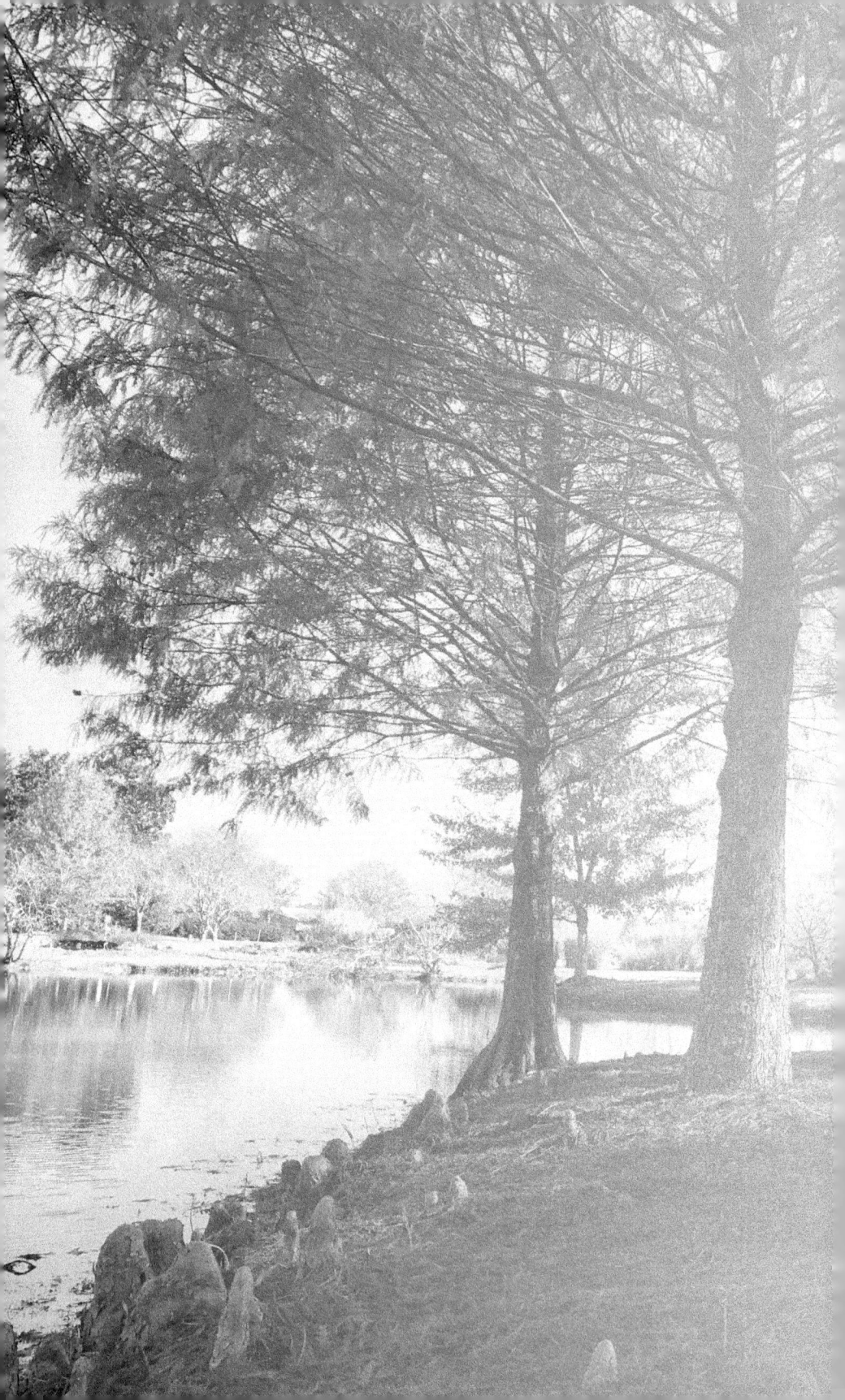

# CHAPTER 28

# FACING MY FEARS

I WRESTLED WITH A BITTERSWEET AWARENESS, though I tried to brush it off, that the time I had left with Mama on the assisted living side was slipping away. Each passing day Mama required more from others for even simple tasks, added to that her hygiene and table manners were becoming worse plus her memory issues and eyesight both added to my growing uneasiness. I didn't have the playbook for Mama's life, but I held onto my faith in God's plan for this precious soul. I couldn't help but beg Him to spare me from moving Mama to the Special Care unit. Moving her meant the end was drawing near. Moving her made me feel as though I failed her. I readied myself for the inevitable moment the administrator decreed the time had come for Mama to transfer to Special Care. Maybe the darkness that overshadowed my thoughts of this pivotal moment was the finality of it all. It may perhaps be the final curtain in my Mama's life.

Her vibrant essence, the very essence that had earned her admiration as a smart and elegant woman, was slowly slipping away. I had a talk with God in plain English...*Her existing heart issues, couldn't they be mercifully replaced with a swift heart attack? Anything, I pleaded with the Lord, anything but the dreaded move to the "unknown" in the back.* My begging persisted and the fateful response was "No, not yet."

The administrator's voice on the phone told me while Mama was sundowning (wandering in the evening) she proceeded to venture outside, in the dark, and because the doors locked behind her, she could not get back in. She had now acquired the label of a "Flight Risk." The decree was handed down - the transfer to Special Care was unavoidable now. Oh, sweet Mama. I found myself searching for an untested courage, bracing myself to confront the very fear I had tried to shun for five years – the Back!

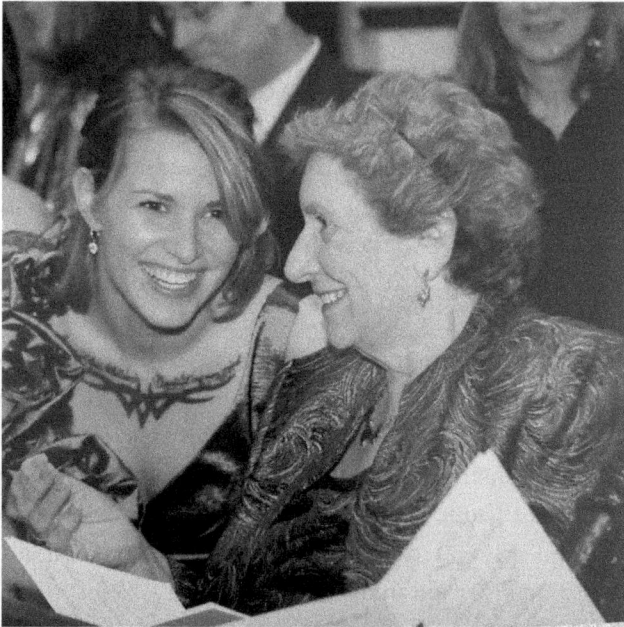

Mama with her granddaughter, Hannah

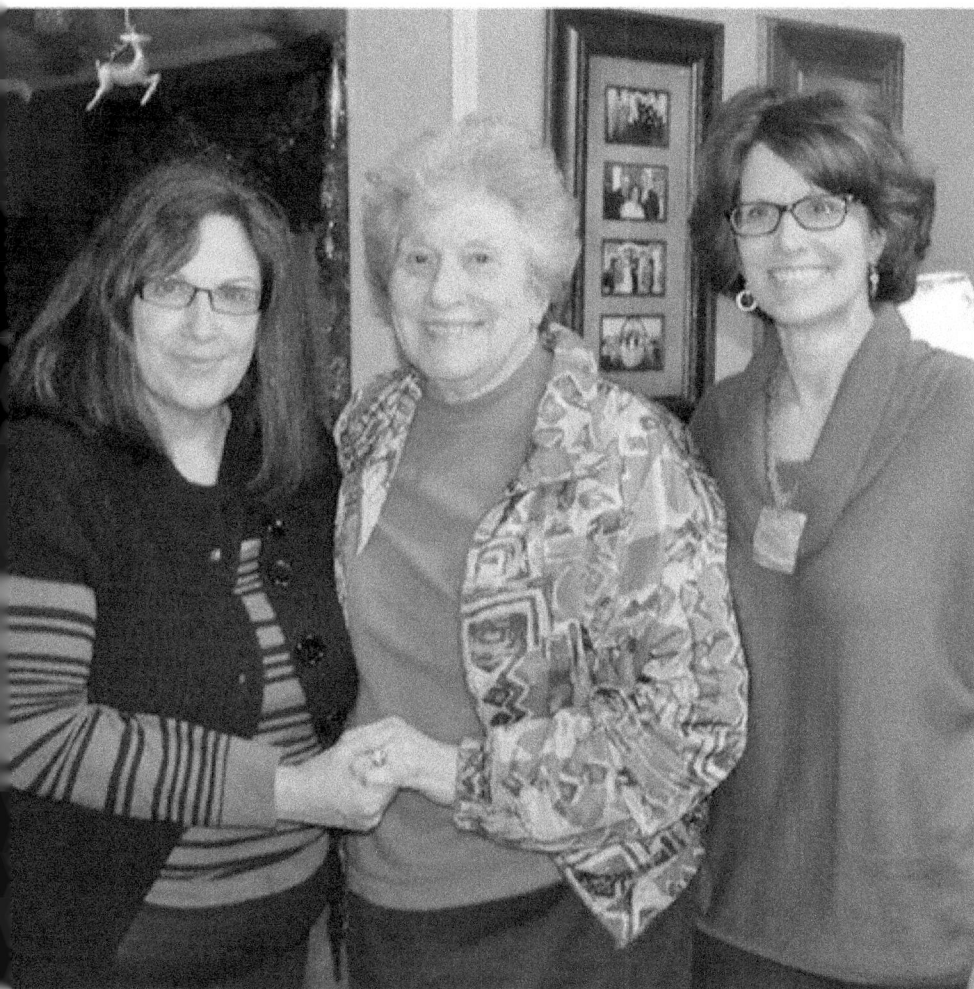

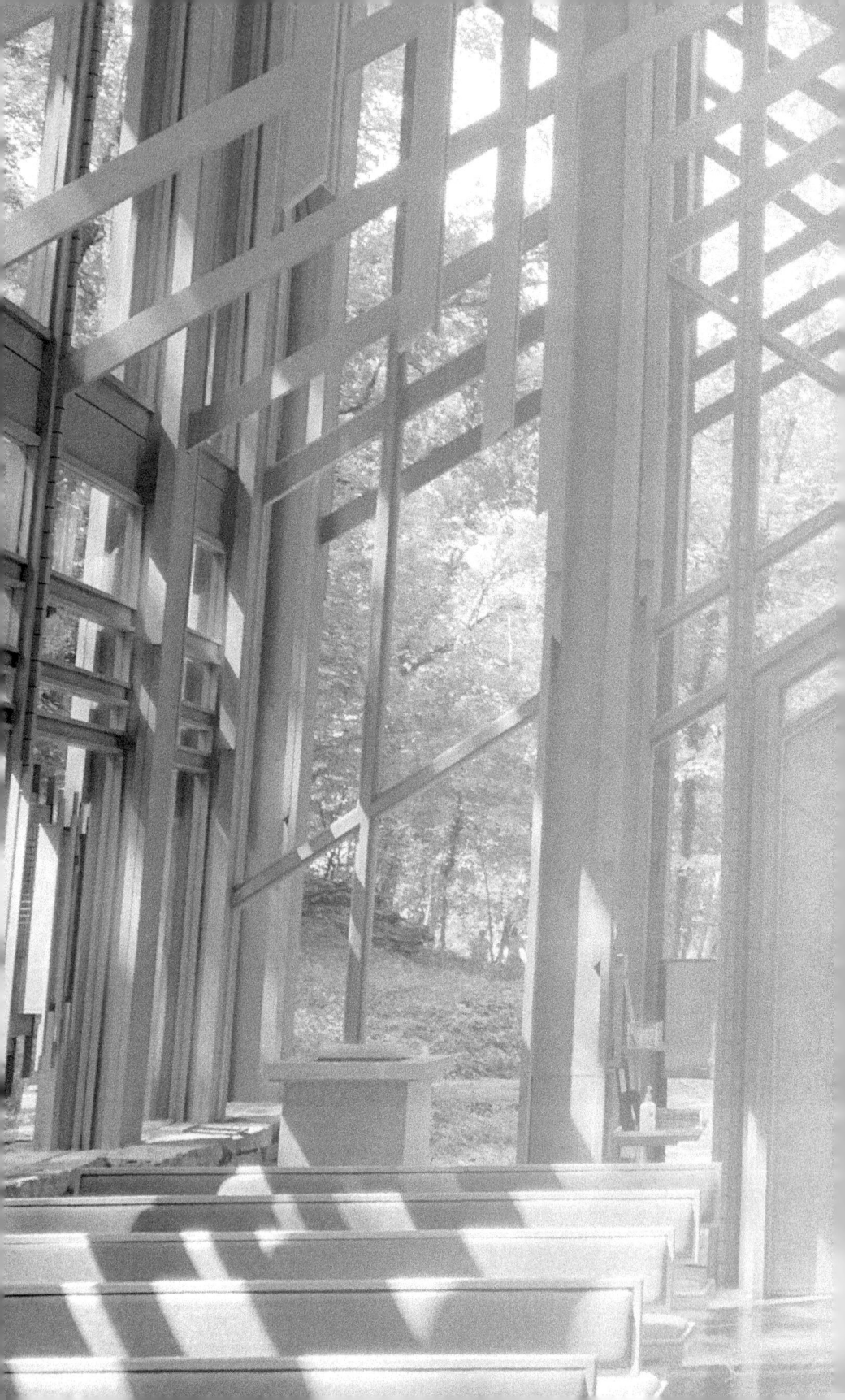

# CHAPTER 29
# A SHOT OF COURAGE

I'VE STRESSED over how this day, the momentous transfer to special care, would play out, and the verse God gave me was about my steps being ordered. He worked out every detail. I had the full support of the staff and He sent me angels who didn't even know what they volunteered for but they offered their assistance regardless. I felt God's presence all around me.

Before my daughter arrived to assist me on the dreaded moving day, the movers I hired arrived in their bright yellow truck and immediately dove into action. It was of utmost importance I kept Mama busy, shielding her from the shift to a new living situation. With her existing level of paranoia, there was no need to compound her distress. While I kept Mama entertained, my friend, Jennifer, directed the movers. This move would have been a disaster without her. She brought some comical relief to an otherwise awful, emotional day.

Another angel was my daughter, Mel. She took Mama out of the facility for nearly four hours, which was never an easy task. She embarked on an adventurous outing by including all of Mama's favorite things...Dairy Barn chocolate shakes and french fries, she drove by Mama's old house, and went to the cemetery to see Daddy's grave along with some of her sibling's graves.

They also visited with Jaci, my daughter-in-law, at her home. Mama had a wonderful time, and it helped us accomplish what had to be done.

<hr />

In "the back" special attention was given to bed checks every two hours. There was a locked entrance, and the nurses' station was conveniently located by the door. Visitors had to ring the doorbell and wait to be granted admission. It was disappointing to me cameras were not permitted in the rooms because I wanted to monitor what Mama was doing in my absence. The facility offered entertainment and meals, with snacks provided at designated times during the day. The population was significantly smaller compared to the front of the Big House. While Mama's new apartment resembled her assisted living space, the overall unit had a different atmosphere. I was grateful it was not as sterile or urine-infused as some nursing homes. The surroundings were comfortable, and the furnishings and decorations were visually appealing. Mama's apartment had been recently painted and thoroughly cleaned, and with her own furnishings arranged perfectly, it looked inviting and Norma Jean approved. I felt compelled to repeat the same scenario I had when I moved Mama into the Big House five years earlier. I stayed with her all day, helped her navigate the lay of the land, met other residents, and introduced myself to the staff. I will never regret giving my time to be there for her. I dare not imagine her trying to navigate all the changes without help. I couldn't expect the staff to devote the necessary time to just one resident. This was a job for the family.

<hr />

I don't understand how some residents can be brought to a facility and literally dropped off and the family never returns to see them. (I saw this far too often). Oh sure, they send a check to the facility every month, but to just leave them? Your person's personality may have changed tremendously, but I believe to my dying breath, they are still in there (body, mind, soul), wanting to be around someone who loves them and cares for them if only for a short while. From one caregiver to another, I'm grateful you found a safe place to put them, but they still need you! If you absolutely cannot have eyes on your family member, consider hiring someone to work a few hours a week. Ask them to retrieve items on their shopping list, check on them, and note any changes they see. Ask the employees if they noted any changes. Let them know who your person is in the facility. I know patients can be mean, cantankerous, unappreciative, and violent, but at least provide for their basic needs (clothes, haircuts, snacks) and call them. Rant Over!

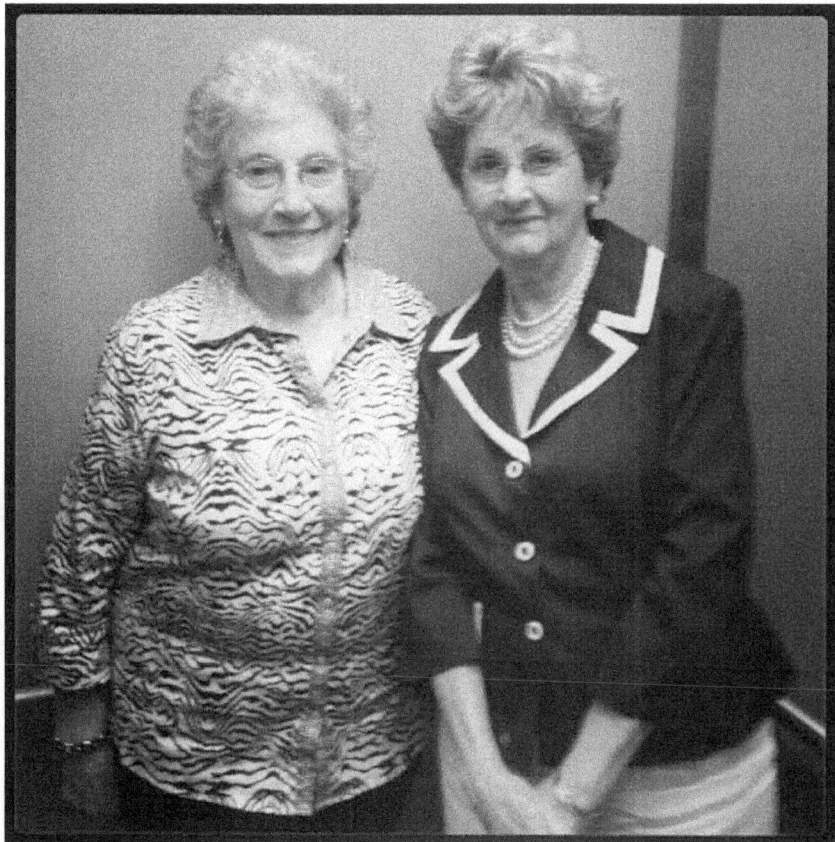

Mama and her sister, Bobbie

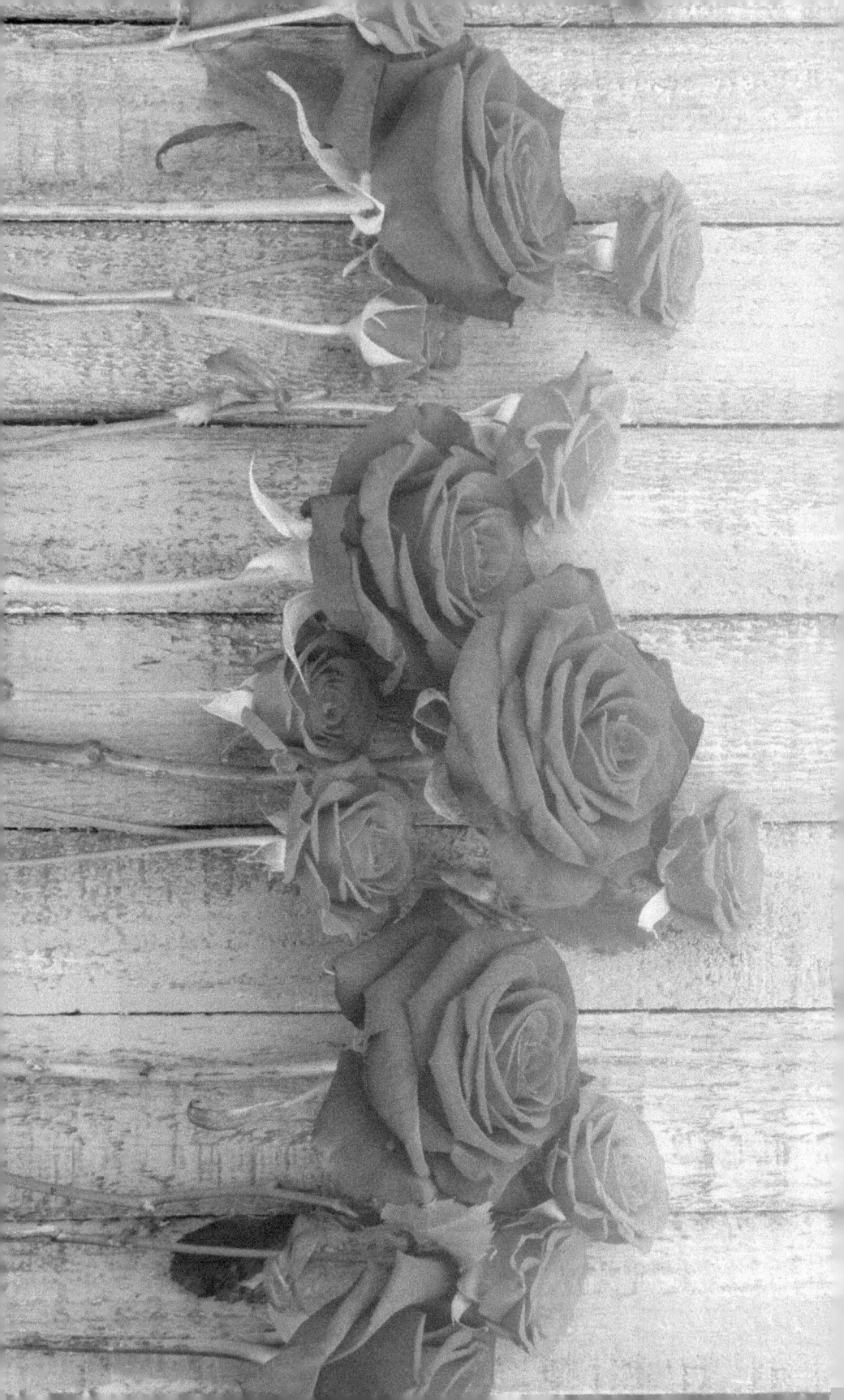

## CHAPTER 30
# NEVER ALONE

I WAS unaware before this transition Mama shuffled her feet when she walked. Without carpet in the hallways and apartments, the shuffle was more pronounced. Mama was seated with a cast of characters at a table for four. She chose to only eat finger foods at this juncture in her dining demise. Her lack of table etiquette didn't seem to bother her new tablemates. The staff was great with Mama. I think her playful reputation preceded her arrival. They immediately played on that. Even with all the shenanigans and laughter, Mama was easily agitated. I don't know if it was because of so many new, different personalities she encountered in the back or the disease, but her agitation was heightened.

<hr>

Her favorite place to be was in the large, light blue TV room lined with recliners. When I first saw Mama in the TV room, it was the second chair to the left of the door she chose and 95% of the time she plopped right there every time. She found comfort in the voices in this room. It seemed to lessen her paranoia of being left out. Even when she was not part of the conversation, she enjoyed hearing people around her and

125

knew she was not alone. I felt we should begin sitting in the TV room regularly where nearly every chair in the room was occupied by a resident.

The TV wasn't played often, but conversations were always happening nearby. Usually residents talking out loud to themselves. Those were hilarious conversations. Like the Enquirer, I got all the inside scoop going on in their little noggins. Somedays, Mama was more engaged than others.

⁓⧉⁓

I enjoyed it immensely when Mama joined me in singing old hymns or patriotic songs and more often than not, some of the staff chimed in the singing. I recorded many of our singing sessions.

---

**I encourage you to take more pictures than you ever have before, record your loved one's voice and video them. It has become a treasure trove of beautiful memories for me and my family.**

---

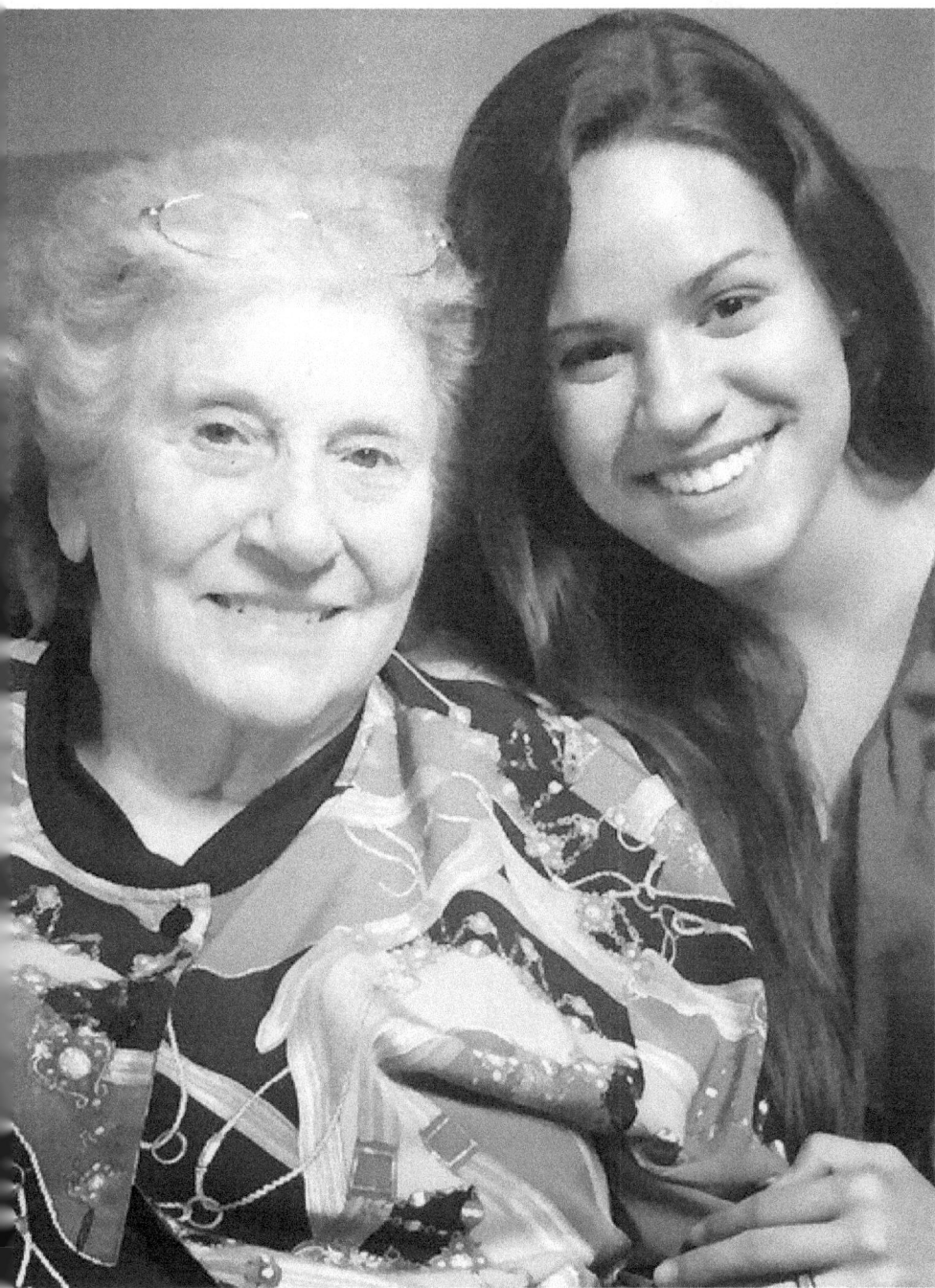

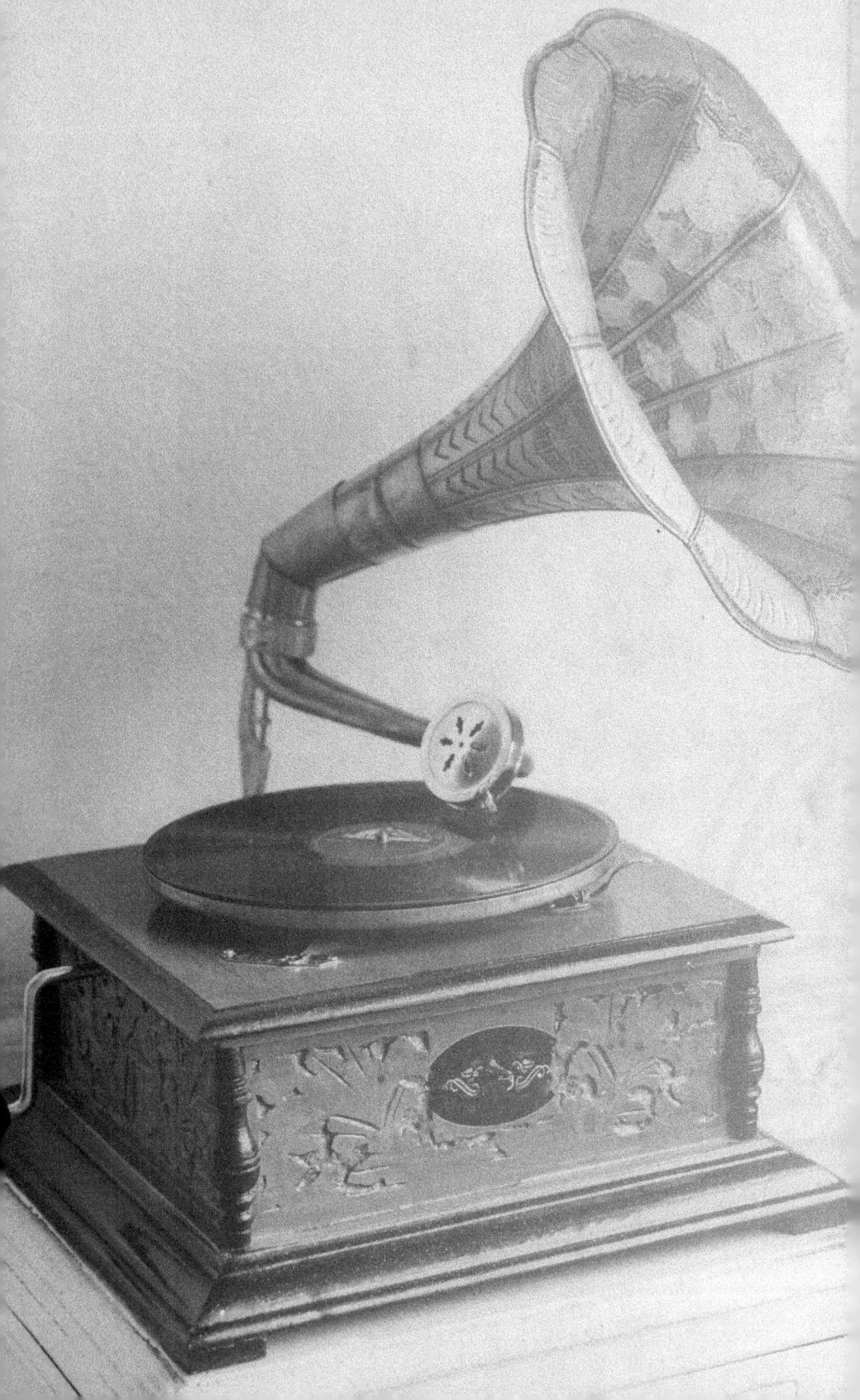

# CHAPTER 31
# FAVORITE MEMORIES

I WAS thankful Mama was still able to walk without assistance unlike many other residents and she enjoyed time spent with my family whether at my house or a restaurant. One particular evening, we gathered at a local Cajun restaurant and Mama was in rare form during the meal, being silly, tickling the children, and saying off-the-cuff remarks.

We all enjoyed seeing a glimpse of Norma Jean at her best. As we began to leave our chairs and walk toward the exit, I noticed how crowded it was and the wait line to be seated was at least 15 people deep. If Norma Jean had run for a political seat, I dare say she had a good chance of winning with all the handshaking, hugging, and jabbing in the ribs she did to the innocent bystanders waiting in the line. She even kissed a few babies. I never knew what to expect from her. Never!

---

As I often did, I visited Mama and found her in the TV room where the staff had a CD playing old songs. The female resident sitting next to me was going on and on about how her husband used to love to dance with her, and she hinted (STRONGLY) she wanted to dance. I asked her to dance, and we did. She LOVED it. She liked to be twirled around.

So sweet. Not one to pass up a good time, I asked Mama if she wanted to dance, and she said, "Yes." She thoroughly enjoyed it, but she was unable to make it through the entire song, the exertion wore her out. I cherished times like this more than words could say. Dancing with my Granny, aunts, cousins, and siblings was one of my favorite childhood memories.

<hr />

In order to go to doctor's appointments, I needed to inform the staff, arrive early enough to get inside the building, and ensure Mama was dressed and groomed. This visit was to see her podiatrist. As we were leaving the doctor's office, Mama surveyed the waiting room and asked, "Where are all my red-headed children?" I was dumbfounded. This statement was shocking and yet touching. Unbeknownst to Mama in her current mental stage, her husband was red-headed, her sixth child was the only one with strawberry blonde hair, and four of her great-grandchildren were red-headed. I could not believe she specified red. I lived for moments like this.

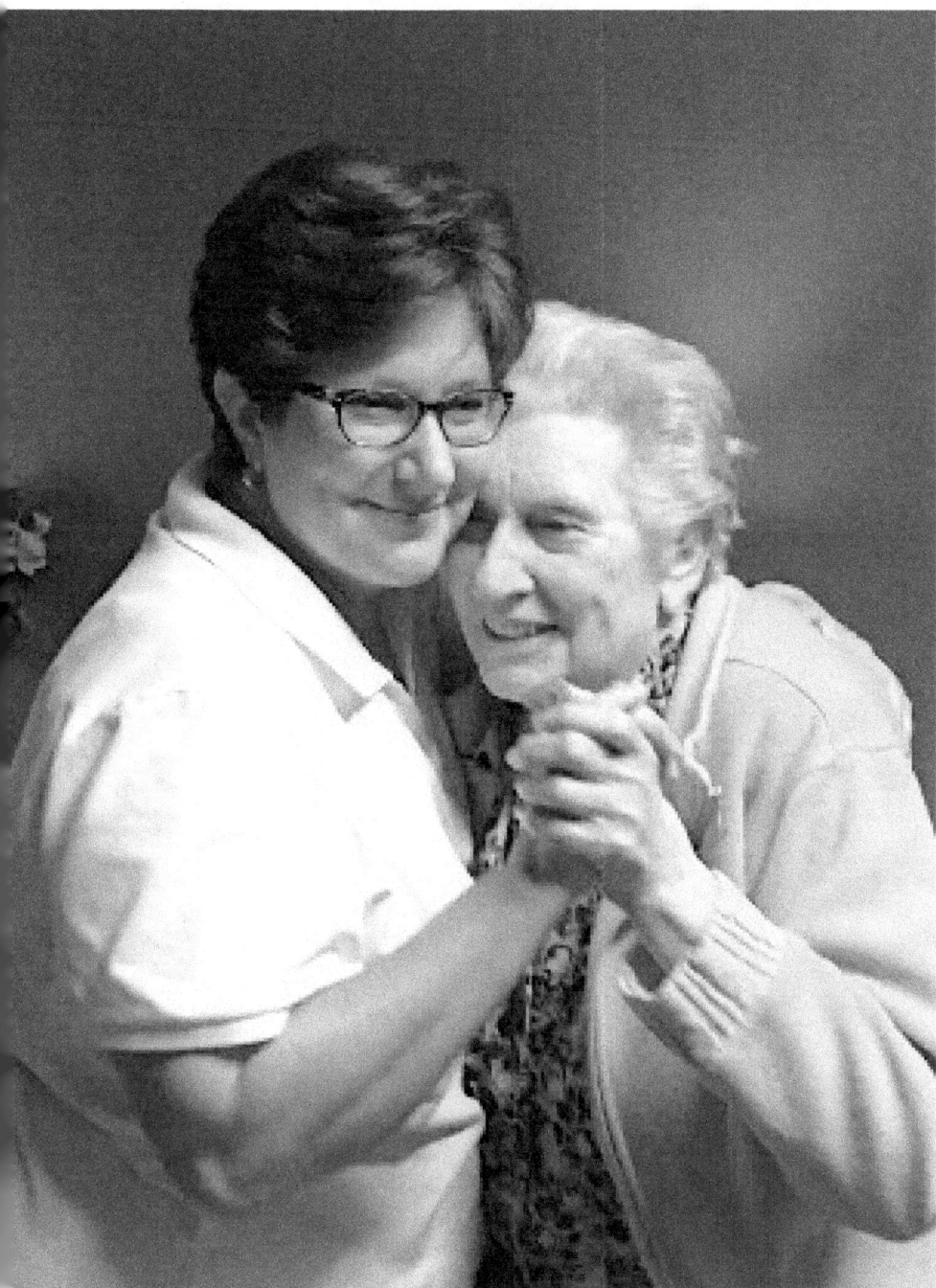

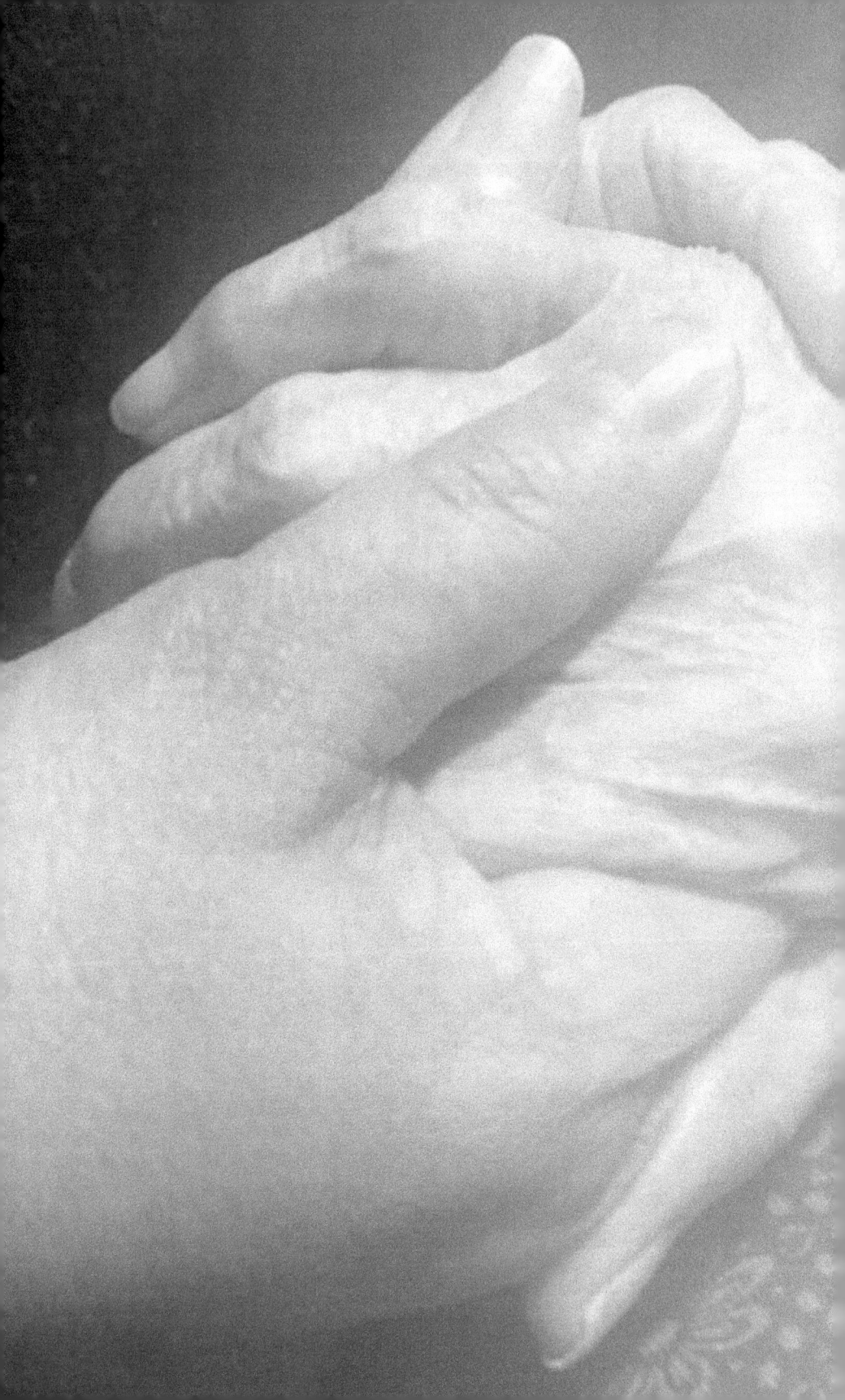

# CHAPTER 32

# MAKING A DIFFERENCE

DURING YOUTH CAMP with my daughters one summer, we talked about God's grace and His unexpected blessings. Soon after returning home, I watched my daughter, Mary Ellen, receive one such blessing.

~~~❦~~~

She received a handwritten, two-page graduation letter in the mail from her cousin, Neal. One of the most touching things he wrote was his recognition of her academic achievements but more importantly, he honored her for all she did for Mamaw, he also quoted scripture about caring for widows and praised and thanked her for looking after Mama. I was thrilled for her to learn a valuable lesson...people are always watching. Since graduation, she became a nurse and continued to assist me with Mama. This unexpected letter was impactful for her, simply extraordinary. Blessings sometimes come in the most unexpected ways.

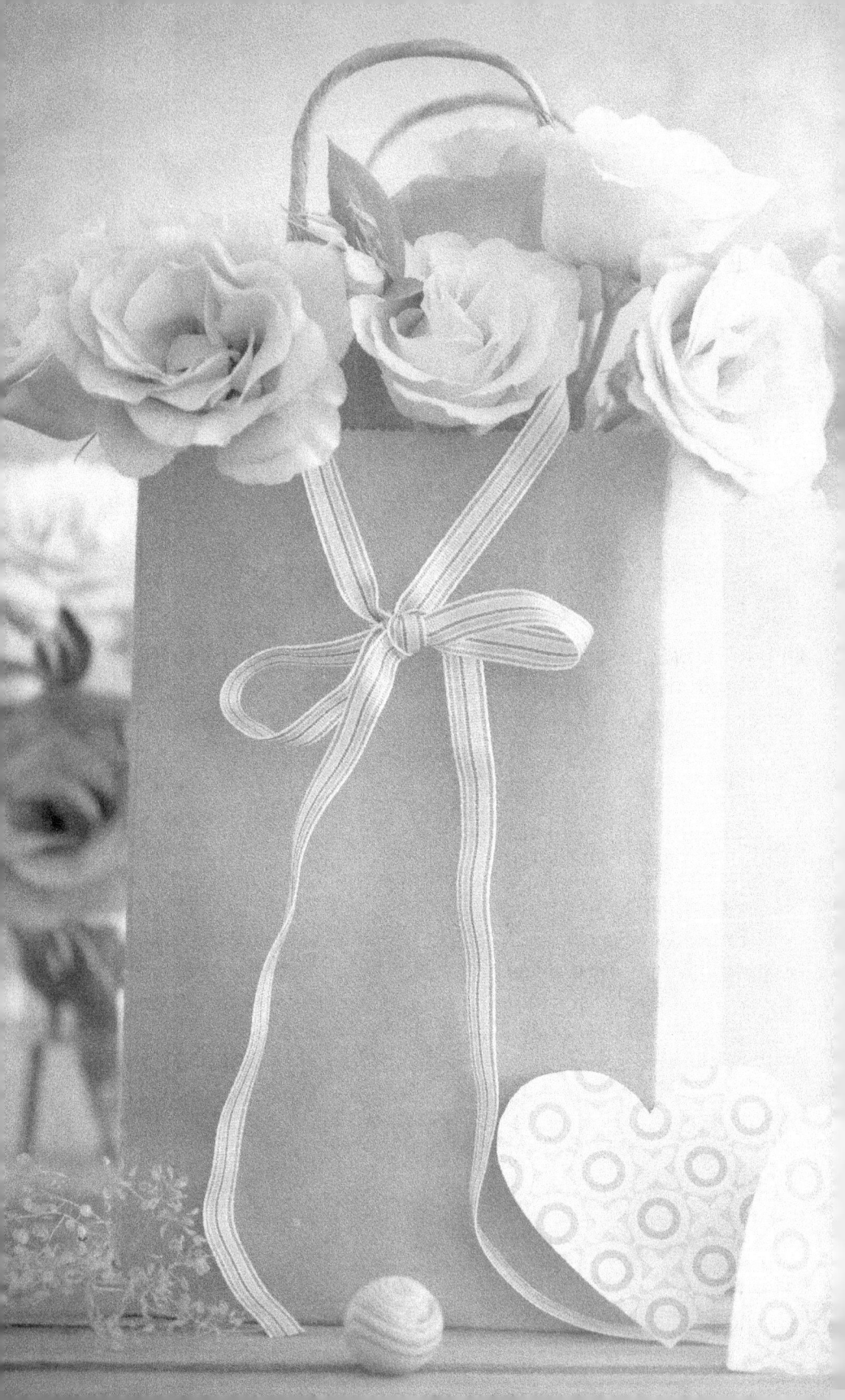

# CHAPTER 33
# CELEBRATING EIGHTY-EIGHT YEARS

HAPPY 88$^{TH}$ BIRTHDAY to the strongest, most innovative, funniest woman I know, my mother. She had many other noteworthy attributes, but since Alzheimer's reared its ugly head, these three qualities stood out so much more.

I already loved her from a daughter's standpoint, but now from a caregiver's point of view. I had become the parent, and she the child. I found myself overly protective of her – her heart, health, mind, and surroundings. In my wildest dreams, I never believed I might be in this position, nor did I foresee Mama's health to be where it was. This, by far, had been the hardest thing I had ever done, yet the most reward-ing, oddly enough.

God equipped me; He held my hand; He guided me through this process. I am thankful for each and every day I had with Mama.

I celebrated Mama the best way I knew how – with music and sweets and family – things that made my Mama happy. Happy birth-day, Norma Jean. You are a fantastic mother and grandmother. You are loved and cherished.

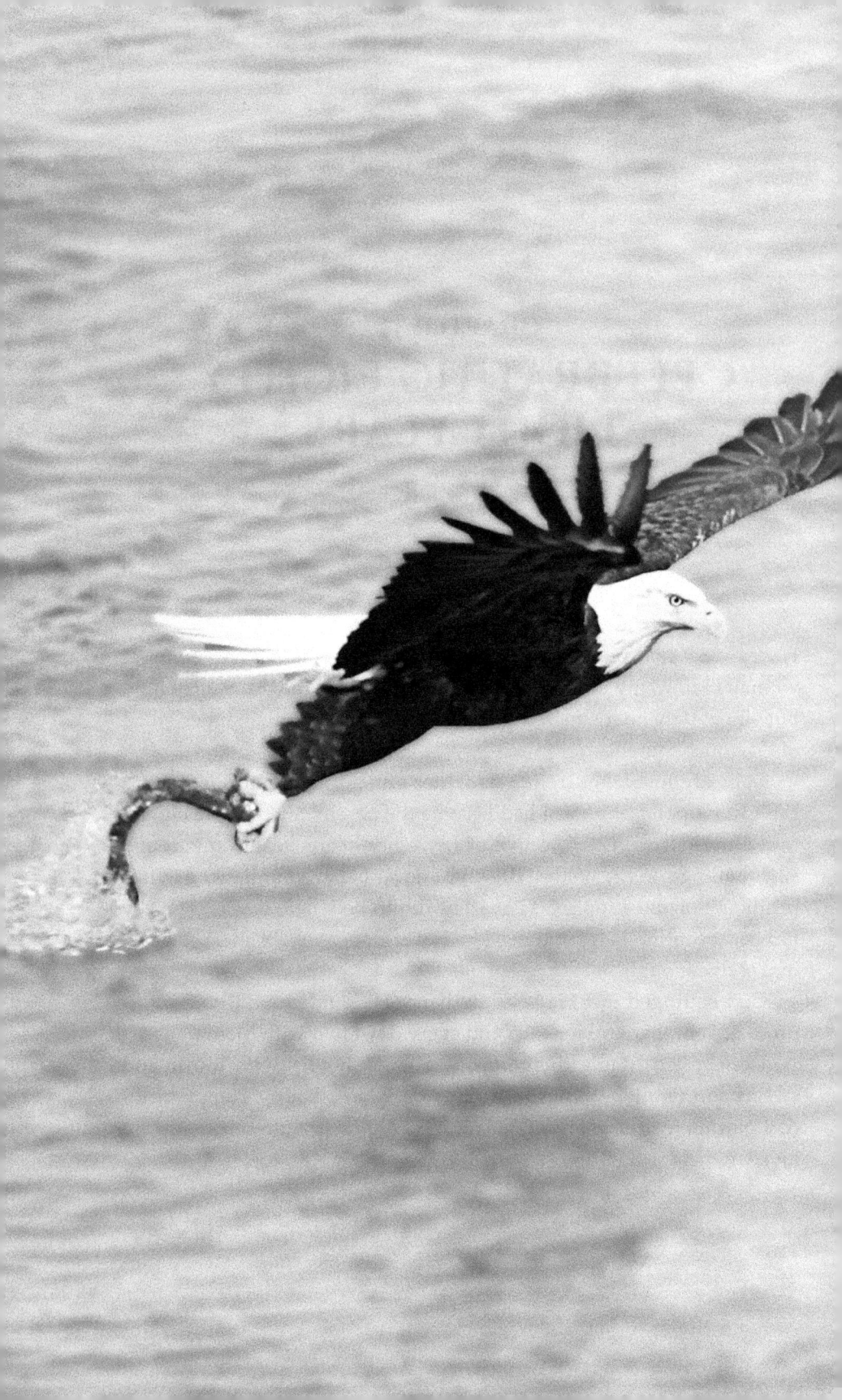

# CHAPTER 34
# SELF DEFENSE 101

A WORD of advice I learned the hard way, literally with a slap in the face or perhaps a punch in the gut. When dealing with Mama, I noted as her disease progressed, she acted out much more frequently. It wasn't necessarily the personality of the caregiver but the ACTIONS of the caregiver she responded to each time.

When we were in the restroom helping Mama get situated on the toilet if she was not warned *in advance* with a gentle voice what would transpire next, any physical movement scared her, and she became defensive! Every time! I personally have been pinched on my inner thigh or upper arm, slapped in the face, and punched in the gut. The first such occurrence totally caught me off guard. Mama had never demonstrated any violence in my entire life. The aides I worked with closely, saw my reaction to Mama's hit and whispered to me to go sit down. I tried to be strong, but I LOST it. So many tears fell that day. It was such a sad day for me. This disease was ruthless! I tried my best to watch and learn from the nurses and aides how to care for Mama properly, lift her, toilet her, and all the things. But this, this just tore me up! I started to see her react the same way to the aides. Those ladies just don't get paid enough in my opinion.

I informed the nurses, aides, and everyone involved in her care, of the warning signs and triggers to avoid similar battles. Norma Jean had quite the right hook!

The second most frequent site Mama displayed her combativeness was in her bed. One of the primary jobs of the aides at night was to change the diapers of the chair-bound or bed-bound residents. Imagine being sound asleep in the middle of the night and someone flipped the light on, and spoke very loudly, often continuing a conversation they were having in the hallway with their co-worker. Without warning or saying her name, the aide pulled her nice, cozy covers off of her and exposed her entire body.

Mama hit, punched, pinched, cussed, and slapped...you name it, she dished it out! She was a fighter. I had never seen this side of Mama, and I was quite proud of her for protecting herself while not knowing what was being done to her. It wasn't until I watched one of my hired night sitters work with Mama, that I learned how to calm her and do it in a more humane manner.

When the evening workers came in, I walked to the head of the bed and gently woke Mama up. She responded well to me putting the back of my hand alongside her cheek. I asked the workers to pull the covers back gently, and all the while, I whispered to Mama and told her what we were doing. When it came time to remove her adult diaper, I put her arms over her chest like an X and spoke words of comfort during the process.

Oh my gosh, what a difference. We continued doing this every night from then on. I am grateful for Kathy D. who demonstrated this technique. What a valuable lesson.

Mama's third most frequent outbursts were usually because of loud sounds. I first noticed this before she moved to Special Care. Mama was sitting in "her" spot by the fireplace in the lobby. A rather vocal lady came to join her and sat in the other fireside chair. She was very talkative. She didn't care if Mama interacted or not. She just kept on talking. It drove my mother crazy; she told her to "Shush" or "Shut up already" or, my favorite, "Don't you have someone else to bother?" The lady never caught on, and the relationship remained strained.

When Mama moved to "the Back," I visited her at supper time after work. If you recall, she had begun playing with her food due to her loss of eyesight and required some assistance. As residents finished their meals, the aides picked up the plates and utensils and brought them to the bin for the cafeteria workers to pick up for washing. The more plates in the container, the louder the noise got with the hitting and clanging of each additional dish. Mama had outbursts when it got the best of her. Might I add, she was the only resident with this reaction. Maybe it brought her back to having a house full of six kids and all the noise we made. Nonetheless, the workers made light of it and shouted back to Mama, "We love you, Ms. Norma." Being how sensitive she became to loud noises, her reaction to loud sounds baffled me knowing her love of music. She loved live bands, and we always had her TV on music channels. She never once asked us to turn it down or off.

⋙⟐⟐⟐⋘

The fourth most apparent time we saw uncharacteristic outbursts with Mama was when she had a urinary tract infection (UTI). As mentioned earlier, I was unaware of how common this was among the elderly, especially women with dementia. The director noticed a drastic change in Mama's personality and nailed the diagnosis every single time this occurred. It amazed me.

As years passed, imagine trying to get a urine sample from one extremely uncooperative, fist-throwing patient. That was a joke and wasn't going to happen. We reached the point where if she exhibited specific behavior changes, we skipped the urine sample and gave her the medicine, which worked every time. Norma Jean came back to "Normal Jean."

Based on what I've witnessed and also been taught by nurses and aides, one of the common symptoms of a UTI in the elderly female population could be a sudden behavior change, primarily confusion, which was how my mother presented most often. Other clues were agitation (check), or aggression (check again.) With my research, I have added to the list dizziness, fatigue, and a change in appetite. Mama never exhibited any of those.

Other than those instances, the fear, the noises, and the UTIs, Norma Jean was a happy person. The more time you spend with someone, the better you know them. You learned when the slightest thing was off. Let me share with you how I discovered the hemorrhage in her eye.

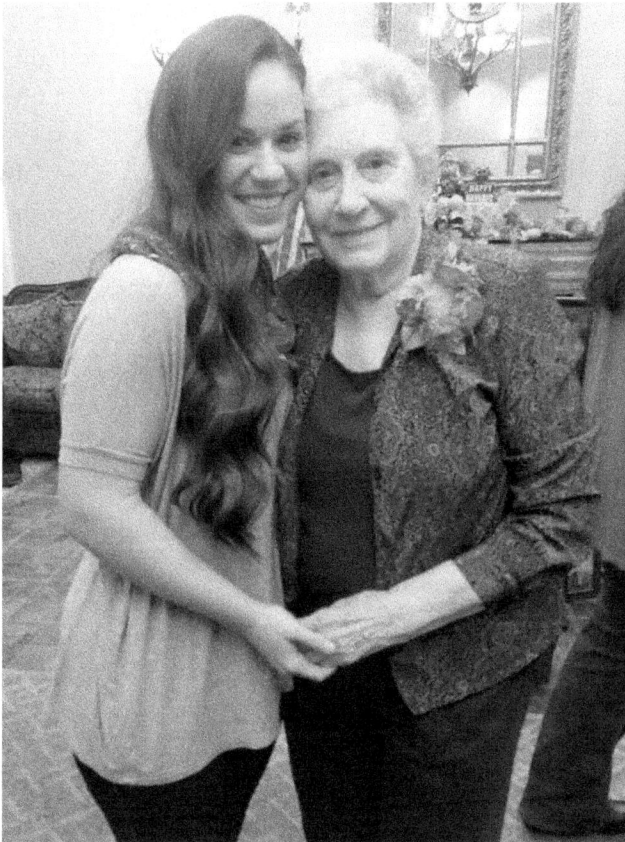

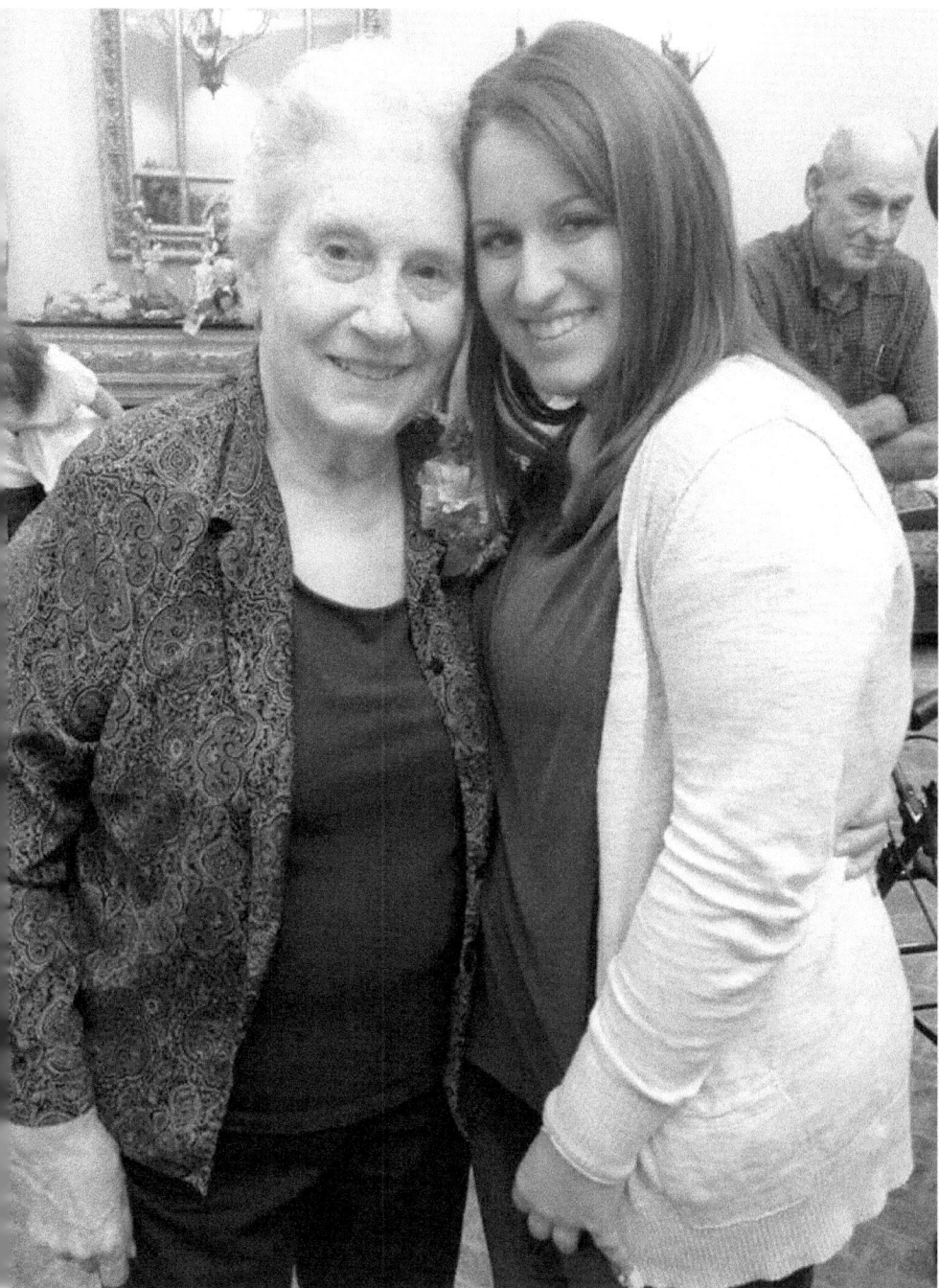

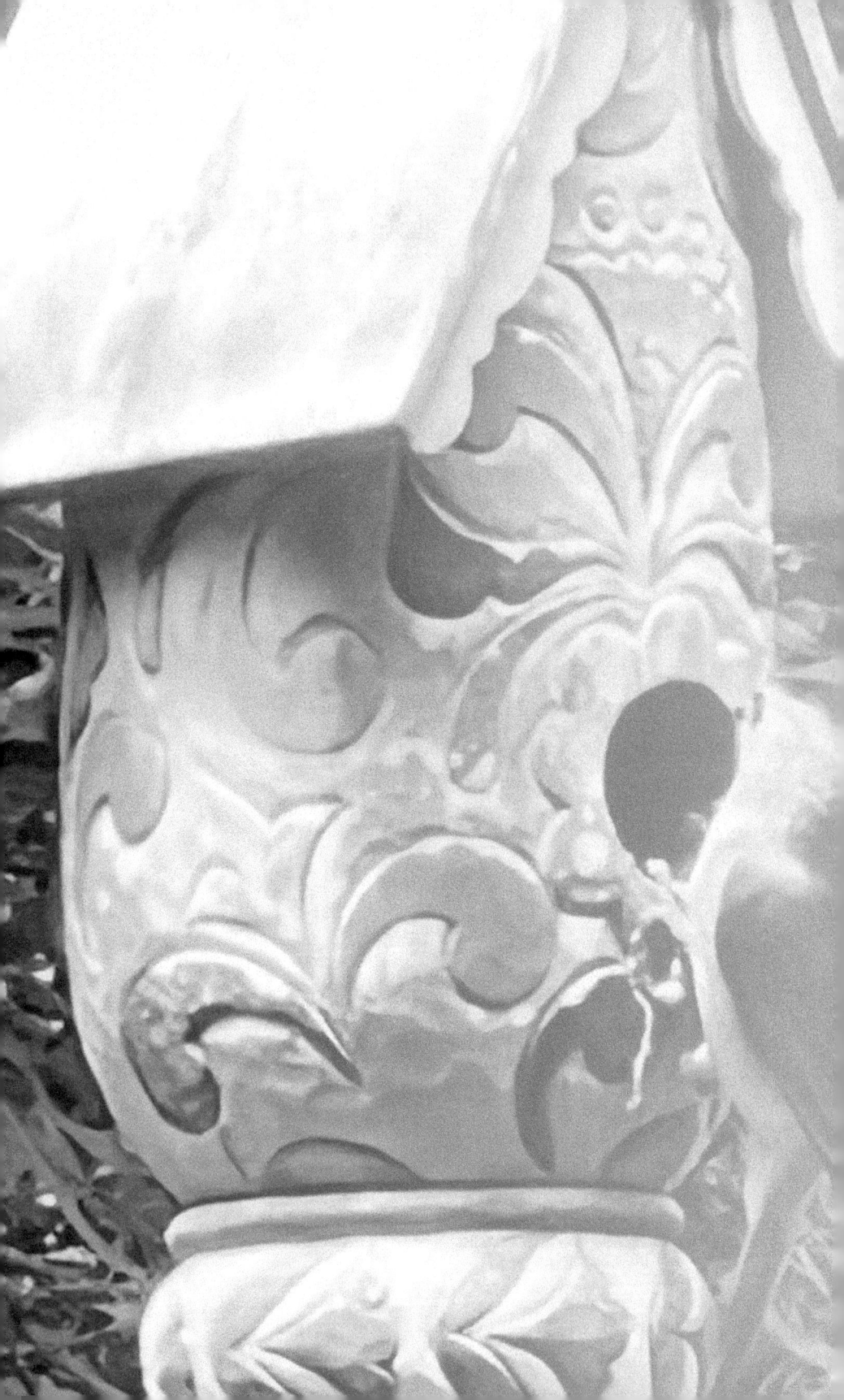

# CHAPTER 35

# I'VE GOT MY EYE ON YOU

As I DID MOST every day, I visited my mother in her apartment at the Special Care facility. She needed to use the restroom, so I brought her in and helped her get situated. I left the door open and sat on her bed right outside the bathroom. We made small talk for several minutes when I realized she was looking about two feet away from where I was sitting.

She smiled and continued chatting. Puzzled, I finally asked if she saw me. She said, "Sure!" I said, "Point to me." She waved her hand in the air nonchalantly. We talked a little more, and I continued to see her looking off.

I finally asked her, "Mama, where am I?" At that moment, she raised her pointer finger and pointed well over two feet away from where I was standing. I tested her several times by moving around to different areas, and she consistently pointed in the wrong place. I was alarmed.

**I've learned in the years of caring for her you never knew what awaited you when you arrived. This was the primary reason I went to see her every day.**

My gut was telling me something serious had transpired. I took her for a stroll down the hall and went straight to the nurse's station and described what I had just witnessed. I told them I needed to make an emergency phone call to her ophthalmologist. After I ended the call, I informed the aides I needed all of Mama's paperwork because the doctor requested to see her ASAP.

Upon arrival at the eye doctor's office, they performed the regular pre-examination routine, including dilation of the eyes. Then they came in and moved her to another room with specialized equipment. I thought, *Okay Inspector Clouseau, I had seen something noteworthy.*

**When you spend as much time with your loved one as I had, you notice the slightest change in them.**

Granted, I didn't know at the time it was such a huge change, but I was thankful I had noticed it early on.

The doctor came in and put the images of her eye on the screen and explained them to me. Mama had a significant ocular hemorrhage in her eye. In my mind, it looked like the shape of Africa. It encompassed over half of her lens. I was speechless. He told me he was sending me to Lafayette (about an hour and a half away), where they will either do emergency surgery or give her injections in her eye. *Ugh! What a dilemma. What should I do? This is clearly above my pay grade!*

I returned to the Big House with Mama, and all the workers wanted to know what the doctor said. Even the director was eager to find out. When I described the picture, diagnosis, and treatment to them, the number one question I was asked was, "But how did you know?" My answer was emphatically, "Because I KNOW her. I knew something wasn't right."

⌘

We arrived in the eye specialist's office the next morning, and although **ALZHEIMERS** was written all over her chart, he seemed to be ignorant as to what this entailed. I reminded him Mama had Alzheimer's. She was incapable of comprehending everything he said and was likely to have outbursts from fear. I was given a chair in the corner. The staff held her down, and the doctor yelled, literally yelled at Mama to be still. Yes, you read that right. Poor Mama was screaming, and the doctor ordered her in his deep voice to BE STILL. Tears welled up in my eyes and spilled over onto my cheeks and I was boiling with anger. He did not talk her through what he was about to do, and *Lord Have Mercy*, she fought him so fiercely. He finally injected her right in the eyeball, and Mama screamed bloody murder. It was absolutely gut-wrenching. It brings me to tears even writing this now. He and the staff walked out of the room, miffed. I rushed to Mama and consoled her. She was completely shaken. Mama was a tough old broad, but this got her. Had I made the wrong choice? This was her macular degeneration doctor. We liked him from previous appointments, but I decided I didn't ever want to see him again.

Honestly, I felt watching and hearing Mama thrashing and screaming was worse than watching your child in a similar situation. A child was not expected to understand scary, painful things and hope-fully, they were comforted by their parents. Although Mama's level of understanding was waning quickly, the doctor should have spoken with her, and the nurses calmed her. That never happened, it wasn't even attempted.

After I was able to calm sweet Mama down, we left for our long drive home. I held her hand and kissed her forehead. I put on some of her favorite tunes. Mama quickly fell asleep. Just like that, my tears started falling—poor precious Mama. I will never understand how doctors specialized in the medical field aren't more compassionate when working with this class of patients. What a nightmare!

Against my better judgment, we returned with Mama to this horrid doctor so he could examine her to see if the shot had stabilized the hemorrhage. It wasn't by choice, trust me! The doctor came in and spoke with me. He suggested she needed another round of shots or have surgery. Before I could tell him I emphatically would not put her through any more injections, he chimed in and said he needed to sedate her even for injections because she was a "loose cannon." *Ya think?!*

Now with her already having Alzheimer's, he went on to say this:

**Putting her under anesthesia would certainly change her current quality of life.**

If we chose neither option, her eyesight in the eye would be lost; only shadows seen. He gave me 24 hours to make a decision.

To say it was one of the hardest decisions I've ever made is an understatement. The reality of her life, as she knew it, was literally in my hands. Although her health was heading south, she was content. *What am I supposed to do?* When you suddenly realized you had to make not only a difficult, but life-changing choice for your parent, it wasn't supposed to be this way. *I want to be a carefree kid again. I didn't sign up for this!*

Later that night, I sat on the sofa with my husband, holding his hand tightly, and discussed my choices with him. After several hours of deep thought, I told James I needed to decide by myself (not involve my five siblings) because, in essence, I was the sole caregiver. No matter how things turned out, I was ultimately the only one who had to deal with the outcome, day in and day out. I made the decision. It was not fun to be a caregiver. It sucked!

I called the doctor in Lafayette the next morning and told him I preferred Mama to have the quality of life she has now and one I know how to work with at this point. I chose to deal with the diminishing vision one day at a time rather than strip even more of her memory away, not knowing what that might look like. The doctor was disgruntled on the phone, but I had complete peace with my decision and had zero regrets.

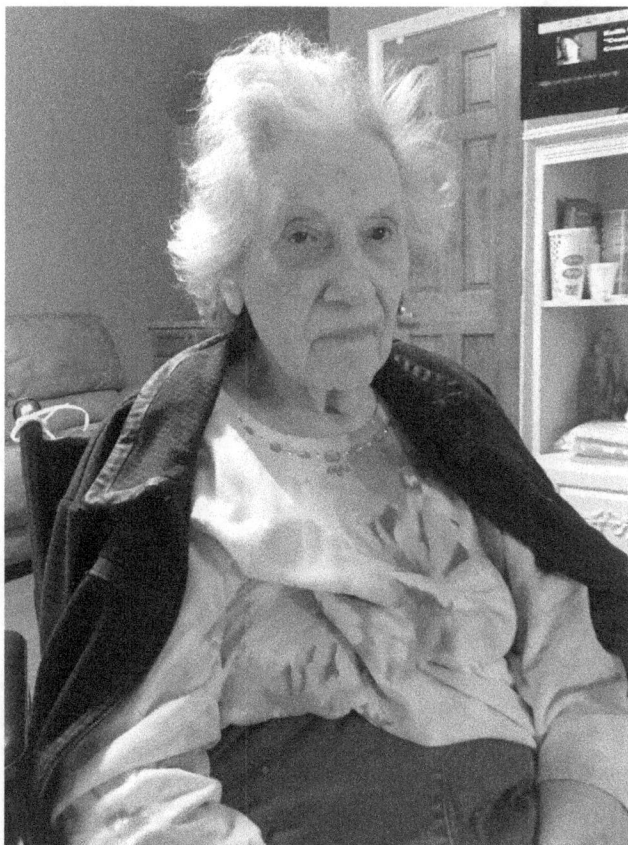

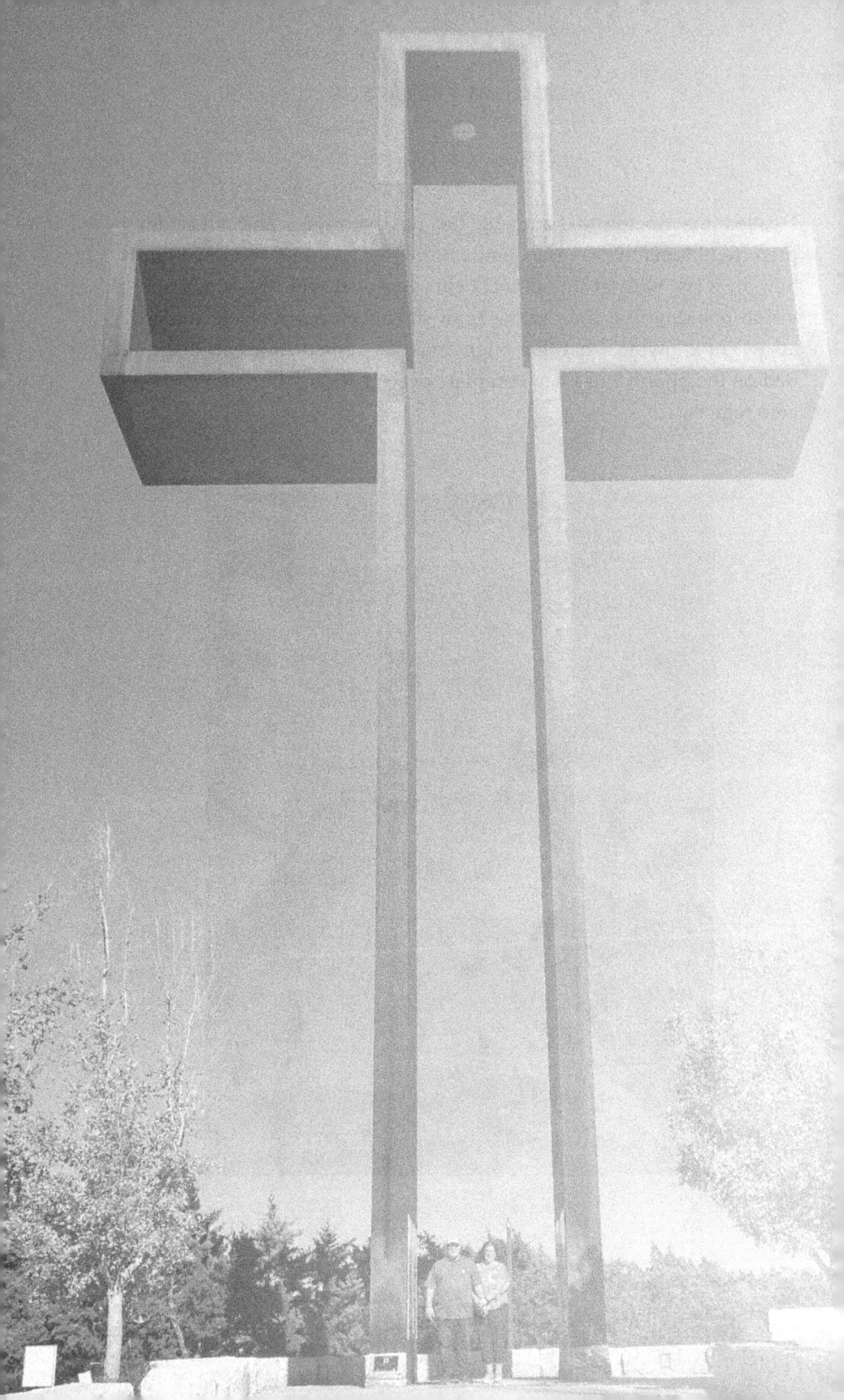

# CHAPTER 36
# PRAYERS OF THE SAINTS

A SWEET GENTLEMAN FROM ST. John Bosco church regularly visited Mama to pray over her and also her sitter for the day. Along with prayers, he brought her communion. I loved to hear Mama recite the prayers she had said her entire life. They were in her heart and mind so deeply. I remain thankful for those who brought her the Lord's supper.

As this gentleman opened his prayer book and began reading the prayers, Mama made the sign of the cross and bowed her head. He went on to pray a second and third prayer from his little book. His third prayer was for her Guardian Angel. It went like this, "Angel of God, my guardian dear, to whom His love commits me here." STOP. At this point, Mama leans forward in the chair and gives three kisses into the air. Now she was one wise woman. I snickered because Norma Jean's guardian angel had been working overtime the past few weeks.

Years later, I was rummaging through some of my forty journals, calendars, and notepads stacked on my table for review for this memoir. I picked up a small, red, thin notebook. I opened the cover and found this very same prayer. How special to have this particular prayer, the same prayer the gentleman prayed, that was clearly part of Mama's daily routine and in her own handwriting. What a treasure. I am highly grateful for a mother who also made a practice of writing down her thoughts and prayers.

A female resident walked the halls daily and told us how many rosaries she said and how she prayed for us and all the sick. We appreciated the prayers and respected her. One morning, I found out Mama had not had a good night, so when this lady strolled into Mama's room, I requested she say a rosary for Mama. She replied with a confused expression, "But honey, I don't have my makeup on!" *Oh, that's how this works; I've been saying my prayers wrong my entire life.*

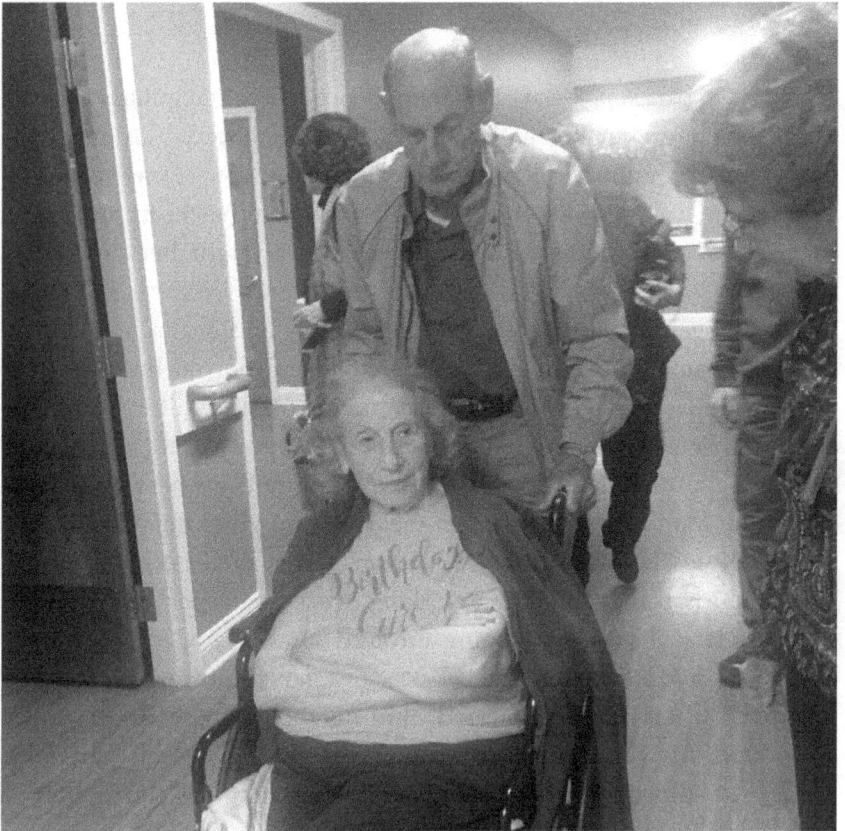

Mama and her brother, Leonard

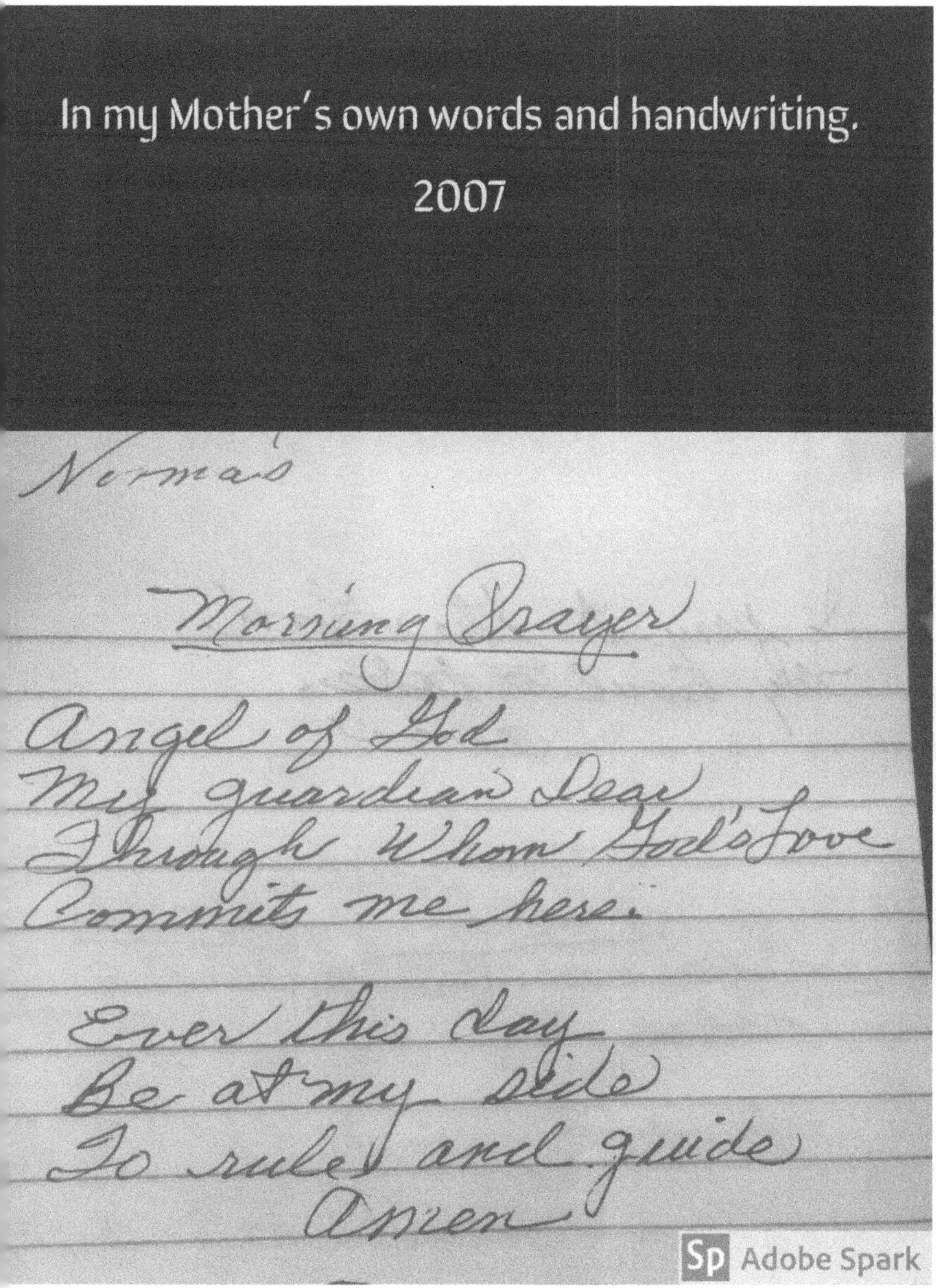

In my Mother's own words and handwriting.

2007

Norma's

*Morning Prayer*

Angel of God
My guardian Dear
Through Whom God's Love
Commits me here.

Ever this day
Be at my side
To rule and guide
Amen

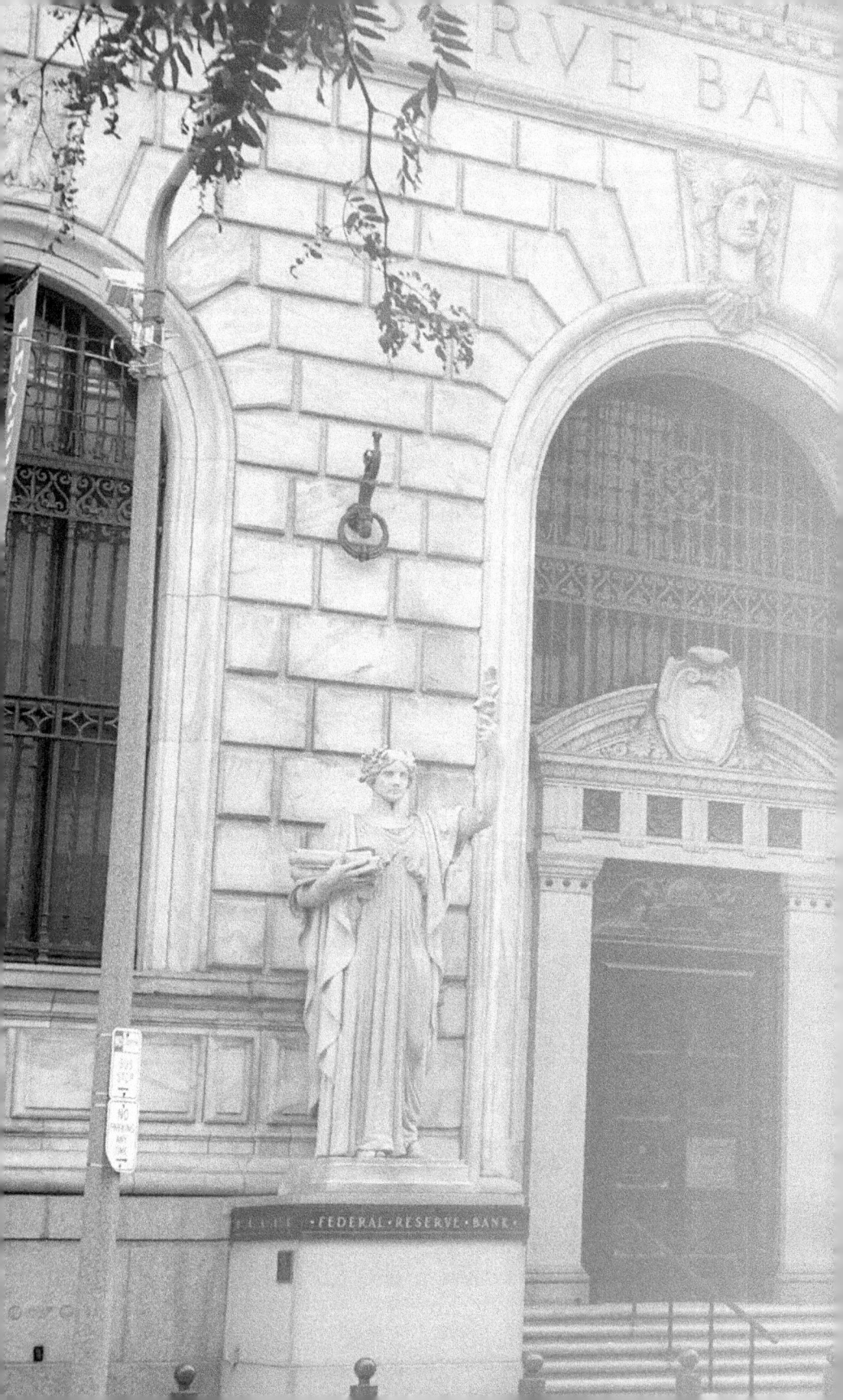

SERVE BANK

FEDERAL·RESERVE·BANK

# CHAPTER 37
# PRINCIPAL'S OFFICE

THERE WERE SWEET, memory-making moments and then there were the moments so outlandish you didn't see them coming and never imagined them in your wildest dreams. I had become accustomed to the reality I was now the parent and Mama, the child. I had to make many decisions that were crucial to her care. I was the only contact, therefore I received calls from the facility if they needed anything. Imagine my surprise when I received one such call from the facility director telling me Norma Jean had an altercation with another resident in the TV room. You're laughing out loud, right? I know! Me too!

***

It turns out a particular resident was annoying everyone, workers and residents alike. She spoke very loud and incessantly. The resident was a source of frustration day in and day out, all day long. Mama had yelled at her to "SHUT UP!" From what I gathered, she yelled several times. When the woman didn't hush, Mama approached her and punched her (school-yard style) square in the face! The victim didn't have any lasting damage, and the director notified her family of the altercation as well. Imagine the roaring laughter that came out of me.

Who ever thought I would receive a call from the "principal's office" about my MOTHER being in a fight SHE instigated? What was even funnier was it happened again. I wonder what other exciting tidbits her file contains!

***

During my visits with Mama, I preferred to leave the door to her apartment open. SNL doesn't hold a candle to the vast array of enter-tainment that came down the hallway and, more often than not, into Mama's room.

One frequent guest always came in and spoke loudly. She was a busybody. Let me tell you how I outfoxed her. Mama was resting, and I didn't want her to be disturbed. When I heard the sound of her trade-mark "shuffling shoes" coming down the hall, I did a trick I learned from Norma Jean; I played possum. I had done this many times, and it worked 10 times out of 10. Awesome. No interruptions for sleeping beauty. I hated telling residents to be quiet or come back later, but by playing possum, I didn't have to. Oh, the games we play.

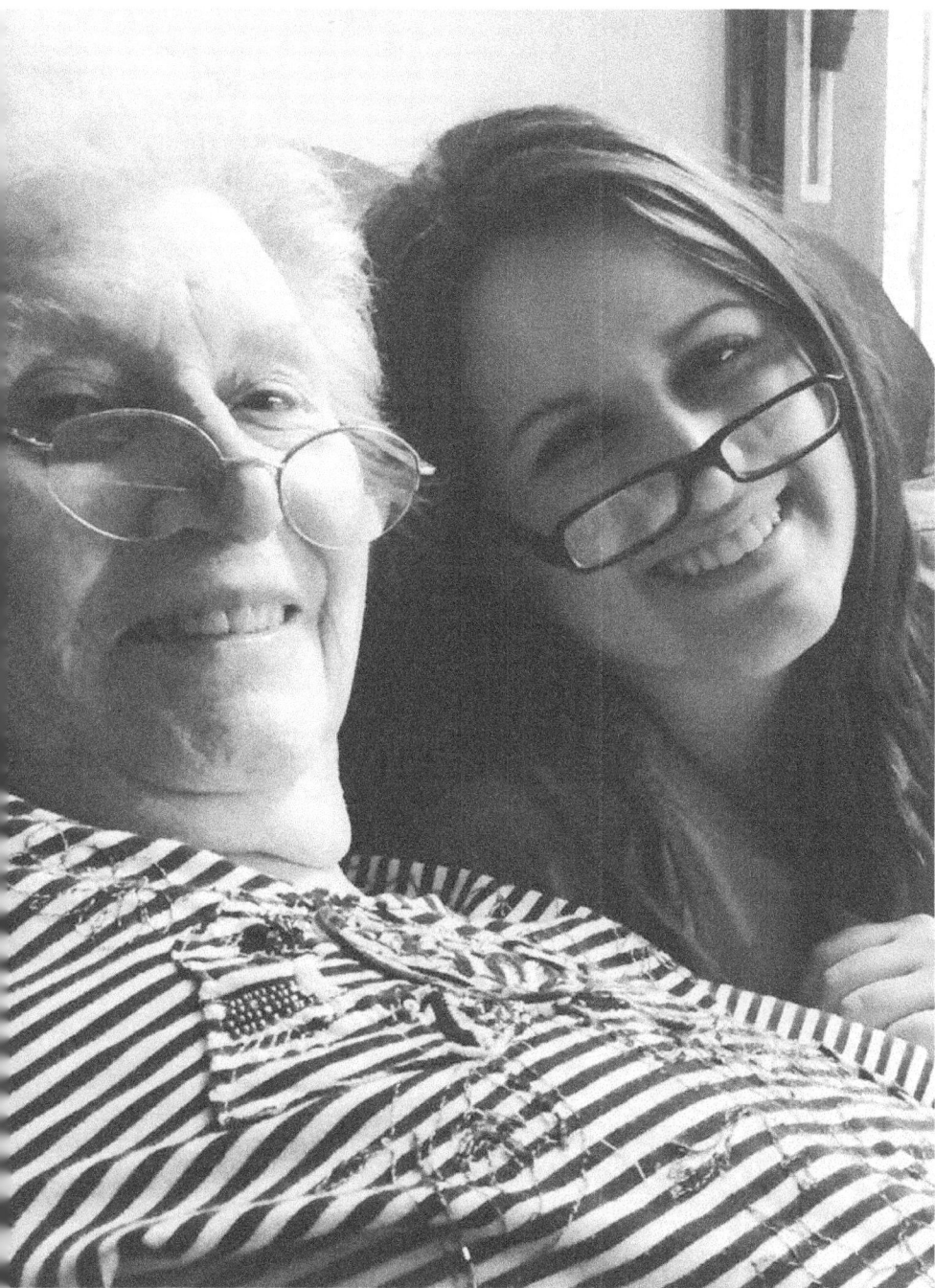

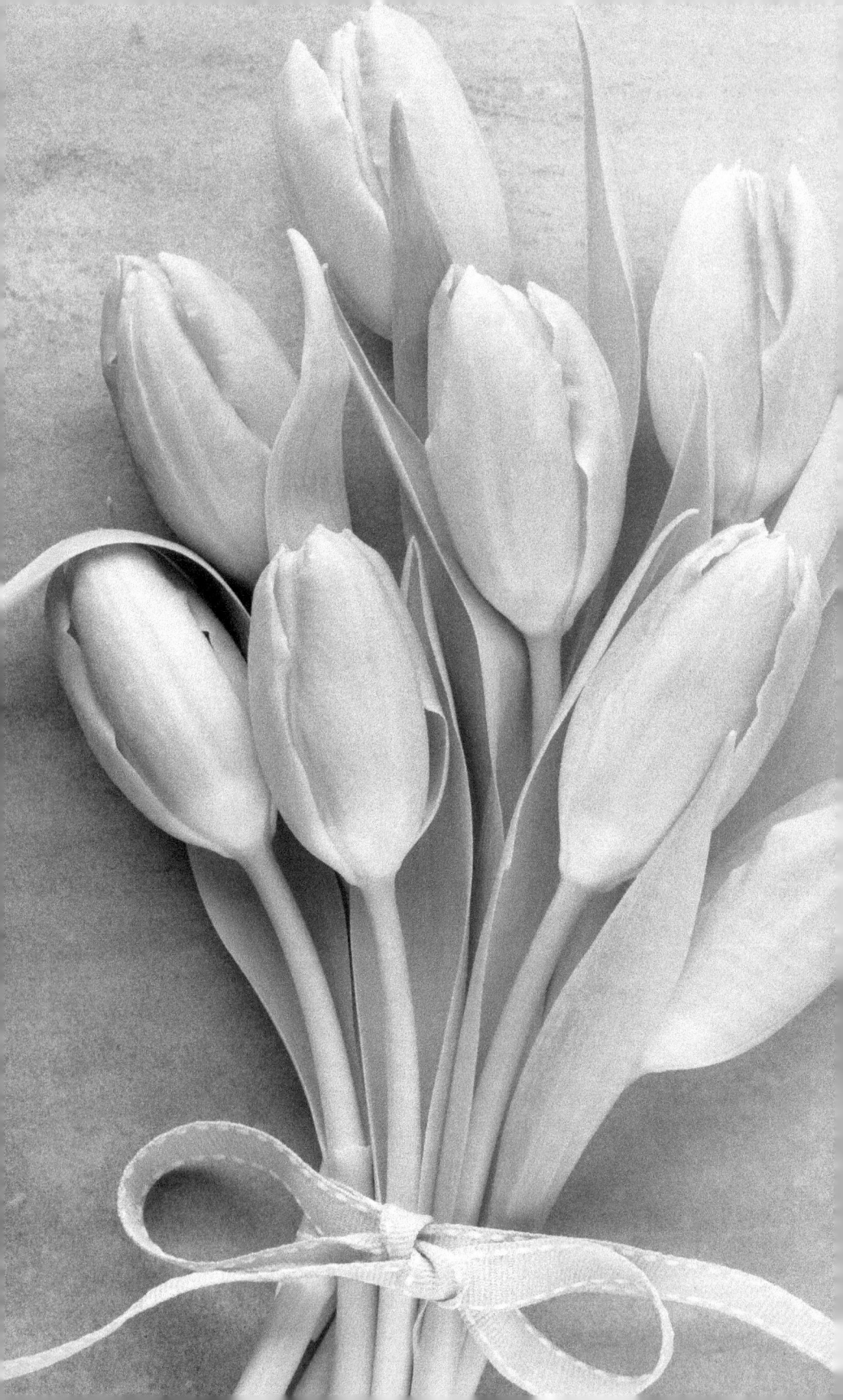

# CHAPTER 38
# IN SICKNESS AND IN HEALTH

A RECENT PROFOUND revelation to me: When you said your marriage vows, specifically the part that included "in sickness and in health," it dawned on me that this commitment extended beyond just taking care of each other during times of illness. It encompassed our children and, more recently, our journey in supporting our parents and in-laws as they faced health challenges, sickness, and, ultimately, the inevitability of death. This revelation was a powerful "aha" moment for me.

You walked side by side through everything in life. Life means, eventually, someone gets sick. While your spouse cared for the children or parents, you had their back. You held down the fort. You prayed for them. You stepped in for them so they could have a break. You were a sounding board for them. Please, be there for them.

So, you say you don't know how to care for someone? Jump in and learn. Trial by fire, as they say. Every small act of care and support makes a world of difference to someone in need. Please don't just sit there on the sidelines being a spectator. It's a joint effort. Those vows are serious business, my friends.

Over the past ten years, Mama was our third parent placed in our care. James and I joined together to care for my Mama every day for 12 years. While James worked out of state, I helped care for his father for the last year of his life (while still looking after my Mama). On the day of my Mama's burial, my mother-in-law came to the funeral sick and was soon diagnosed with pneumonia. She was hospitalized for two weeks. We have been caring for her and juggling hospitalizations, rehab, nursing homes, and assisted living on the heels of Mama's death. As of this writing, it has been five years.

⚜

I hope this sparks a necessary conversation between you and your spouse. Are you willing and able to bring your parent into your home? Would you still be able to work outside the home? If you have children at home, how would this affect their current lifestyle? Do you have finances set aside for spans of one to fifteen years, if necessary? Watch your friends and family members who are walking through this now. Learn from them, the good and the bad. Ask questions. Get prepared.

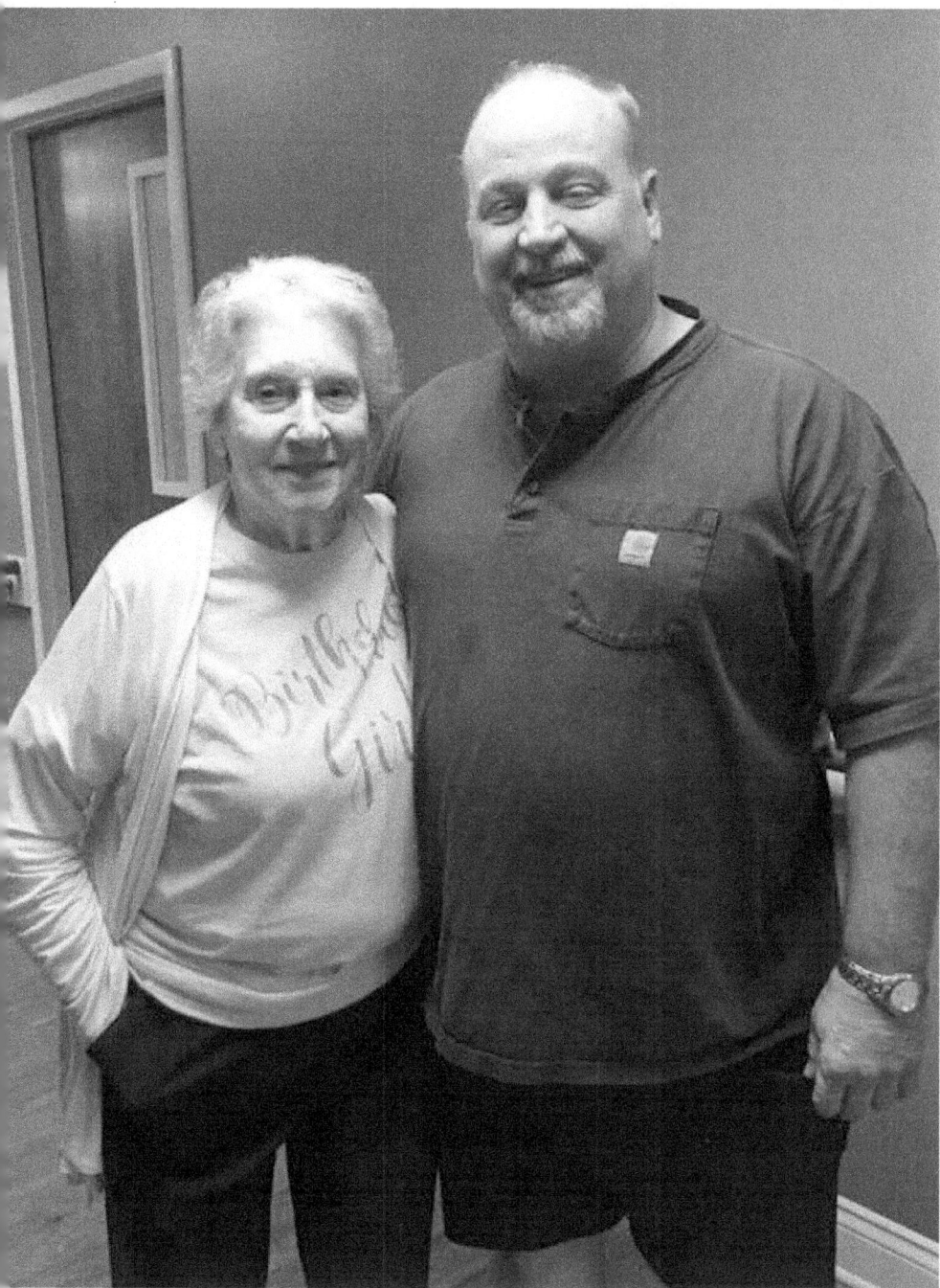

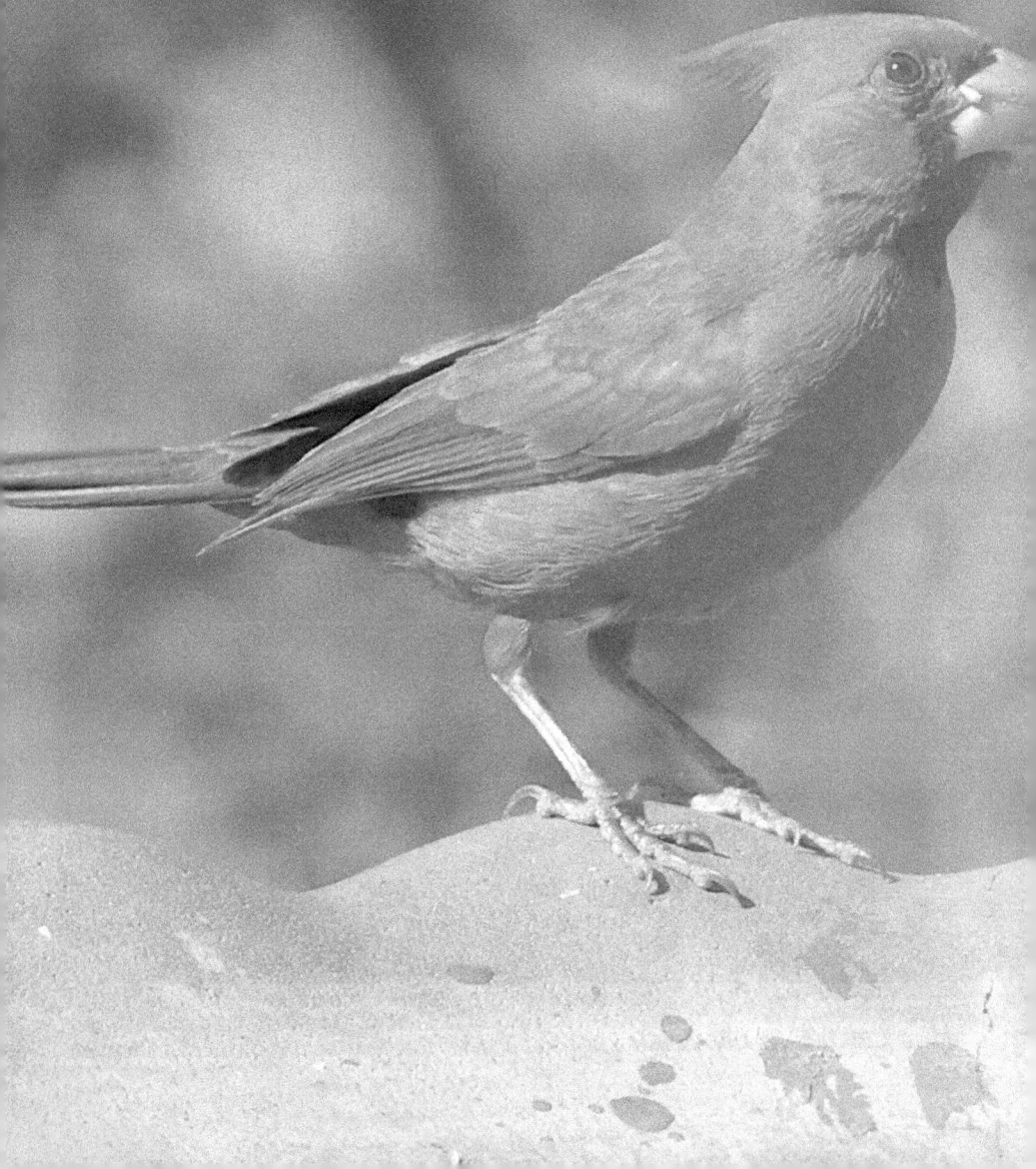

# CHAPTER 39

# MARVELOUS MATRIARCH

I AM grateful my mother met four of my five grandchildren. This was especially important to me because my father never met my husband much less my four children. Daddy was taken away entirely too young, but God left us with a powerhouse of a mother for the next 40 years.

I love that my grandchildren were unaware of Mama's Alzheimer's because of her innate playfulness on display around children. The children were never offended she couldn't recall their names, but instead, she used endearing names like *Sweetie*. They just thought she was funny. The children gladly pushed her down the hallways in a wheelchair or raced alongside her while she rapidly peddled her feet. She bounced them on her knee with copious amounts of laughter coming from the little ones. She sang familiar songs to them, gave lots of tickles, and shared her stash of candy.

<hr/>

This reminded me of one particular day I went to the Special Care unit and walked past the nurse's station on my way to the TV room. As I approached the open door, I stopped abruptly. What did my little eyes see but my mother bouncing a child on her knee? The hilarity of the situation was, that I had no idea who this child was.

I walked into the room and felt a huge, smug smile suddenly spread across my face. The little boy was having a great time riding Mama's horsey. I relished this moment. Gosh, I love this woman.

Norma Jean sang a little song to the child, the same song she sang to three generations of children in her family. "Giddy up horsey, giddy up horsey, Whoa! Whoa! Whoa!" She was very expressive in the latter part of the ditty. I inquired to whom this child belonged. It turned out he was the grandson of another resident. He had visited his grandma, but Norma Jean snatched him up. The boy's mother was enjoying the "rodeo" show.

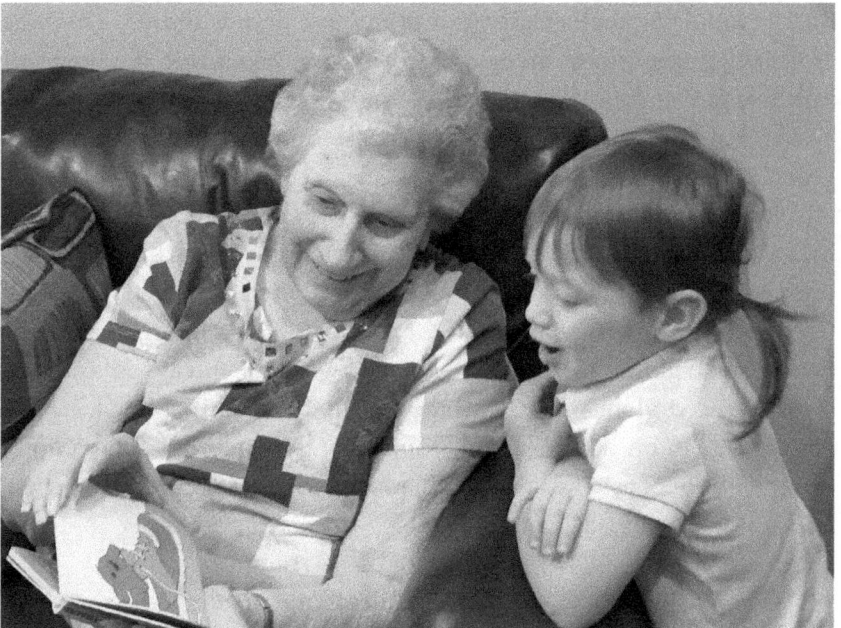

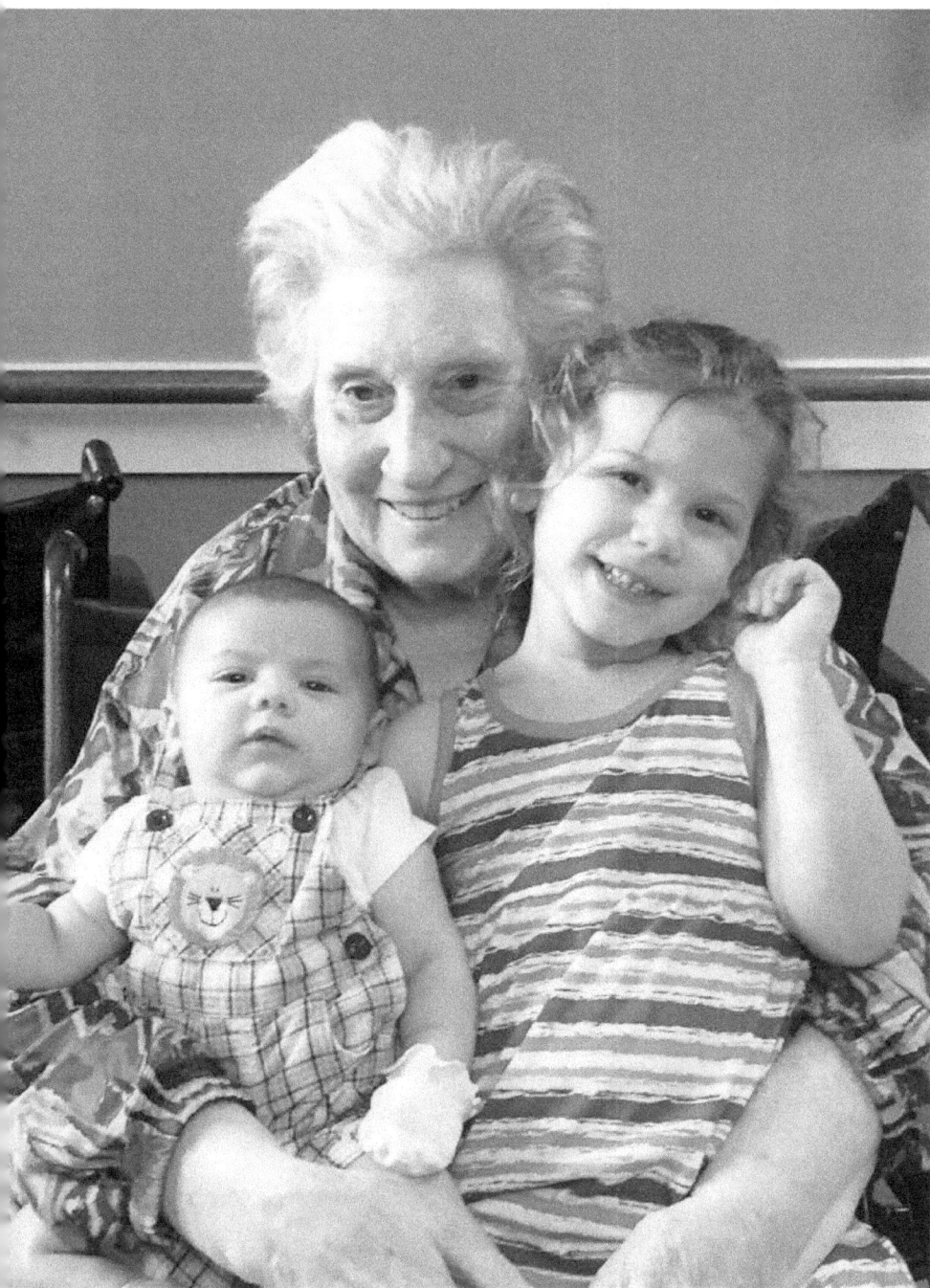

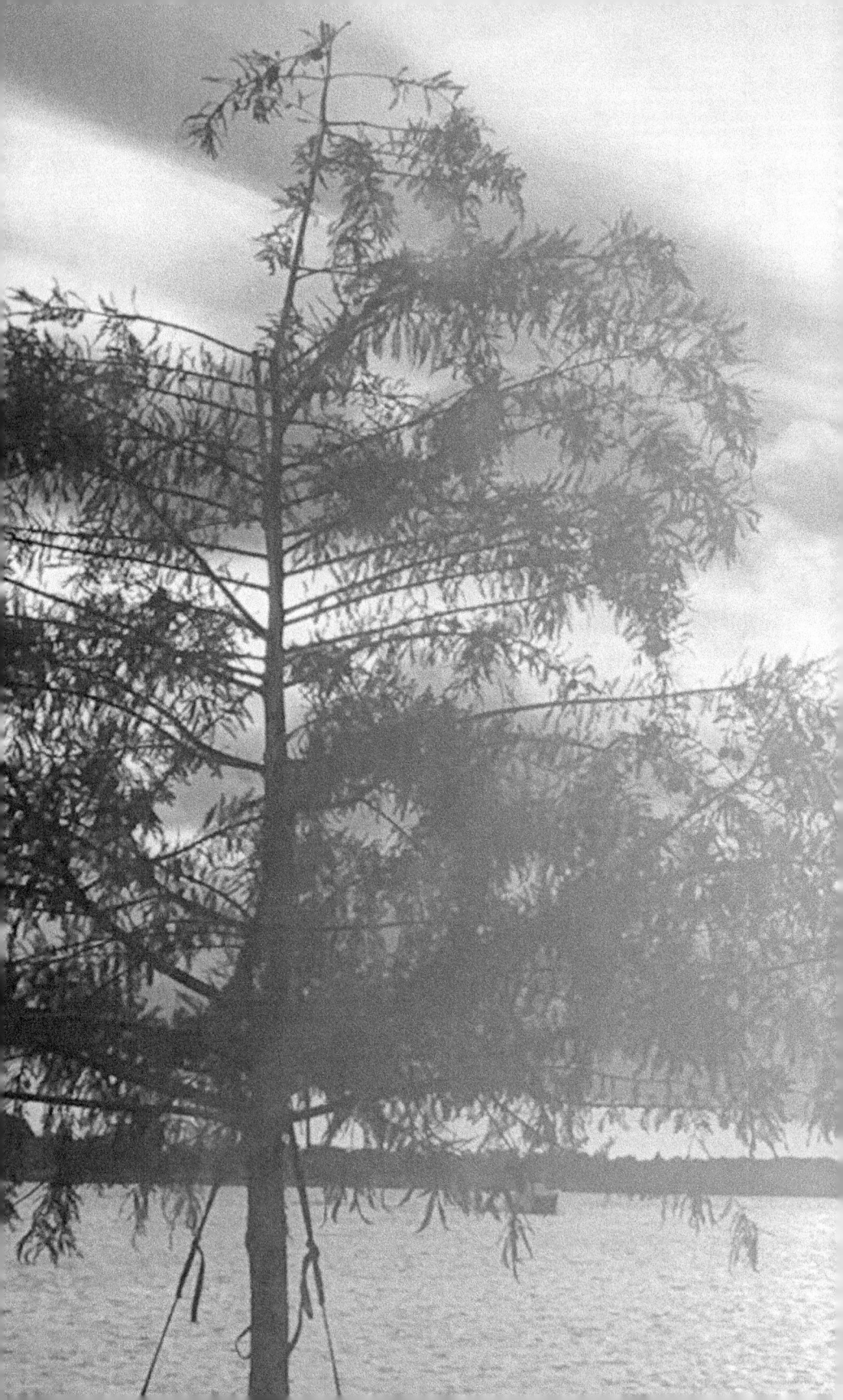

## CHAPTER 40

# REFLECTIONS

MAMA LOVED to nap in her recliner. She leaned to one side of the chair and her crossed legs perched on the opposite arm of the chair. She was agile and very flexible. I sat quietly on her couch opposite her. As I glanced over at my mother, I found myself reflecting on her natural beauty, unwavering strength, remarkable resilience, and her uncanny ability to overcome. She was the whole package, and God, our Father, had chosen her to be my mother.

This is a reminder to look beyond the person seated in front of you and look at their heart. They are still there...even to the end. I promise you. They miss you as much as you miss them. They did not ask for this disease. It is not any easier on them than it is on us.

My personal soapbox: please don't ever talk about them in front of them. Whispering about them is frowned upon, too. There is no way to know how much they hear or comprehend. Promise me please, you will never do that. If a professional begins to do it, redirect them.

While I was at work, I met with a new client, an older lady who was very friendly and pretty. Her eyes had not yet faded with age and I could still see a sparkle there, along with her beautiful smile. This lady had all the finishing touches on her hair, makeup, and nails. She was dressed very nicely. She made me think…this was how Mama *used* to be. Mama always took pride in her appearance. She had hair appointments every other week, did her own manicures on her beautiful, long nails, and completed her style with an outgoing personality. What a cut-up and loyal friend she was to many. Her smile was the most beautiful thing about her.

That was my mother just ten years ago—ten short years. So much had changed, yet I thought she was still beautiful. Perhaps, not always on the outside because some weeks, let's just be real here, she doesn't want to get her hair styled and rarely even has lipstick on. Full disclosure – somewhere along this journey Mama's naturally curly hair became straight without so much as a wave and I never had success using a curling iron with her. It bothered me to no end she didn't look like herself due to her inept caregiver/stylist. Beauty salons had become a thing of the past with all her personality changes and unfortunately, she was stuck with me.

I learned to redefine my definition of beauty and to look beyond the skin, hair, and nails and look to the heart and soul of a person, in particular, my mother's. She was quite the entertainer and loved people. She was indeed a beautiful soul. I also learned to count my blessings and my friends. Remember to stop and make memories with not only people you love, but people you just met. Look beyond the cover of the book. The beauty may be hidden below the surface.

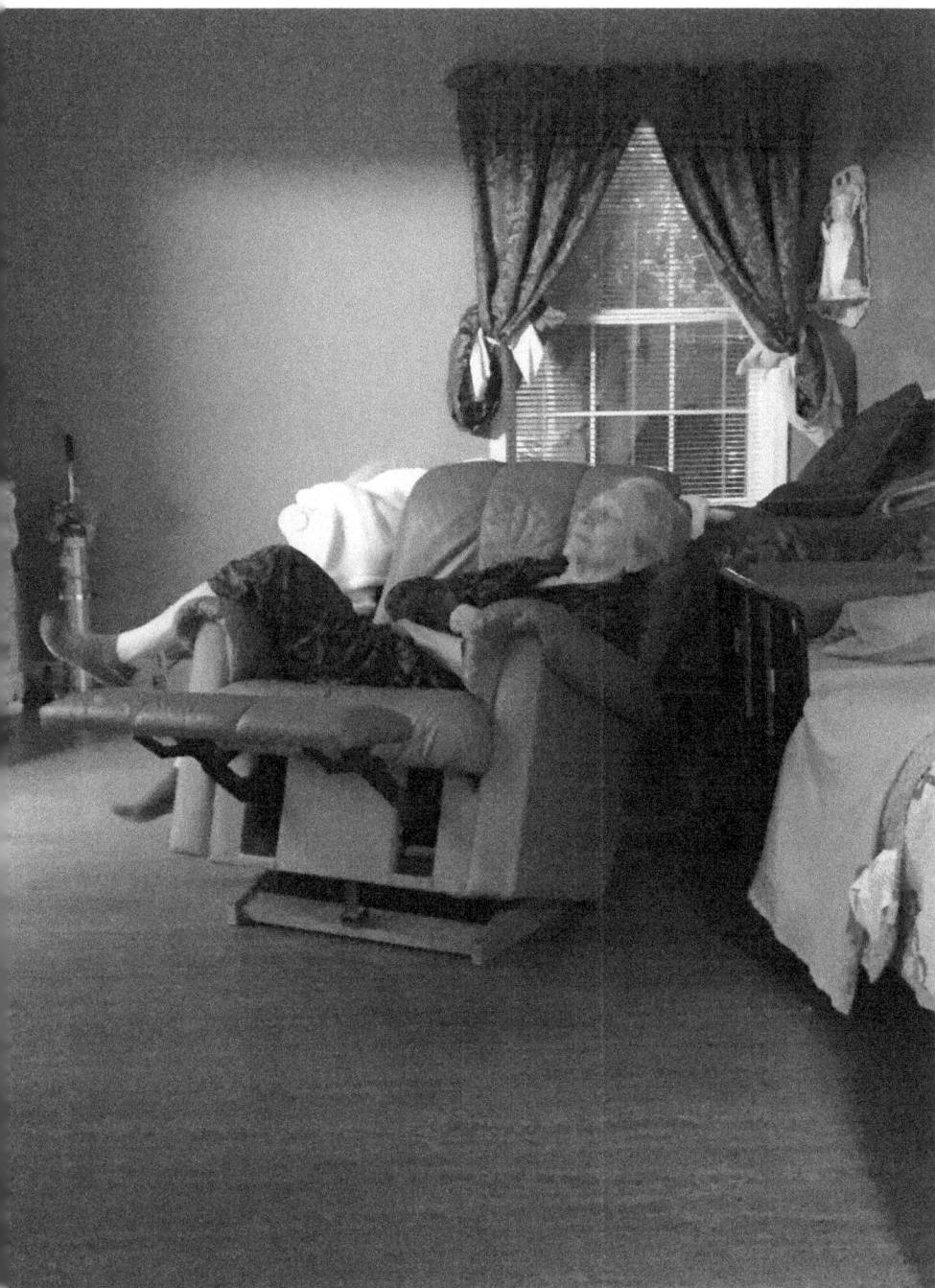

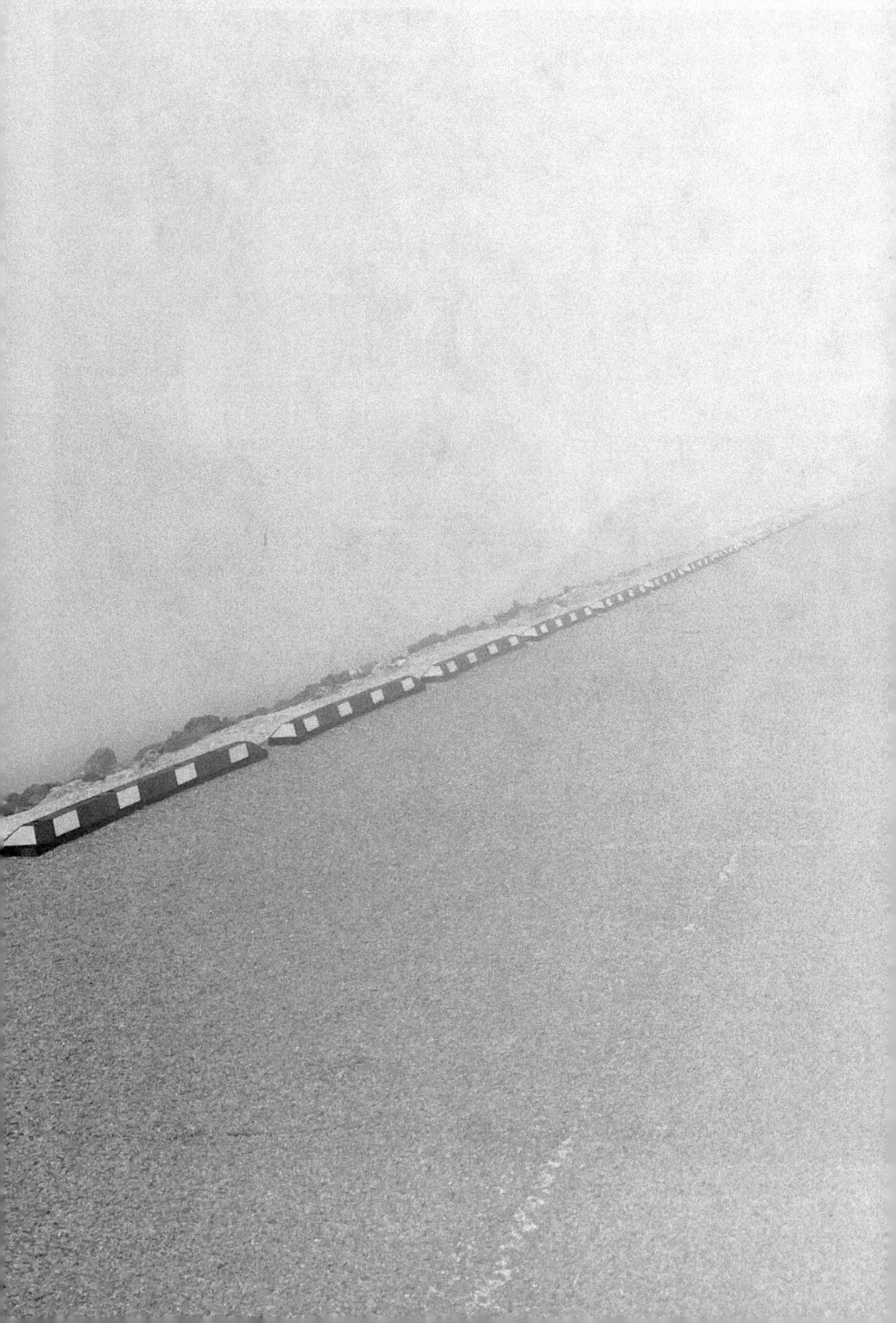

# CHAPTER 41

# NORMA JEAN'S
# ROAD SHOW

I SHOULD HAVE TAKEN Norma Jean on tour! I brought Mama for a doctor's visit and we walked inside and sat down in the waiting room. The room was at full capacity. Mama sat quietly for a few minutes and then loudly announced, "You people have done an outstanding job decorating this place." I whispered to her, "Mama, these people are patients, too." She responded, "Well, they are REALLY good then." A few short moments go by, and Mama shouted, "Well, does anybody want to come sit on my lap?" Oh, the looks, smirks, and laughter that erupted in the waiting room. Even the receptionist behind the glass window started laughing. I believe Mama may have been prompted to say that because she saw two children waiting with their parents. Sadly, no one volunteered, but it made me chuckle. Never a dull moment with Norma Jean.

⊰⊱⊰⊱

During one of my regular afternoon visits with Mama, she randomly asked me if I slept in the same bed as my husband. *(Insert smirk)* I held back my belly laugh and answered her, "Yes." After I composed myself, I asked Mama what made her ask me that question. Her response was

169

unforgettable. "You got to keep the cold stuff with the cold stuff and the hot stuff with hot stuff." Mic drop!

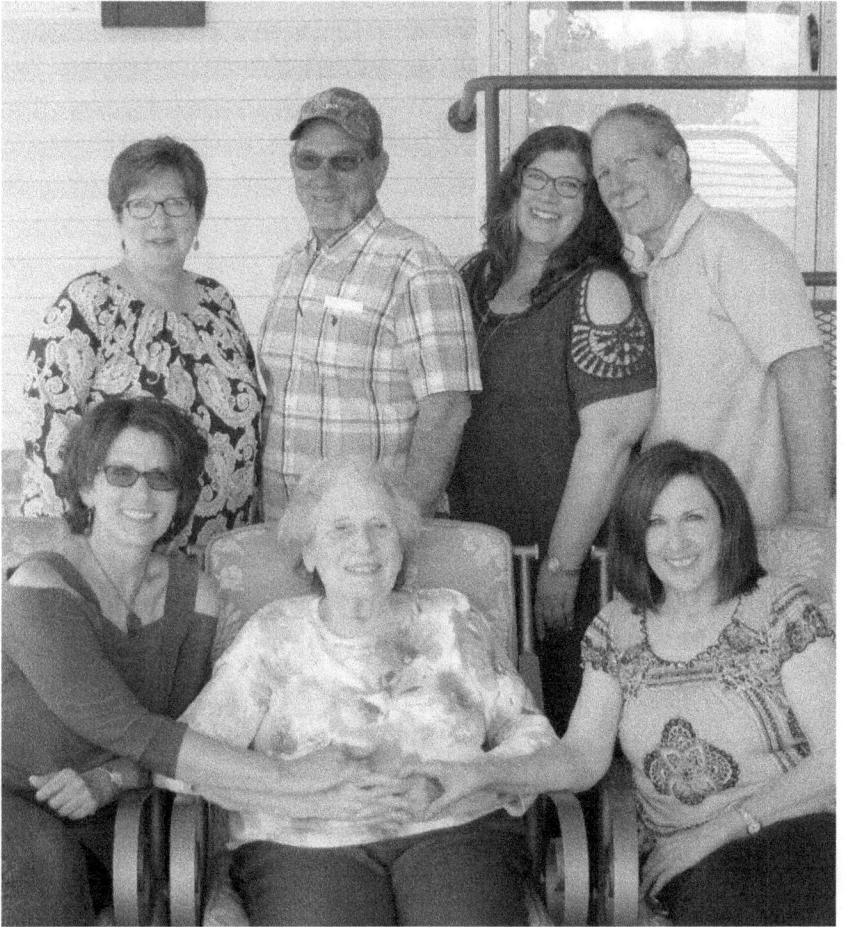

Mama surrounded by her six children

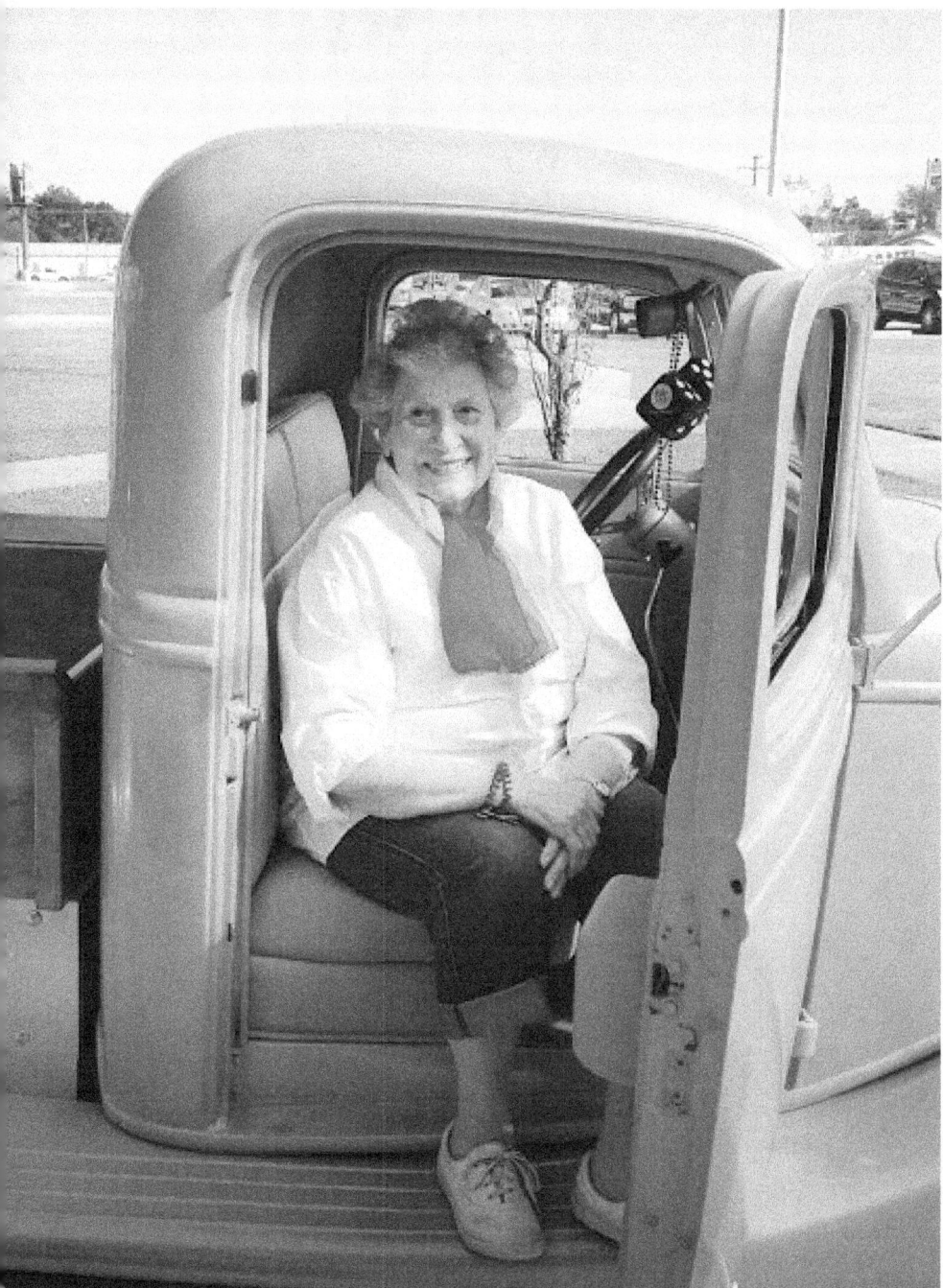

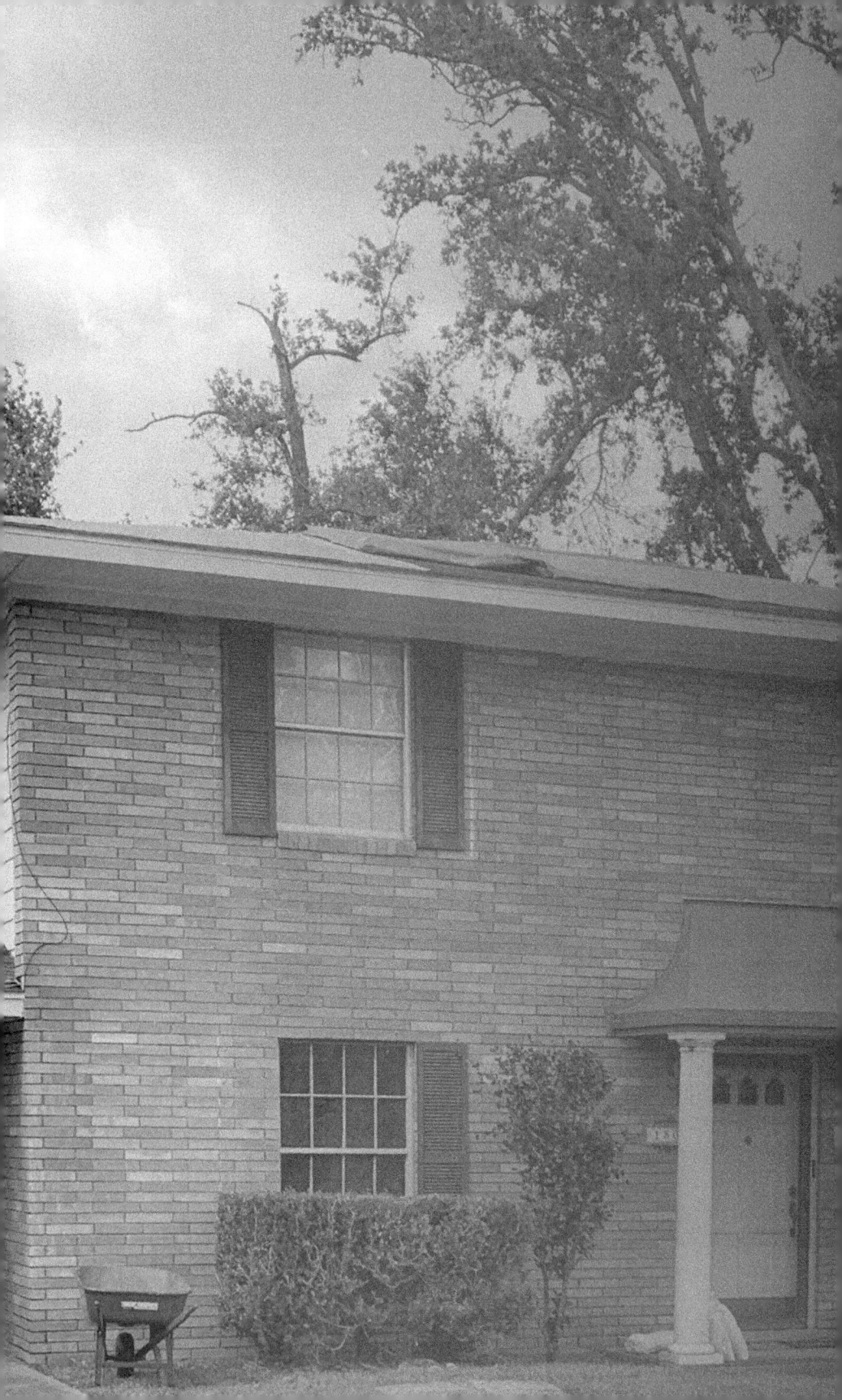

## CHAPTER 42
# A HOUSE BUILT ON LOVE

I TOOK Mama out for a drive and decided to show her the different homes she had lived in while residing in Sulphur. The first stop was our two-story, brick childhood home. Mama "downsized" and sold it in 1996.

Despite her struggle with her memory, whenever we went for a ride, my mother always seemed to recall the streets and houses of friends and family with remarkable precision. She begged me to drive by specific homes, some from 60 years ago. However, this particular time was markedly different from those previous experiences. I turned down our old street and asked her if the street looked familiar. She replied, "No." Our street was comprised of a rock road and only five homes. I drove closer to our childhood home and asked the same question again getting the same response from Mama. I turned around at the dead end and again passed in front of our old house. As we sat in the car, on the street, in front of our old home, I asked Mama if she recognized it now. *Oh, how badly I wanted her to remember it.* Her response was, "No, should I?" I asked again, and still the same response. I finally told her it was our old house.

The look of astonishment on her face was both saddening and oh-so-precious. She stared in utter amazement. She had no idea she could have ever owned a home as beautiful as this. I told her it was the house Daddy built, and they raised six children there. She was truly flabbergasted. "That was my house? Did I live there? It is so beautiful."

She was in awe and began to point out everything she loved about it. The large oak trees, the driveway with the apron (concrete extension), the landscaping, and the gabled roof portico. As I sat behind the wheel, I turned my head away from her while my tears flowed freely. It was priceless to see her reaction, and yet, saddened she had no memory of our lives there. I could only imagine her and Daddy's plans when they were dreaming up what kind of home they wanted and how pleased and proud they must have been when it came to fruition. When I think of my parents planning this home for their growing family, I think of Miranda Lambert's song, "The House That Built Me." It's one of my favorites. We slowly drove away as I called out the names of all our neighbors, none of which rang a bell with her—sweet, sweet Mama. You were so precious to me. I'm learning life lessons the emotional way, not hard, just emotional.

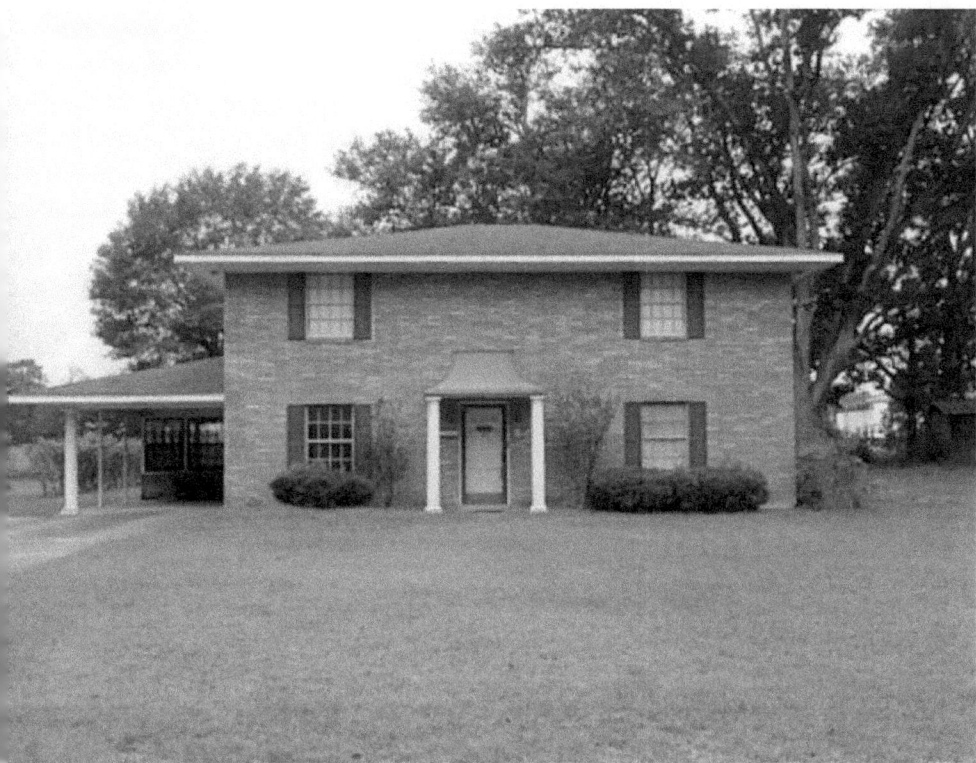

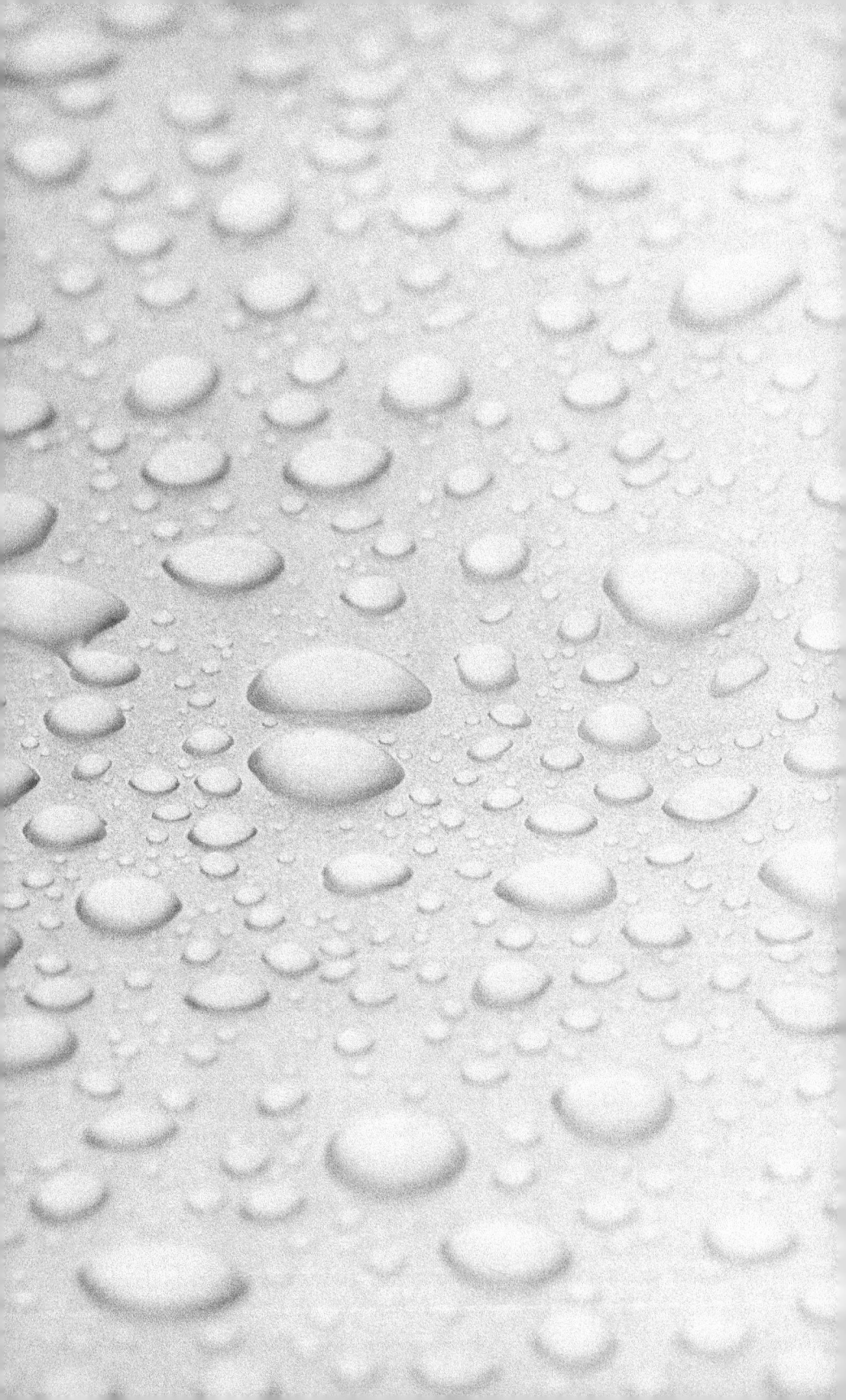

# CHAPTER 43
# PERSONAL MATTERS

MY BELOVED FATHER-IN-LAW, Bubby, was brought to the hospital with issues with his heart, potassium, and blood sugar. He was admitted and stayed for three days. I took the night shift to allow my mother-in-law to rest at night. After she arrived at the hospital mid- morning, I drove over to check on Mama, feed her lunch, then catch a quick nap and repeat. Soon after being discharged, Bubby was brought back to the emergency room.

Again, he stayed for three nights. I was on instant replay; stay the night with him, have the most endearing conversations, and then leave to care for Mama. When it rains, it pours. My sweet mother-in-law, Ann, was hospitalized for five days with cellulitis. Less than a week after Ann was released from the hospital, we decided to put Bubby on hospice. I've included information on hospice in the **Resource** section of this book.

With my husband working out of state, I stepped in to help as much as possible while simultaneously caring for Mama.

**Even when you believe there is no way on earth you can stretch yourself any thinner, you can, you just learn to let things slide because in the grand scheme of things, your loved ones take precedence. They need you! You could very well be their lifeline.**

The summer brought some much-needed visits from my family. Two of my sisters, Suzy and Lydia, came in to give me a break, and Billy, my son, drove in to see all three of his grandparents. While my sisters stayed with Mama, I rested at home and then spent time with my in-laws.

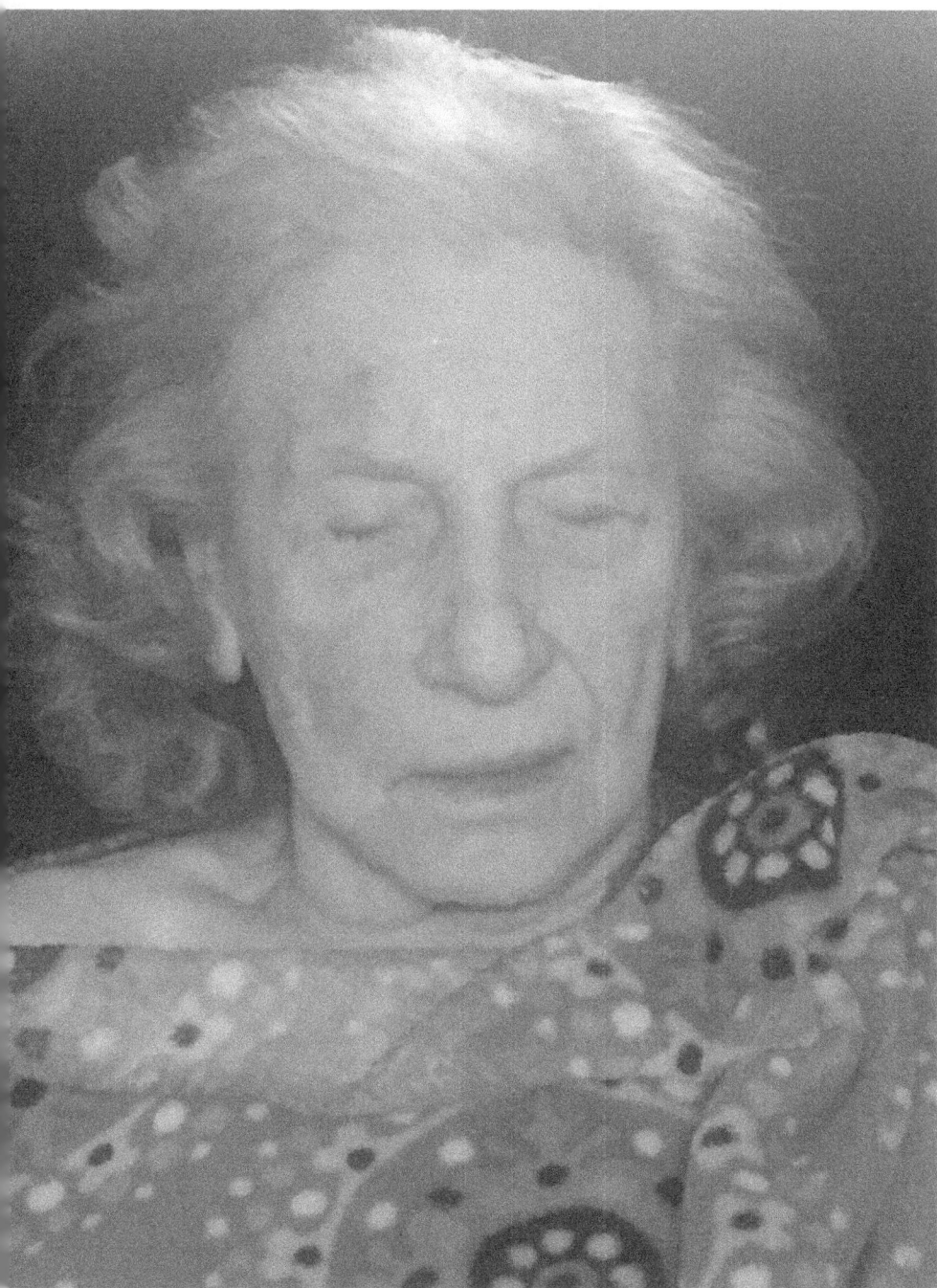

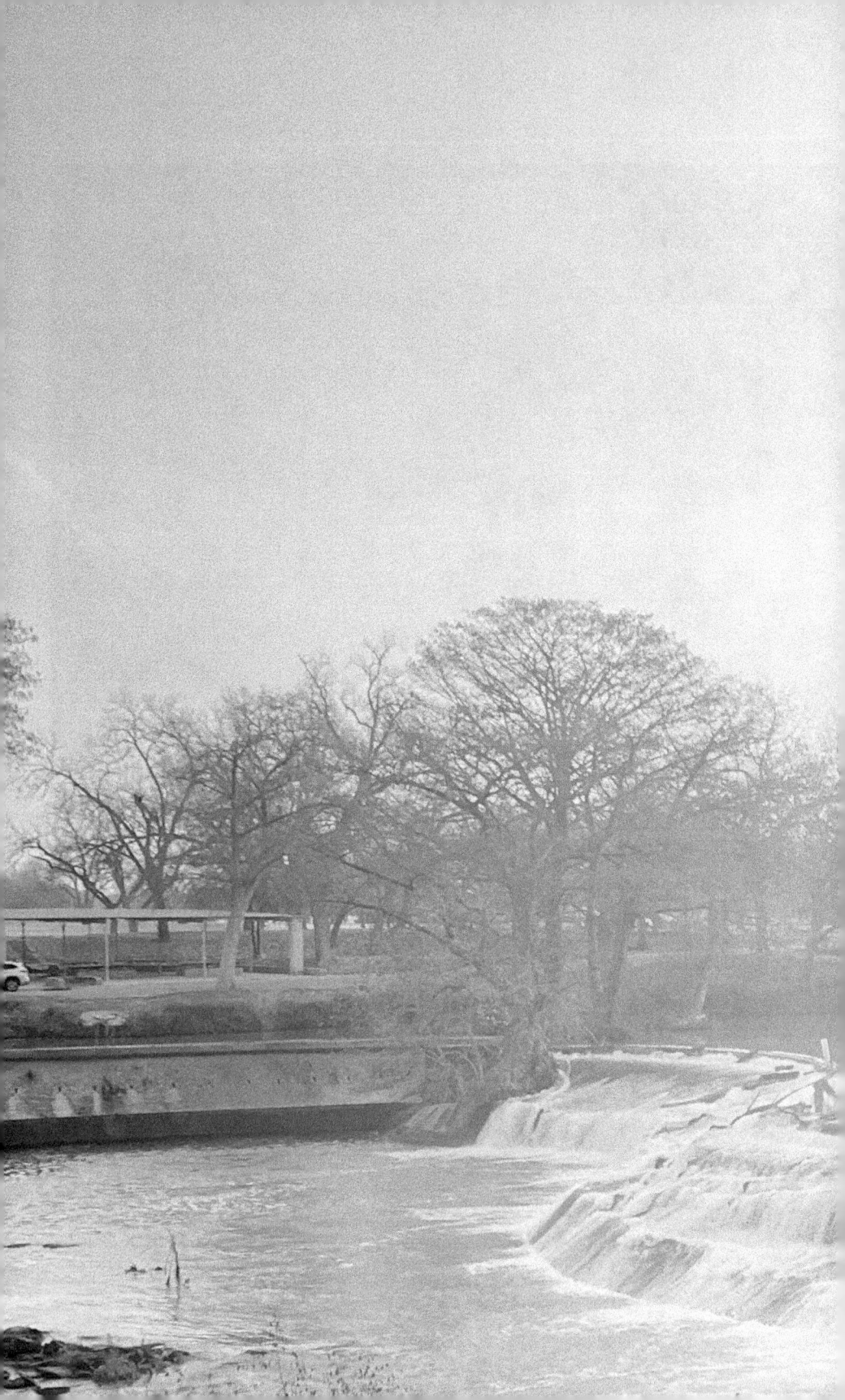

# CHAPTER 44

# WHEN THE CAREGIVER NEEDS A CAREGIVER

WHEN YOU ARE A CAREGIVER, you tend to put your needs to the side not because you choose to, but because there is no other solution. It's a very common occurrence among this population. Several years ago, I found myself in a precarious, ongoing health crisis. I was regularly choking on a granola bar or rice and fries, to cite a few, but bread was enemy number one. Knowing several family members had a history of choking issues, I wasn't overly concerned. Only two of them had resorted to getting their esophagus dilated; therefore, I decided to wait and see how it played out. Besides, my plate was quite full.

Time passed, and the disorder intensified to include choking on water. What scared me was when I choked so severely, my daughters grabbed the phone, with bated breath, ready to dial 911. That happened at least three times. My heart broke to see the fear in their eyes. My symptoms continued to escalate and I began choking in my sleep. I can't even adequately describe it, but it was scary as hell. I sprang straight out of bed and attempted to take breaths, which resulted in a deafening, inhaling sound but without a whisper of an exhale. It felt like I couldn't breathe! I looked at myself in the bathroom mirror, hands clenched on the counter, horrible thoughts racing through my mind, and it was terrifying. I can't revisit that scenario without getting upset. You could hear me trying to breathe all throughout the house.

I struck the walls or doors with my fists as my plea for help when I was genuinely frightened. I didn't want to die alone, much less in a bathroom (just being real). Friends, it was awful.

My husband was present for one such episode. He saw me struggling and assured me I WAS BREATHING, but you could have fooled me. I recognized he was a first responder, but I still doubted whether his assessment was accurate. We may never know what "that" was, but it'll be too soon if it ever happens again. It was about that time I decided to finally seek professional help.

***

DIAGNOSIS: RARE

My local gastroenterologist couldn't provide a diagnosis without the proper testing, so ready or not, here we go. After the testing, my physician told me I had Achalasia, a rare disorder. It's found in 1 in 100,000 people, and they believe it is associated with an auto- immune disease. My issues consisted of the muscles in my esophagus not contracting (due to a nervous system breakdown), and therefore it could not move the food "down the pike." In addition, the flap at the bottom of my esophagus (lower esophageal sphincter, also called LES) primarily stayed closed, consequently causing everything I ate AND drank to back up in the esophagus, resulting in an uncomfortable fullness in my throat. Add the choking I mentioned initially. Talk about the trifecta. Are you getting the picture?

There has been no cure for Achalasia thus far. Doctors only offered procedures to diminish the severity of the rare disorder. I found a qualified, knowledgeable, experienced doctor at the Cleveland Clinic capable of giving me substantial relief. After receiving the test results, I was informed it was worse than I thought, and my condition was more intrusive with each passing day. This disease controlled my life.

***

So why didn't I call and schedule the surgery already? Because I was waiting on God. I believed in modern-day miracles and supernatural healing. I had been healed in that manner three times in my life: rheumatoid arthritis, infertility, and IBS. I prayed God would speak the Word and heal me. I prayed for His will to be done. I didn't want the easy way; I wanted His way. I prayed God directed my steps and my husband and I had peace about the decision.

Shortly after the new year, and after three personal spirit-filled days spent with God in my living room, I felt a peace from God that I should call and make the appointment. Several months later, we flew to the Cleveland Clinic, had a day full of testing, and the following day I went under the knife for the surgery called Heller Myotomy with Fundoplication.

When I woke up in recovery, my husband and son were there beside me. They reported during the surgery, the doctors were shocked to discover two things: My esophagus still had food in it even though I had not consumed anything but liquids for four days; secondly, my esophagus was acting as a second stomach since food wasn't able to go down and, therefore, it had become severely deformed. Four years later I am still doing great. This procedure was life-changing.

I'd like to share a few thoughts if you will allow me.

1. Please don't assume just because a person looks fine on the outside, they are. They could be dealing with serious struggles not visible to the naked eye.
2. Appreciate what you have, again even those things you can't see. They can be taken away from you through no fault of your own.
3. Waiting on direction from God is the best insurance policy you can have. You cannot put a price tag on peace.

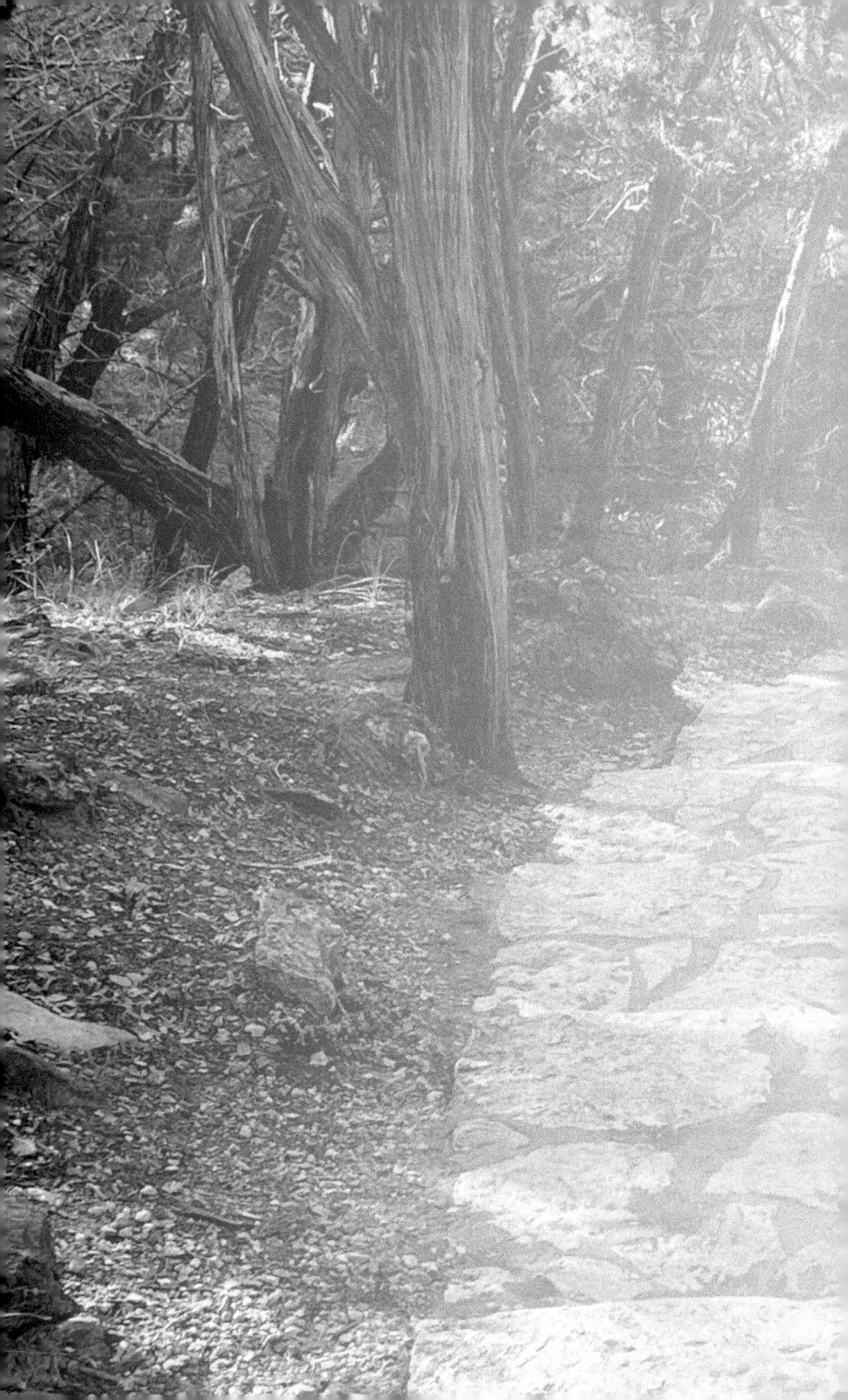

# CHAPTER 45
# HIDE AND SEEK

I LOVED my mother's sense of humor and when she was talkative or comical, I attempted to FaceTime my sisters so they could not only enjoy hearing her voice but seeing her as well. Today was Cathy's turn to receive a call. Mama was in rare form, so it was a perfect time. Mama had both of us cracking up the entire conversation. I encourage caregivers to utilize the technology that is available to allow their families a lifeline to their parents.

Record your conversations, keep all the voicemails, and snap pictures. Have zero regrets.

⸎⸎⸎

Most of the time spent with Mama, even though awake, she kept her eyes closed and rocked her head side to side while she listened to something beautiful playing in her mind only for her to enjoy. Why do I make this assumption? Because of the smile across her lips.

Last night was an extraordinary gift to me. Mama spoke for an entire hour. She had her eyes wide open and had many stories (ramblings) to share. She was quite expressive, and I loved every word that poured out of her mouth.

During the many times we have rested in the TV room, I began to notice a handful of the residents pulled their blankets completely over their heads. I thought it odd, but then again, this was the special care unit and you never knew what might transpire with the residents. After breakfast, I brought Mama to the TV room to rest her eyes but not get too comfortable. My goal was to have her sleep the entire night. She was very quiet on this rainy day and then it happened. She pulled her blanket over her head. Her head, shoulders, and every hair on her head were covered. I couldn't believe it. Then it dawned on me. There was no way she picked up this oddity from the other residents. She couldn't see them. She could hardly see anything with her ocular hemorrhage, so perhaps she felt like she was living in darkness anyway. After that day, Norma Jean pulled the blanket over herself at least once a week. She was a card-carrying member of the 'Hide and Seek' gang.

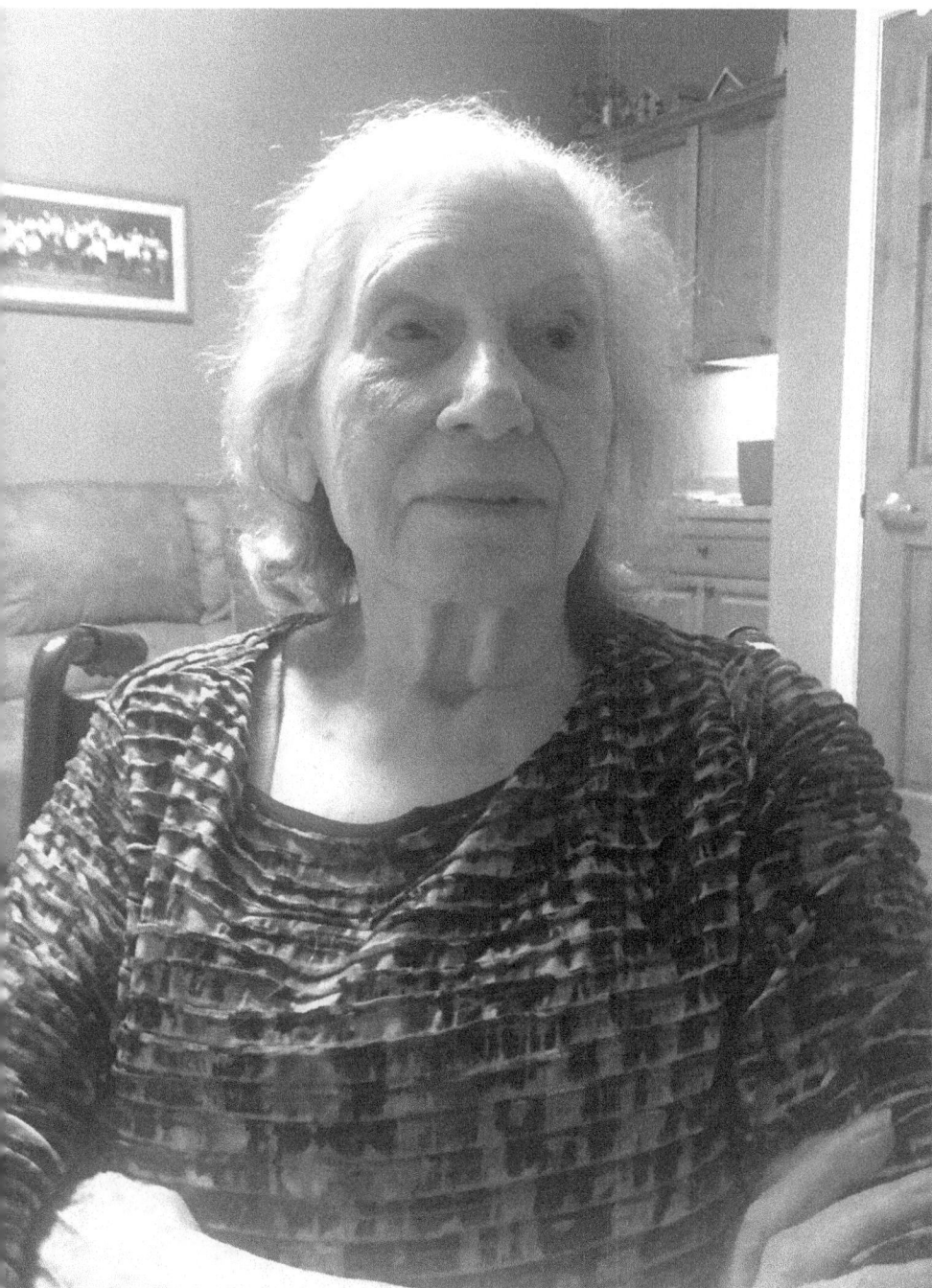

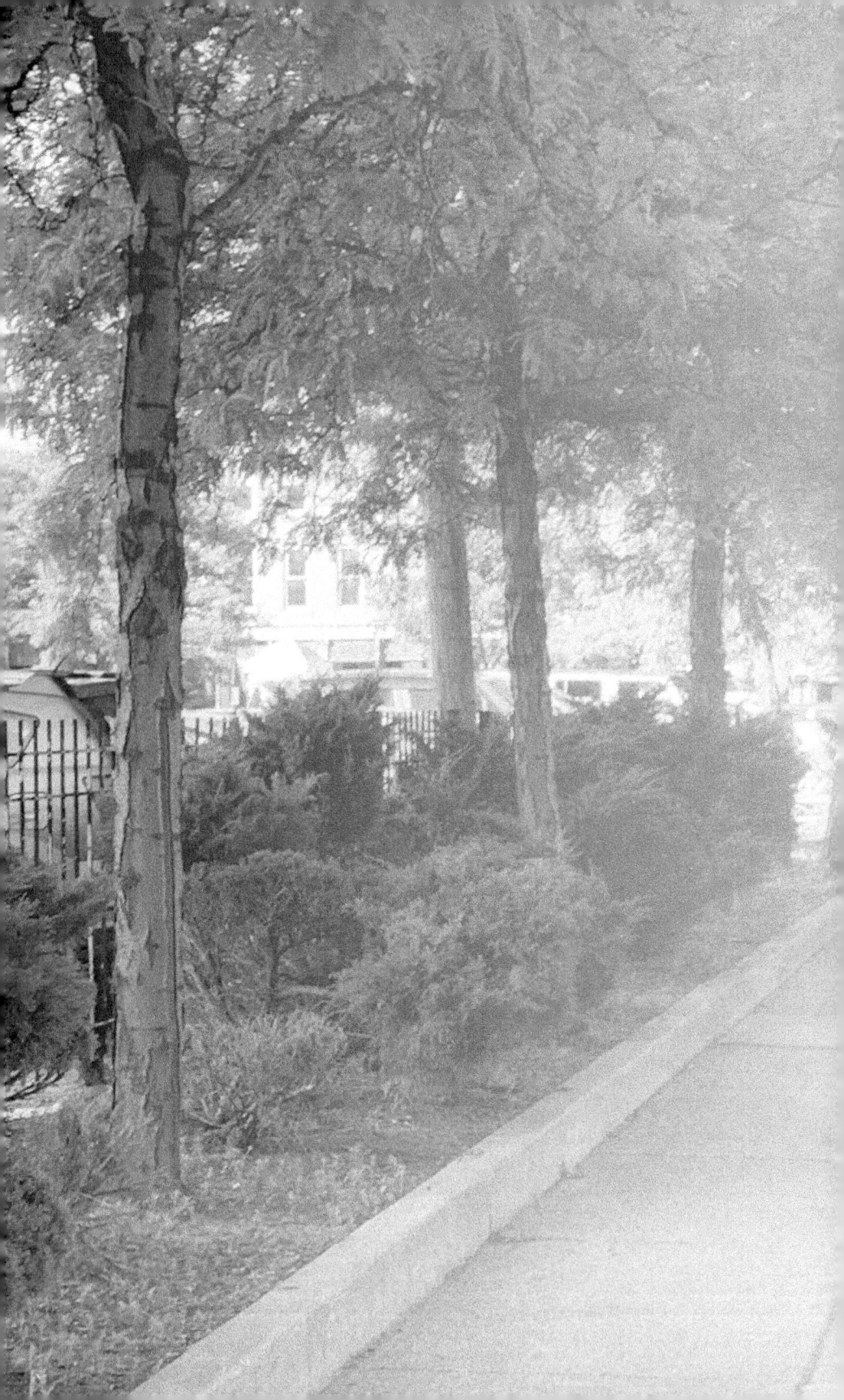

# CHAPTER 46
# WHO DONE IT?

TYPICALLY, when I was at the Big House, I took time to visit with the aides, other families, and of course, the residents. While speaking with one of the aides, she mentioned a young girl came and picked up Mama and checked her out of the facility. *WHAT?* They assumed it was a granddaughter or niece. Mama only has two granddaughters living in the same town who are *my* daughters. They go visit often and nearly everyone knows them. This caused me to start processing this disturbing information. *Who was this person? Where did she take her? Why, after all these years, did this happen? Why didn't they call me or at least ask who she was and her relationship with Mama?* I knew nothing. Thus began my wild goose chase.

I found out the approximate age and hair color of this mystery woman. My detective skills were rusty, but I had to find out the true identity of this person. I made sure the staff knew NEVER to let that happen again. After quizzing everyone in the assisted living and special care units, I finally figured out it was a friend's granddaughter who met Mama when she lived in the assisted living unit. Still, to this day, I don't know what possessed this young lady to do this random act, but I am happy to report it never happened again.

# CHAPTER 47

# TEST OF MY FAITH

THERE WILL LIKELY BE times when you feel you unequivocally CANNOT handle yet another thing on your plate since caregiving is consuming the majority of your day. I felt that way, too. My mother, my family, hurricanes, my in-laws, my esophagus issue, and oh, let's add one more thing.

I noticed my head had the oddest sensation while I was at work or driving. It felt like my scalp was divided equally into four sections, think puzzle pieces. For no particular reason, it felt they shifted. It stopped me in my tracks every time. I never felt dizzy or nauseous. It was never accompanied by a headache or vision problems.

This sensation went on for several weeks before I consulted my doctor. She immediately sent me for a brain MRI after she watched me step down from the examination table and witnessed one of my events. I had the MRI immediately. I was at work the following day when I received a call from my doctor telling me they made an appointment for me at M.D. Anderson (one of the best cancer hospitals in the country) to see a neurological surgeon. I had a brain tumor!

Naturally, I burst into tears, *big surprise*, and my co-worker ran to my side. We prayed. I asked God, "Why? I am already in over my head. I'm not strong. Please, Lord Jesus, I beg you to let the scans be wrong." The rest of the day was a blur, and I asked to go home early so I could have a horribly, ugly cry and process this news.

I turned the engine on to my car, and the song playing on the K-Love station was God's intimate message to me. *"It Is Well with My Soul"* was one of my favorite songs, and today, it took on a whole new meaning. God's message came through loud and clear. I knew, I knew, I knew, I would be okay.

Two weeks later, accompanied by my husband, I met with the neurologist in Houston. It was the best outcome I could have asked for other than the fact they found there were TWO tumors. They were benign. The doctor labeled them medullary meningiomas. He said there was spinal fluid between the medulla and the tumors, and both tumors have a nice round shape. *Great it's a matching set to the rest of my body.* The brain was not angry or swollen. The tumors were not the cause of my head sensations. He reported it was not interfering with anything. The doctor believed it could be hormone-related and possibly have had them for some time, even since puberty.

He predicted my tumors to be in the 7 to 10 percentile which never grow, never interfere, and never have to be dealt with. He laughed and said, "You will probably be 89 years old and still housing the tumors, same size, same shape." I was scheduled to report back to M.D. Anderson once a year for an MRI of my noggin.

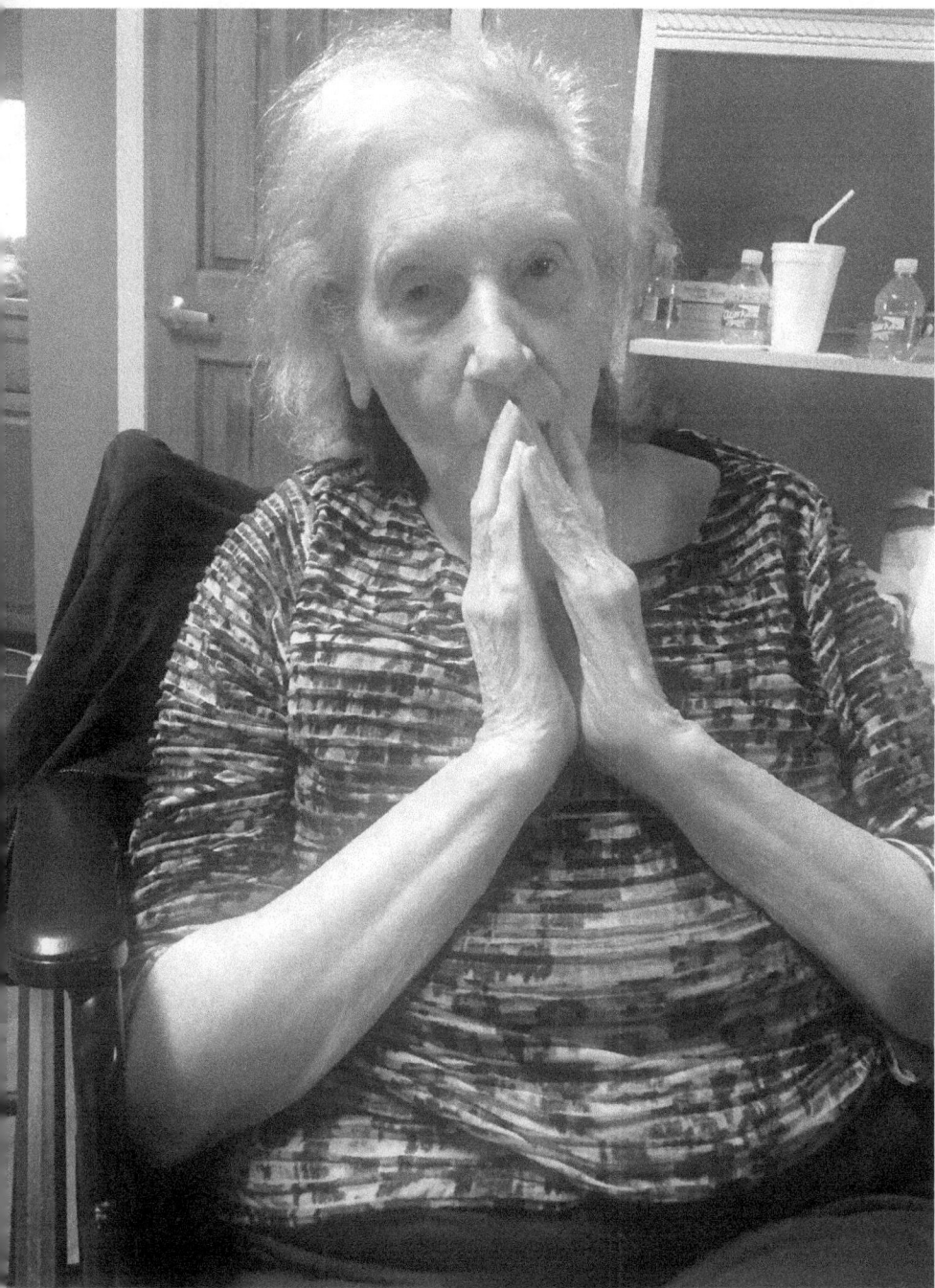

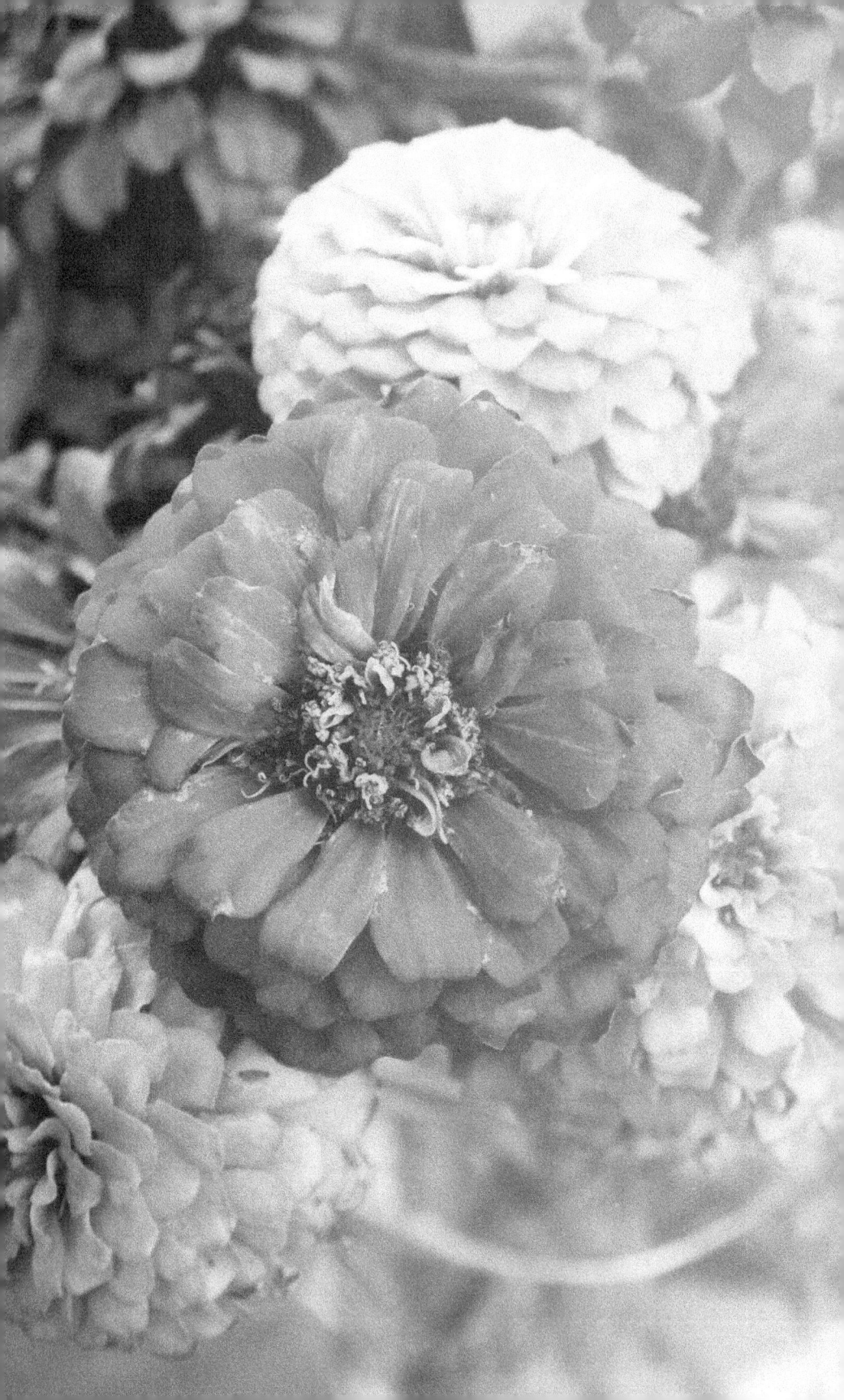

# CHAPTER 48
# A HALLMARK MOMENT

I DROVE Mama to the doctor for a check-up, (I felt like that's all I ever did anymore), and when we returned, there was a beautiful vase of flowers on Mama's nightstand. With her birthday this week, I was sure it was from one of my siblings. You could never imagine what I am about to share.

I opened the envelope for Mama and began reading it to her. The card read, "Our Secret Love is No Secret Anymore." *What in the world?* If this wasn't a Hallmark moment, I don't know what was. This card was mysteriously sweet. The card was signed by a person who was very familiar to me. He was an old friend, a widower, and a lifelong friend of my parents and uncles.

I ran out of the room pushing Mama in her wheelchair and asked the staff about the delivery. They said the gentleman just asked for her room number, dropped it off, and left. I have yet to hear a word from him. Of course, at this stage Mama had no idea who he was so she couldn't fully appreciate the sentimental letter. I did not want to contact him and cause him embarrassment, but it was the sweetest gesture.

I had been with Norma Jean almost as much as if I lived with her. I knew her friends, her enemies, and her comings and goings (except for that one time). I honestly never saw this coming. Sweetest thing ever.

⧽⎯⎯⎯⎯⎯

For Mama's 90<sup>th</sup> birthday, Chrissy penned this story for the birthday girl. I love her heart and her beautiful writing.

*Meet my Mamaw. She is one of the most beautiful people you will ever meet. I've heard stories of her basketball days and of her and my Papaw's love story. We've had our own share of memories of making French toast early Saturday mornings, followed by yard work soon after, but today is a memory I will cherish for the rest of my life.*

*As I visited my Mamaw today, I knew she would not remember me or who I was, but none of that mattered because I wept as I lay in her arms while she held me. I wept because, for the first time in a long time, I closed my eyes while cuddled up in my grandmother's arms, and it felt like she had never left me like it was just another Saturday morning.*

*Some of you have met this amazing woman and been blessed by her sweet spirit, but I get the most incredible blessing of being called her granddaughter.*

*I love you more than you will ever know Mamaw. Chrissy*

⧽⎯⎯⎯⎯⎯

The highlight of my day was when Mama's 90<sup>th</sup> birthday party was over, and most of the room was empty of guests. Mama was asking my daughters rather loudly, "I just want my daughter!!!" Mama had all four of her daughters there, but she made it clear the other three were not the daughter she was searching for. She hasn't remembered me in a while, and she's long forgotten my name, but as long as she knows I'm her daughter, all was well in my world. What an unexpected gift from God today. And yes, you better believe I came running to her side.

The day was drawing to an end. Mama enjoyed her party and was ready for bed at 4:30 pm. The family helped me out in every single area. I'm forever grateful for the love shared and memories made that day, all to honor Norma Jean. The cousins ended the day in true Cajun style, going to eat seafood and dance to the Cajun music at a local restaurant.

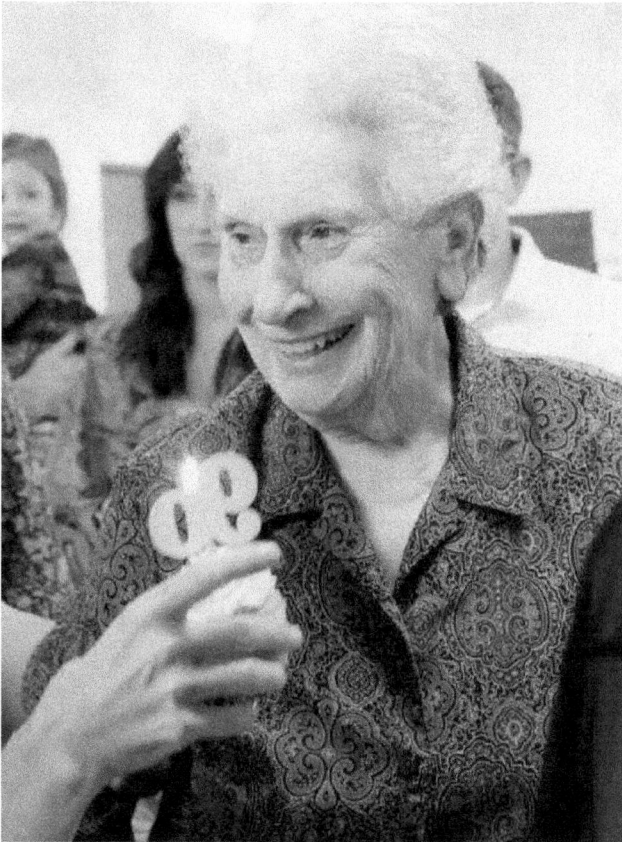

Happy 90th Birthday, Mama.

# CHAPTER 49
# UNRESPONSIVE

JAMES and I went to Cracker Barrel for supper and we thoroughly enjoyed it because frankly, I had been cooking very few home-cooked meals those days. Today was like any other day. I had spent most of it with Mama.

During our meal, I received an alarming call from the Big House my mother was unresponsive. *What? What does that even mean? Did she have a heart attack? Was she dead? What?* I never encountered that terminology before. They just told me to get to the Big House, STAT! While James drove, I called Cathy. I told Cathy what I knew about Mama's situation and to please start the phone tree, calling the other four siblings.

~~~∞~~~

I arrived at the back door of the special care unit, wide-eyed and teary. A couple of the aides I considered friends escorted me to Mama in her apartment. She was lying down in her bed and appeared just to be resting. I knelt down next to Mama and in a tender voice, I spoke to Mama, assuring her I was there. Upon learning her vital signs were stable, an influx of questions began. *"What happened? Where was she? What caused this?"* The aides relayed the story.

Mama had just finished supper in the dining room and suddenly Mama passed out, but not like fainting. They tried to rouse her but were unsuccessful. She was not responding. She was slumped over in her chair. The nurse started rubbing her chest vigorously with her fist, and Mama regained consciousness. Stop right here. Mama had a DNR in place, Do Not Resuscitate. *Why in the world did this happen?* If this was God's plan for her to leave quickly and painlessly, then so be it. A whirlwind of thoughts exploded in my mind. She was now frail and lethargic.

⌘

I made a phone call to Mama's church to have the priest come and give her the Last Rites and he arrived within the hour. Mama woke up at one point, looked at the priest, and asked, "Are you coming back tomorrow?" Oh, Mama, she was something else again. Her antics gave me something to laugh about amid the river of tears. She quickly drifted back to sleep. Mama slept all night and was in bed for nearly three days. The episode just wiped her out. She talked every now and then, but it was mostly radio silence. This gave me a generous amount of time to pray and prepare myself for the impending future. My amateur research showed an unresponsive event was when a person was not moving and did not respond when you called them or gently shook their shoulders.

With my recent, first-hand experience with hospice while caring for my father-in-law, I decided now was the time to put Mama in the care of hospice. Mama's beautiful apartment was transformed in the blink of an eye. A hospital bed, an oxygen tank, new XL twin sheets required for the hospital bed, a new bedspread, a huge stack of diapers they provided, and a lock box with end-of-life medicine to keep the patient comfortable. Hospice covers most medications used for the primary diagnosis of a patient being placed in hospice. Hospice staff members

200

showered Mama several times weekly, clipped toenails, and ordered and provided diapers and bed pads.

<hr>

Mama's sister also had Alzheimer's and lived in assisted living in another state. It was interesting to learn she and Mama even had the same exact apartment number. They had a lot in common in their journey with this disease. No two Alzheimer's patients will be exactly alike, but they definitely have some similarities. This makes two of Mama's siblings that had Alzheimer's. When her sister passed away, her memorial service was held in our hometown. All of my siblings came home and we attended the service together. I am glad all of my brothers and sisters and my cousin were able to come visit Mama in her apartment after the service. Her unresponsive events were cause for great concern.

<hr>

I took advantage of having family in town to take care of Mama's funeral preparations knowing her days on earth were fewer and fewer. Why should I postpone making arrangements? At this age, her passing was inevitable. My sister, Suzy, her husband, Dave, and I went to the funeral home and spent four hours with a funeral planner. We were glad we had chosen the pre-planned version because it was intense. Not emotional, just volumes of information to process. So many decisions! I've included some tips on funeral planning in the **Resource** section.

<hr>

January was quite a memorable month full of struggles and new territory for me. To sum this month up, Mama was unresponsive twice in 10 days, she consequently slept for two to three days afterward, and she stopped talking for a day and a half. This saddened me the most. *What if I never hear her voice again in speech or song?* I treasured our little chats. I knew her better than I ever had. The absence of conversation was tough for me. Tougher than when she forgot my name or our relationship. Mama had seen all of her children and some grandchildren this month, and then sweet Mama rebounded, at least for a while.

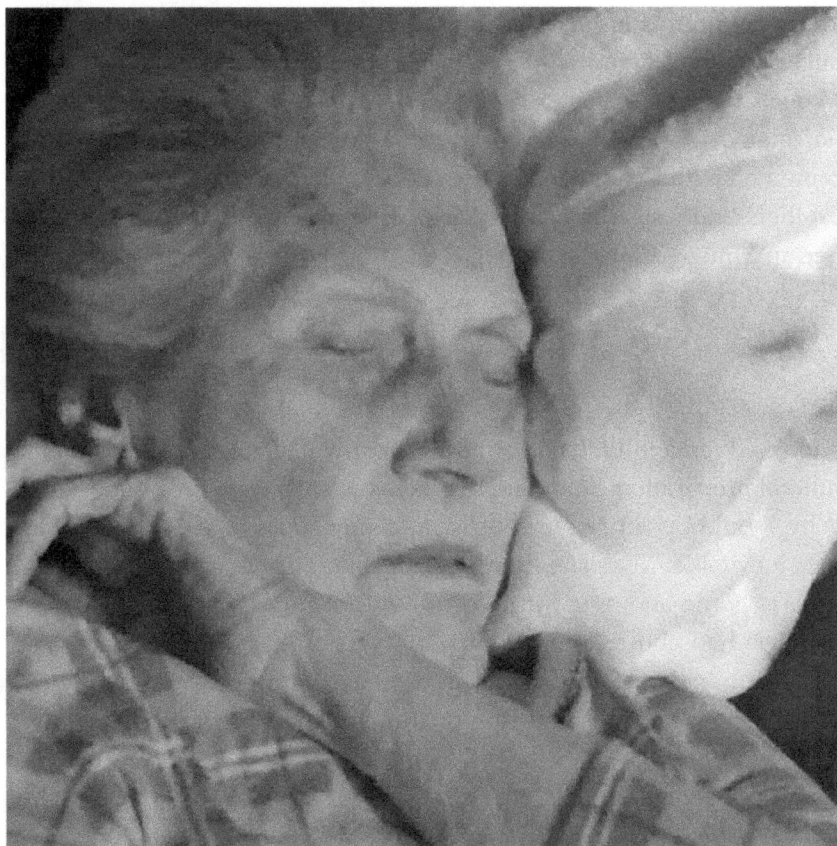

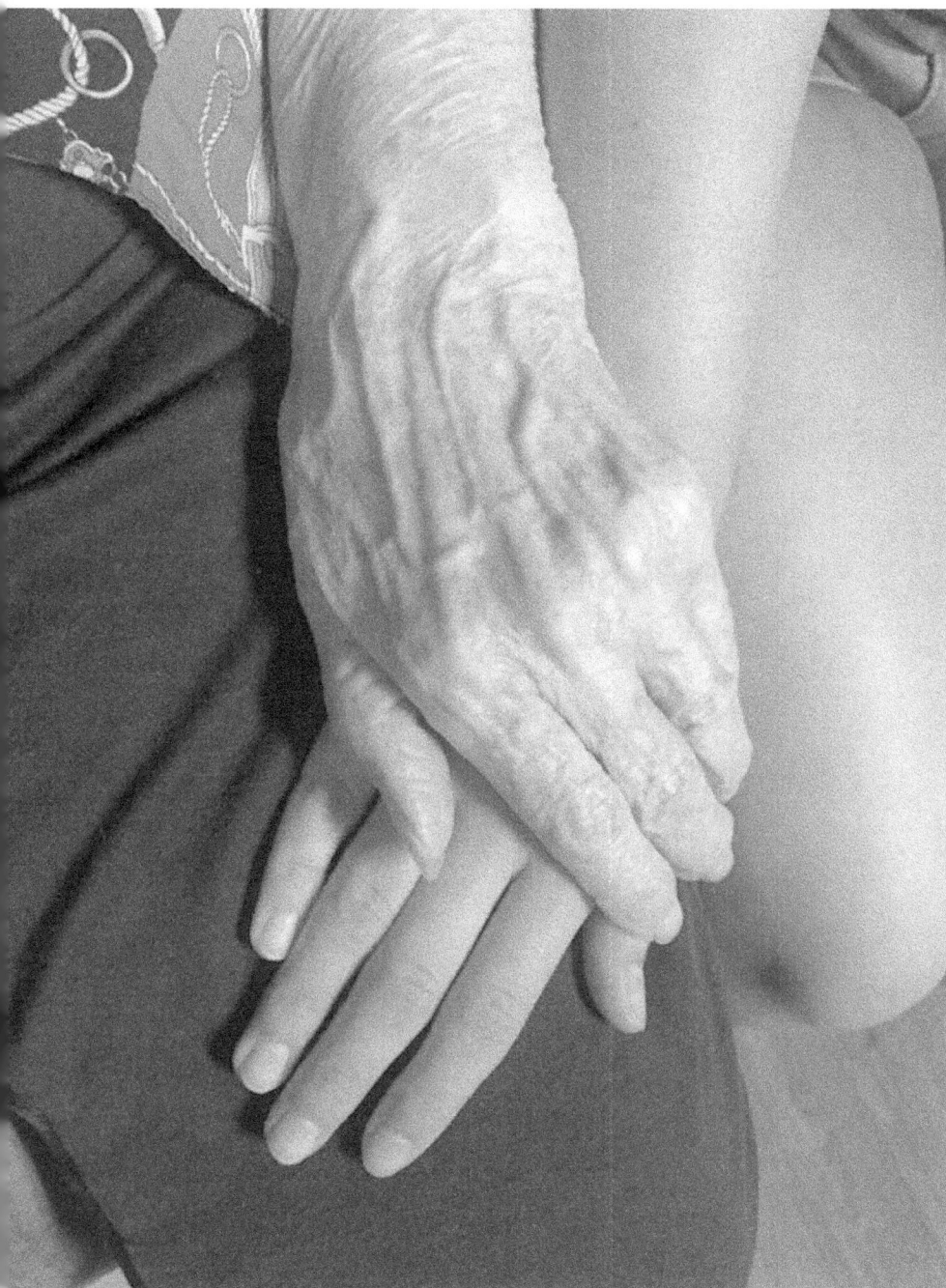

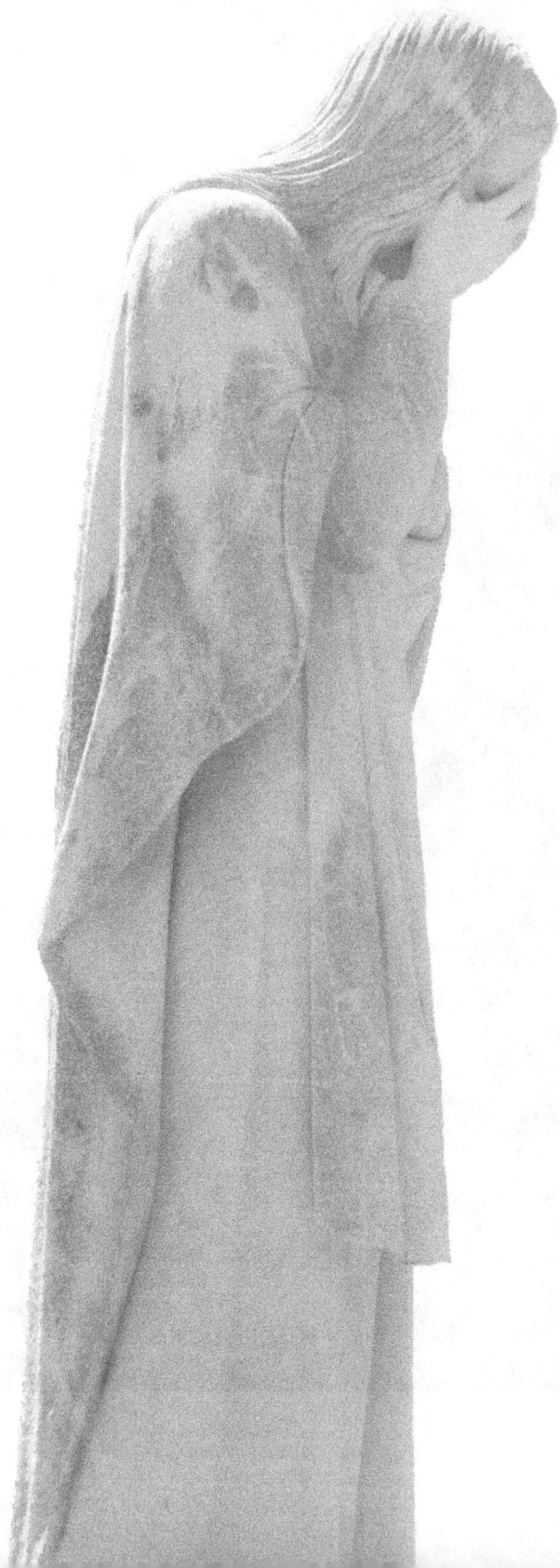

# CHAPTER 50
# HEAVY- HEARTED

I DROVE straight over to the Big House after work to check on Mama and feed her supper. I waited for the outside, locked door to be opened, greeted a few residents and workers in the hallway, and then rounded the corner with a bird's eye view of the dining room, specifically Mama's table. She was leaning to the side of her chair, nearly laying her head on the table. Nurses and aides surrounded her. I saw her head fall forward, and as I ran to her, she was losing her color. Poor Mama was cold and clammy, and her body became limp.

In a blink, I had two conflicting emotions, sadness and relief. She did not respond to stimulation at all. The nurse began rubbing Mama's chest with her fist. Again, **not** following the protocol of the DNR in place. I was infuriated!! When Mama regained consciousness, her color came back slowly but she slept for two solid days.

With the sudden onset of Mama's decline in her health, my thoughts weighed heavy on my heart about her impending death. I believed as her caregiver, I had cared for her to the best of my ability.

# CHAPTER 51
# CELESTIAL VISITS

SEVERAL DAYS after Mama's third unresponsive event, it was a dreary afternoon, but Mama surprisingly blessed me with random comments such as, "I'm talking to Verda" (her deceased sister). I asked her when, and she responded, "Early this morning." Yep, that sounded like my Aunt Verda. She was always an early riser.

During supper, Mama looked me square in the eye (and remember, her vision was null and void for the most part) and said, "We need to do this more often." I asked if she meant me coming more often (secretly, I hoped that's what she was referring to) or did she mean eating more often. She never replied, so I stuck with my first inclination.

Before supper ended, she started mumbling. I asked who she was talking to and she replied, "Your brothers." When I questioned her trying to get their names, she said two of *her* deceased brothers' names, "Milford and Lubert." I assure you, she had an eventful day, and witnessing it firsthand brought me immense joy.

I am thankful for my time with my mother. Listening to her quick wit, her enjoyment of hearing others laughing, her random visits with those who have gone before her, and much more. There were a lot of quiet days, but today was a banner day for me. I felt like I was part of a family reunion.

—⁓⁌⁍⁊⁎⁓—

You talk about a cliffhanger. Since Mama would soon turn 91 in a couple of weeks, I asked her if she was getting ready to go to heaven. Her response...wait for it... it's a cliffhanger, friends. She responded with, "No," to which I quipped, "Why?" She said she was, and I quote, "Waiting." My mouth flew open, and I scooted to the edge of my seat and asked her, "For who or what?" Nothing, nothing at all. She was finished talking. It was climatic and a cliffhanger all in one fell swoop. I may never know.

Don't worry. I trust God's perfect timing, but I get rather curious now and then. Today was just one of those days. I just had to ask. Her answer could be comprehended as, "No, not today." I do know when God called her home, she was ready. She had been ready for 20 years. I look back over the past 20 years and at the many lives she touched. She never stopped and wouldn't stop until her last breath.

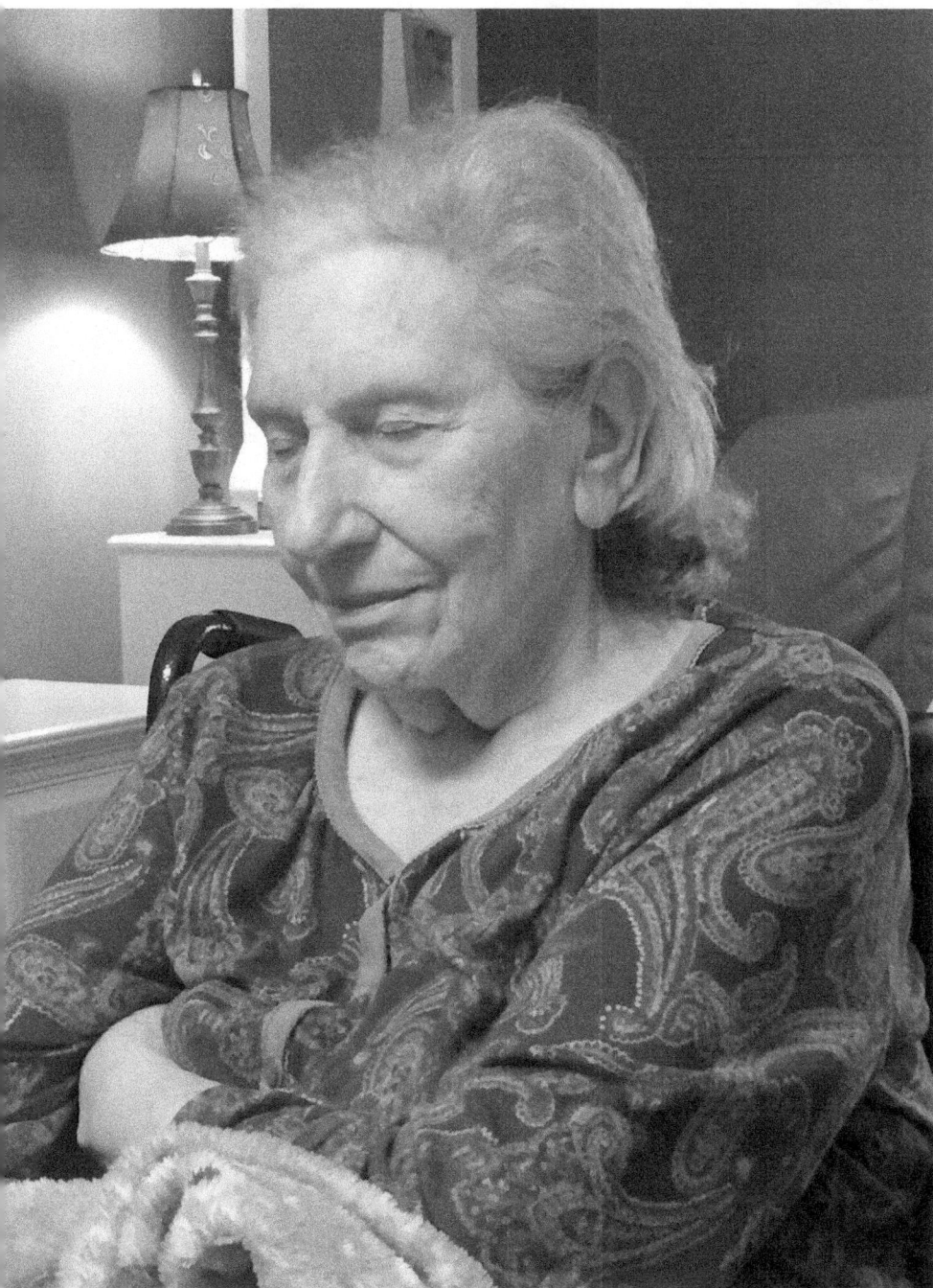

# CHAPTER 52
# SAME SONG, SECOND VERSE

SAME SONG, second verse, could be better but it's worse. I received a call from the Big House. Mama had fallen in her bathroom. I called the hospice nurse, and they came to check on her and brought her a wheelchair. Thankfully, as we began using the wheelchair, Mama seemed to enjoy it. She used her feet to get her exercise and pedaled at a pretty quick pace down the hallways. During most days while I worked, Mama was on her own. Aides helped her shower, dress, and go to the bathroom. They put her in the wheelchair, and she "drove" all over the halls pedaling her feet. At times, something enticed her to go inside someone's apartment and visit. More often than not, it was the sound of the television broadcasting a Catholic rosary being said, or she heard music that appealed to her. This particular day, she was 'driving' down the hall and stopped in a female resident's room only a couple of doors down from hers. She was in her room only momentarily when she came back out of the door. She had positioned the wheelchair parallel to the hallway, and as she started to turn the wheels, she collapsed and fell halfway out of the chair.

Mama sat there slumped over for a few minutes without another soul in the hallway. Suddenly, the little female resident who said all the rosaries and loved to dance, found Mama and immediately knew to go find help. She shuffled her little feet as quickly as possible. Soon after, two aides came, and a group of onlookers gathered. You may wonder how I know all this. When Suzy and I met with the director, she showed us the video. *What was going on, sweet Mama?* My thoughts were racing. I was grateful they did not try to revive her by rubbing their fists on her chest. They finally understood I meant business. DNR, DNR, DNR! *Do Not Resuscitate!* From that moment on, I kept a very close eye on Mama and was with her as much as possible throughout the day until she fell asleep.

Several weeks later, I went after work to visit Mama, feed her supper, and stay with her until she was asleep. When I arrived at 5:30, I found her asleep on her leather sofa. I sat near her for 15 minutes, trying to rouse her, gently calling her name while stroking her arm. After several unsuccessful attempts, I stepped out of her room and questioned some of the aides about what type of day Mama had. They all reported, "She was tired." We all have those days, I didn't think anything of it, especially since she was 90 years old.

I drove home and less than 30 minutes later, I received a phone call from the Big House telling me Mama had fallen and hit her head on the baseboard. "It was not good. She needs to be brought to the ER." When I reached her room, she was already black and blue around her eye and required stitches. I am thankful James met me in the emergency room. Mama was extremely hard to contend with in that environment. Her fear and confusion displayed itself as combativeness and foul language. The doctor put eight stitches near her brow. Thank goodness, he had the patience of Job. We brought Mama back to the Big House and I stayed with her the next 24 hours. Once we returned to her apartment, Mama slept for two consecutive days. When Mama was awake, she constantly played with her stitches. This prompted me to move my chair right next to her bed to try and catch her hand before it reached her face. It was exhausting!

The following day, I asked the facility to see the video. It was alarming only 15 minutes after I left her something this horrific could occur. This was the precise moment, especially after viewing the video, I decided I needed to ramp up to using private sitters for 24-hour care and a wheelchair at all times. Mama struggled with her eyesight already, but this video showed her weaving down the hall like a hard-hitting, three-day drunkard. Once she started losing her balance, she slammed into the linoleum floor and baseboard. You could hear her moaning, but she wasn't moving.

A week later, the hospice nurse came by to remove the stitches. She turned to me after examining Norma Jean and reported Mama had already pulled all the stitches out of her eyebrow. *Norma Jean, what a hot mess!*

---

After this fall, I stayed at the Big House nearly 24 hours a day. I was scared to leave her alone. My daughters were so good to me. They brought coffee and supper and visited with me often. It was very easy to go stir-crazy staring at the same four walls day in and day out. I was thankful I had my laptop and was able to work remotely. I could never fully express how much my girls' kind-hearted gestures meant to me.

---

Mel gave me the sweetest card. What a beautiful way to lift my spirits and encourage my walk through this caregiving journey. She wrote,

*Ma,*

*There were so many times when you could have walked away and said I'm tired, I can't do this anymore, but you didn't. You fought the battle and are continuing to fight it, and I can see you're tired, and somehow you are still continuing. I honestly don't know how you do it.*

*You are strong, kind, and the most compassionate person I know. 1 Peter 5:10 says, "In His kindness God called you to share in His eternal glory by means of Christ Jesus. So, after you have suffered a little while, He will restore, support, and strengthen you, and He will place you on a firm foundation."*

*I fully believe restoration is coming soon, Mama. You need it; I know you're running on empty, and God knows, too. Like Dory on Finding Nemo says, "Just keep swimming, just keep swimming."*

*Mel*

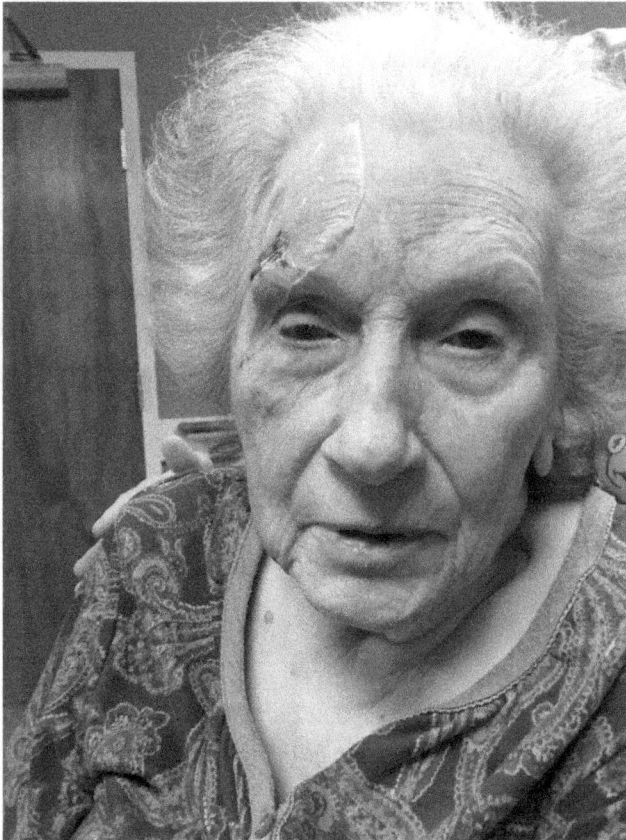

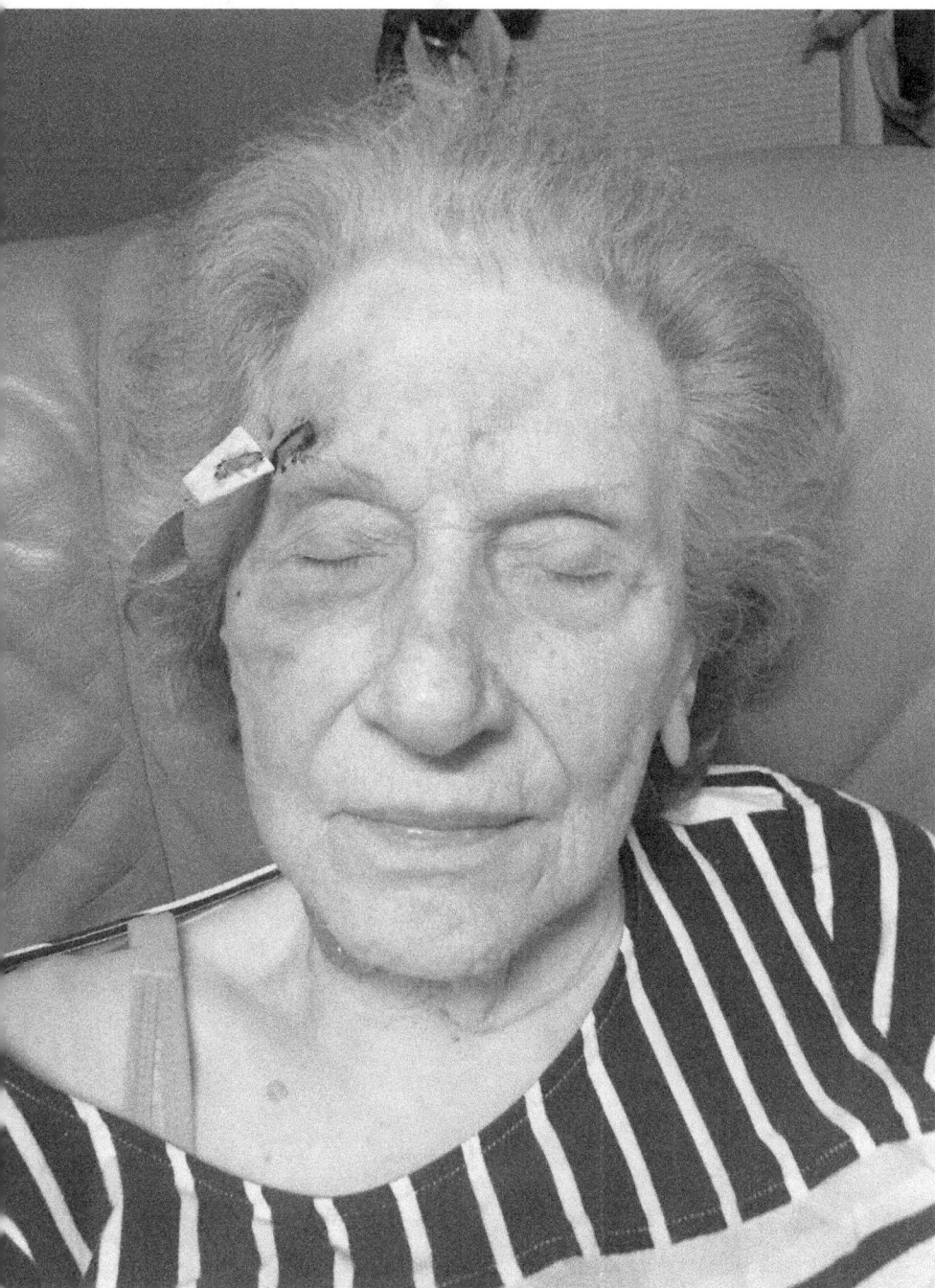

# CHAPTER 53

# THE LOW DOWN ON
# SITTERS

IF YOU HAVE NEVER HAD to hire sitters for the most precious person in your life, then allow me to give you some tips.

I only interviewed people referred to me by personal friends. I asked for at least one other referral from each applicant. With the sitters working in a facility versus a private home, they were required to pass the facility's screening as well. I offered to pay for the screening. Interviews were conducted in Mama's apartment. Her apartment was very nice, clean, and beautifully decorated. I don't think anyone would be opposed to sitting there making some money.

I typed a list of specific duties sitters were required to perform. I could tell immediately some of the older applicants didn't fit the bill; they were barely able to even catch their breath after walking down the hallway.

⁙⁘⁙

Having been with Mama every weekday and on the weekends, I possessed an intimate understanding of the necessary requirements for sitters. I was well acquainted with Mama's routine, was actively involved in her well-being and had been for a span of nine years. I questioned the applicants extensively about their experience. I chose to have them work 12-hour shifts, and I paid them the going rate, which at that time was $10/hour. The sitters were paid weekly. I was shocked at the number of employees at the facility eager to pick up extra hours, even those in management. If you think their job pays well and is easy money, think again. The large majority worked so hard and were paid so little. I am thankful to those who joined the "Norma Jean team." I knew Mama loved them and was thrilled to have them come along side me to give her the best possible care.

After interviewing a half-dozen women, I was intrigued by the actions of a few. Some were very polite. They asked if they could approach Mama, and with a nod of my head, they began to interact with her. I loved watching this exchange. It spoke volumes to me about their character. Mama wasn't always talkative and often just stared into space, rocking her head from side to side. That didn't seem to hinder these few. They were very kind. It warmed my soul.

Others came in and never even looked at Mama. They were only interested in how much I was paying and only accepted cash. That was a huge red flag to me. I was accountable to the government for every penny I spent of my mother's money, and I needed a paper trail for the money I disbursed to those sitters.

Another valuable lesson I learned was to listen to the applicant when talking about her previous jobs. Some were too open and gossiped about their patients, using their names and including information about their health and their extended family. *Excuse me! That was personal. You should not be sharing any of that information.* They definitely did not make the cut!

<hr />

After I made my selections and hired the sitters, I arrived at shift change, morning and night, at 7 o'clock for the entire year until Mama passed.

**It was imperative communication was at its best between all the players who were involved in the care of my mother.**

I didn't want any hiccups in the shift change, so I made myself present. I also wanted to hear first-hand how the shift went, if there were any changes in my mother, or any other anecdotes I needed to hear about. I asked a lot of questions so I could get the answers. Those shift changes also allowed me to develop a solid relationship with the sitters. Often, I stayed an extra hour after Mama was asleep and visited with them. With no family nearby, they became like sisters. It was evident they dearly loved Norma Jean.

<hr>

I have included a document in the **Resource** section where I had each sitter read, sign, and date so they knew exactly what was expected of them. It included my contact information, Mama's schedule, and details, lots of details about her personality and needs. I also had a huge dry-erase board with a large calendar where I listed who was sitting for each shift. I filled in for the shifts where I couldn't find some-one, which usually accounted for two or three shifts a week. I've included a photo of the dry-erase board in the **Resource** section. The board also facilitated my desire to have everyone be on the same page regarding Mama's care. The board served as a checkpoint with the staff and hospice as well. It was an amazing communication tool.

We kept track of Mama's bowel movements, appetite, any changes in her health, sleepless nights, UTIs, aggravation, combativeness, etc. My name and my husband's name and numbers were written on the board. Mama's hospice nurse was listed on the board, along with her phone number. I usually included a scripture verse or uplifting message. I instructed them to list any supplies that were needed. That board was my control center.

<hr>

The worse part about having 24-hour sitters was making up the work schedule every month. I printed a blank copy of the calendar and had each sitter mark which shifts they wanted to work. Several of them always worked the same days. Others were very sporadic. I had the board fresh and clean with all the new assignments before the first of each month. I placed a copy on the control center board and printed a copy for each sitter to take. I always breathed a little easier when that task was done. My weekly tasks were to write their paychecks. No two weeks were alike for the sitters. It was a juggling act at times and I was always happy when the checks were disbursed.

<hr />

I had learned about the proper way to lift patients in and out of wheelchairs, etc. I learned how to groom, potty, and shower Mama. I definitely was not a bystander, and the staff and private sitters appreciated it. Unfortunately, as a result, I needed to visit my chiropractor regularly.

<hr />

Today, Mama was given the best gift. The family across the hall were caring for their mother who had always been a friend of our family. It was wonderful on those long, unending weekends, to meet with her grown children in the hallway and just chat, compare stories, and pray for each other. It gave both of us a chance to step outside our day-to-day arena and enjoy some much-needed conversation. When their mother passed, they gave me her lift chair to alleviate all the lifting now required with Mama. What a welcome blessing. Everyone who was involved in Mama's care was appreciative. When Mama passed, we gifted the chair to another family in special care.

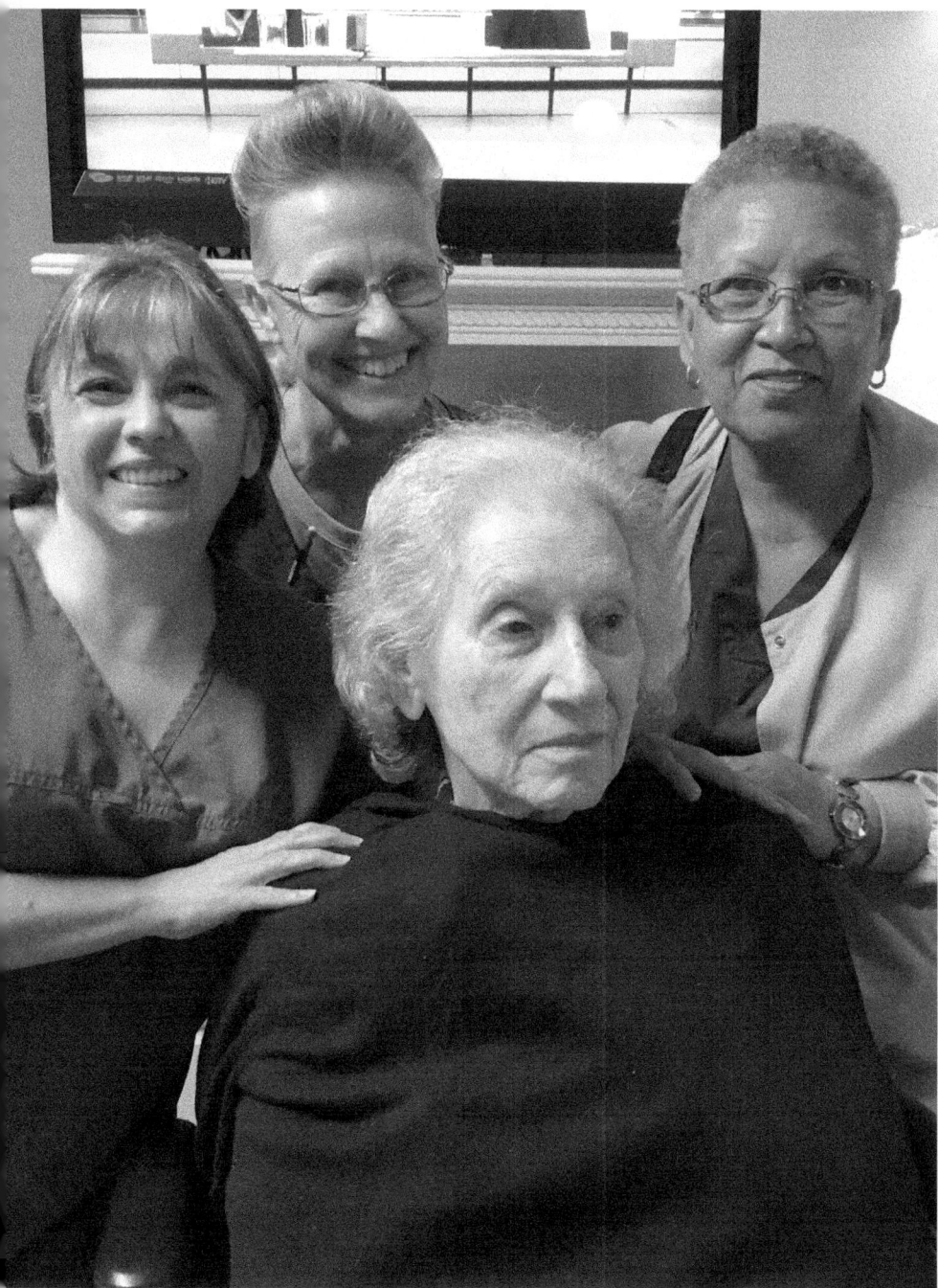

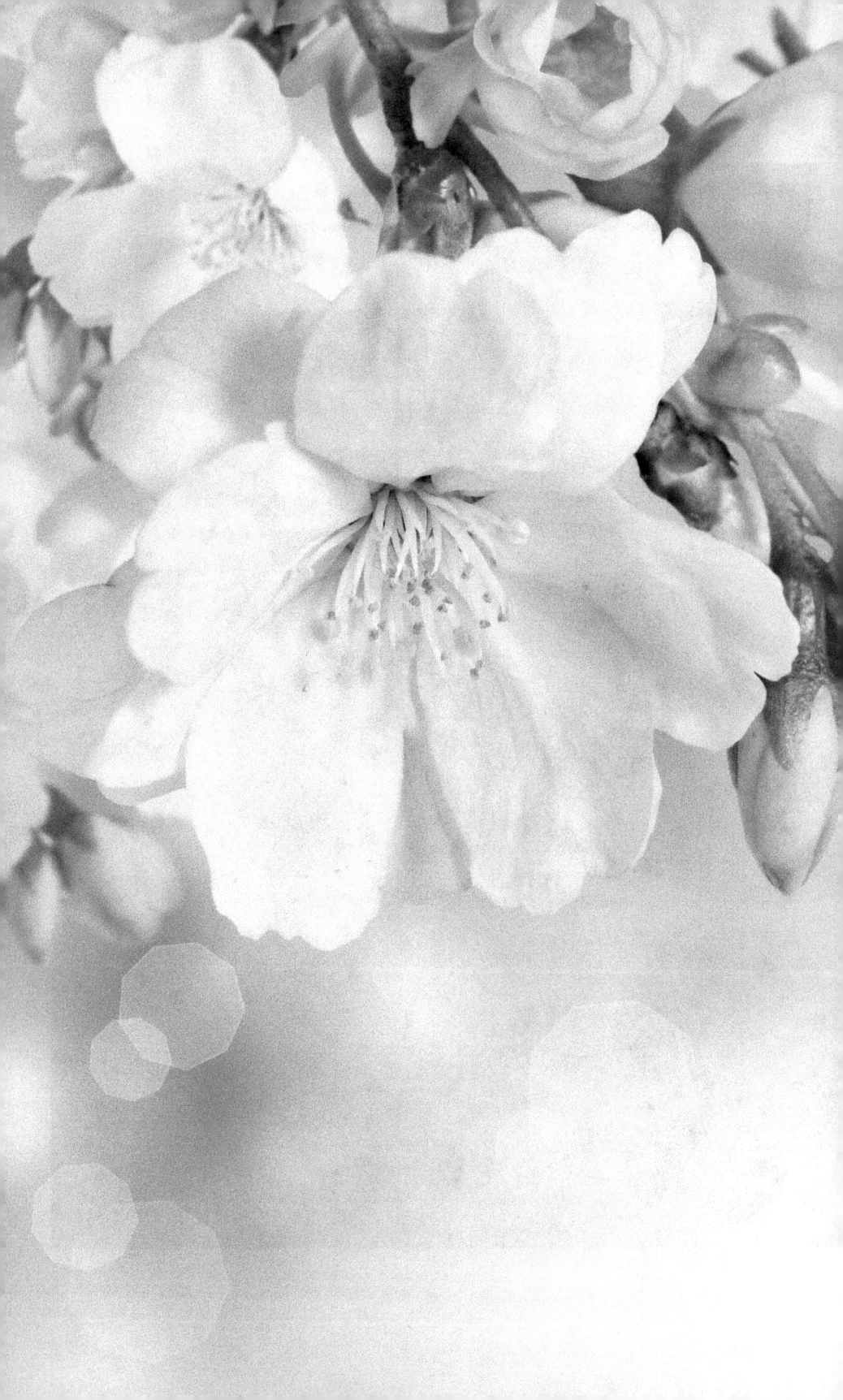

# CHAPTER 54
# OH, MOTHER OF MINE

ON MOTHER'S DAY, I was attending a conference out of state and it was one of only two days I recounted not being with Mama on her special day. One blessing in disguise with Alzheimer's was she didn't miss me, and she never knew what day it was and was not upset at all I had not spent Mother's Day with her.

I could not count all the lessons she taught me throughout my life. Still, I can tell you I've learned the most significant, valuable, life-changing lessons most recently, walking with her through this horrific disease. I am more inspired by her than ever before as I witnessed first-hand the heart and soul of this human. I know I have her sense of humor, love for people, devotion to God, ability to sing, and the joy of cooking. However, I do not have her gardening or sewing skills, nor her ability to make something out of nothing, her "workhorse" energy, or the ability to play piano. I can live without a few of those.

What I strive to remember from this season was her strength, not just physical, but mental. She had the heart of a warrior. She was incredible. Her ability to compensate for her shortcomings and then rebound and come back better than ever was uncanny.

When she had a deficit in some area of her life…her eyesight, her ability to walk, her Alzheimer's, somehow, someway, she compensated beautifully, and most people never knew the difference. She was grateful for the smallest things, so much so she repeated most things three times. "Thank you, thank you, thank you, or love you, love you, love you." She wanted you to KNOW she really meant it. She kissed hands, she kissed cheeks, she kissed arms, she kissed lips, she kissed foreheads…she just showered love.

I often prayed, "God, please have mercy on my precious mother and do not let her suffer. Take her to her eternal home in heaven and give her the rest she longs for. Thank you for allowing the six of us to have her for our mother *and our father* for the last 39 years."

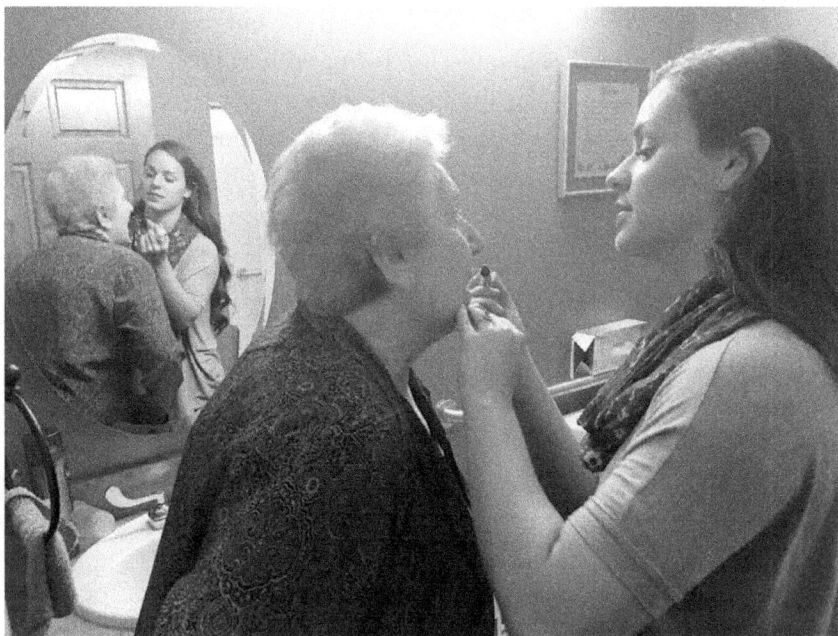

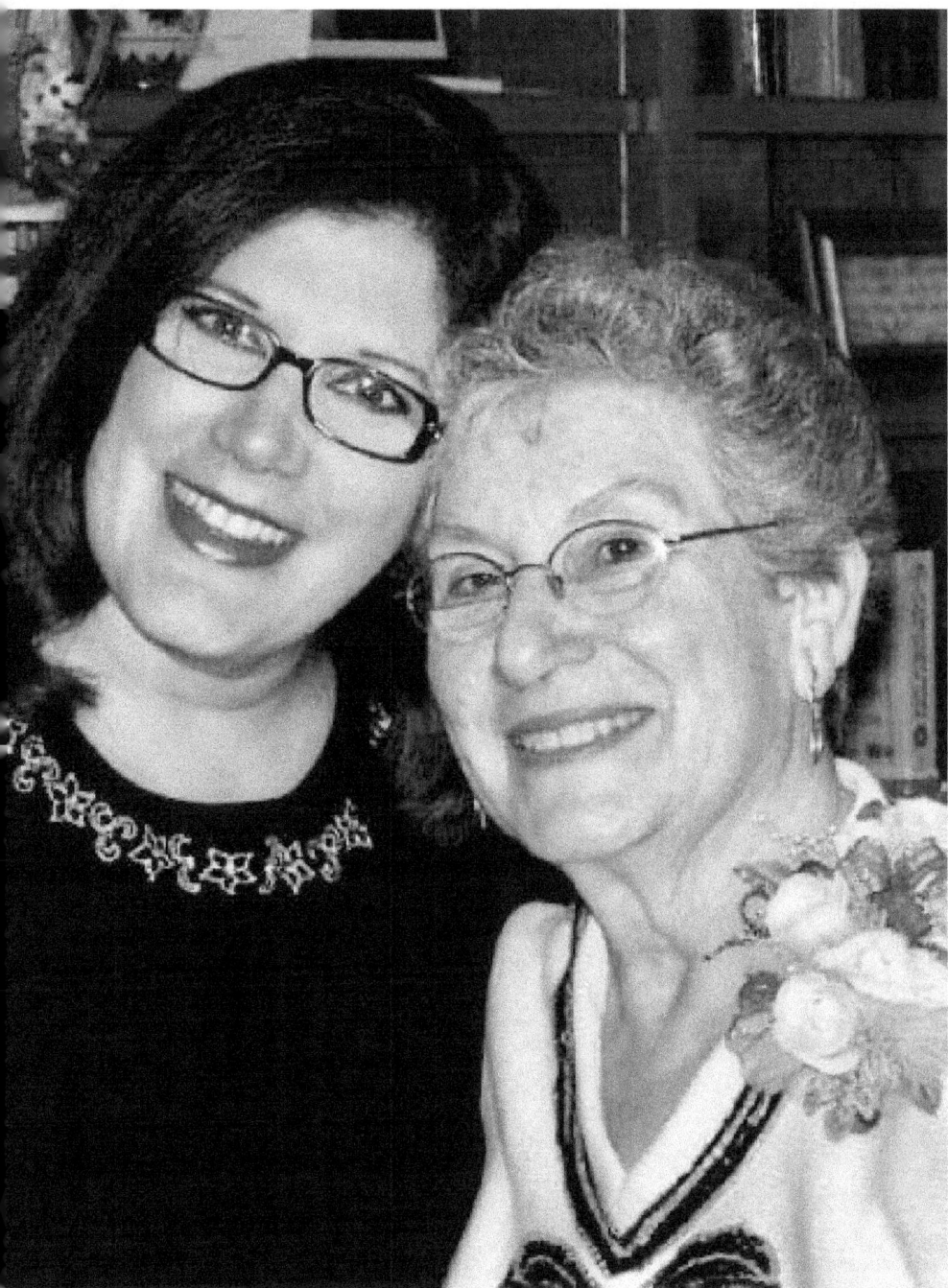

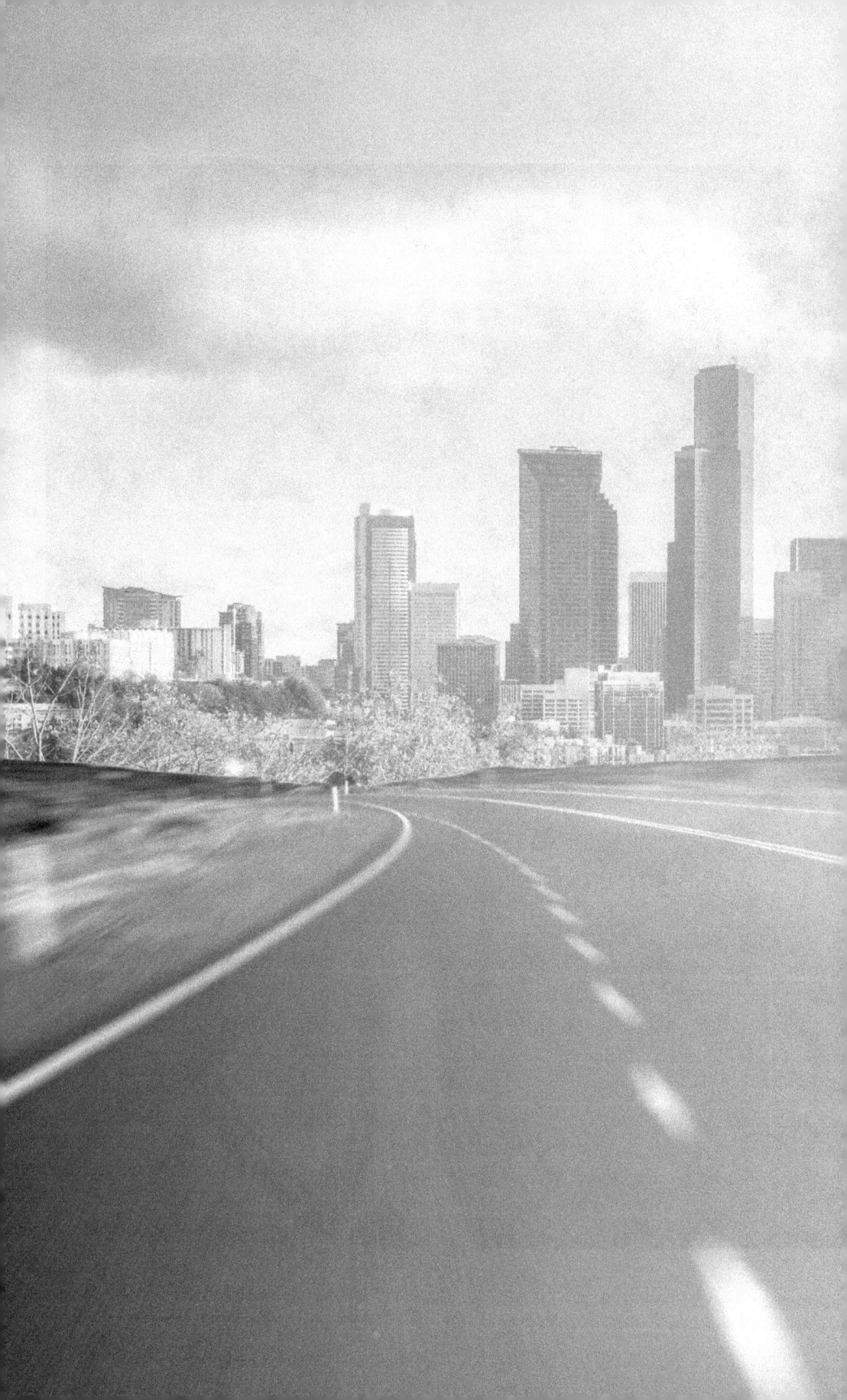

## CHAPTER 55

# NEW DIRECTOR, NEW RULES

IN THE FALL, I had been requested to meet with the new director of the facility as well as two other managers. I was informed in order to keep Mama from being moved to a nursing home, Mama's sitters needed to help in transferring and toileting her. To be more specific, any time one of those tasks needs to be done, the sitter and only **one** employee should be involved. We were all aware Mama always required two people, but now one of the two people had to be the private sitter.

---

**"When an individual consistently required the assistance of two employees for transfers and toileting, it goes beyond the scope of assisted living and enters the realm of nursing home care."**

---

When I initially hired private sitters, I was informed by the previous director their primary duties involved observing and never leaving Mama's side, as well as feeding her at mealtimes. However, the new director indicated these guidelines had undergone a revision. After reading over the mandated revisions, I typed up a new Sitters Requirements form (see **Resource** section) and asked each of them to sign it. If they felt as though they were physically unable to continue as a sitter, they let me know immediately. As much as I didn't want to, I needed to replace them to do what is best for Mama and keep her in this facility as long as possible. After this surprise meeting (I felt like I was ambushed), I did lose one private sitter, but the others agreed to stay.

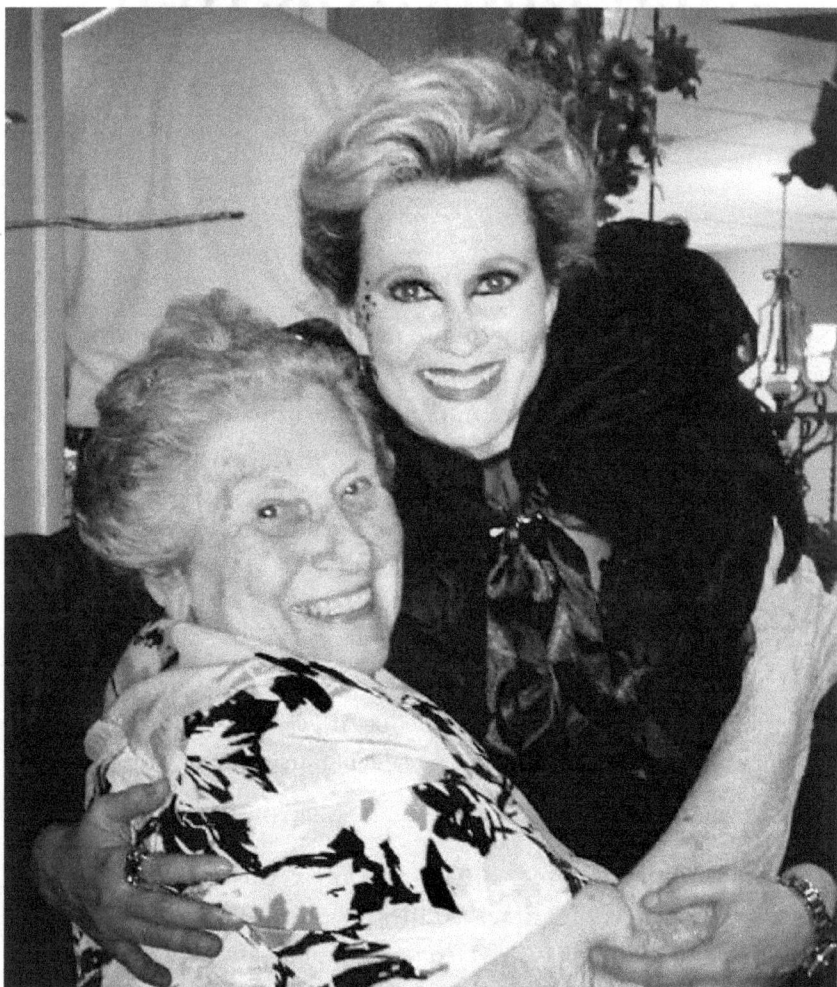

Mama and Kelly, the Activities Director

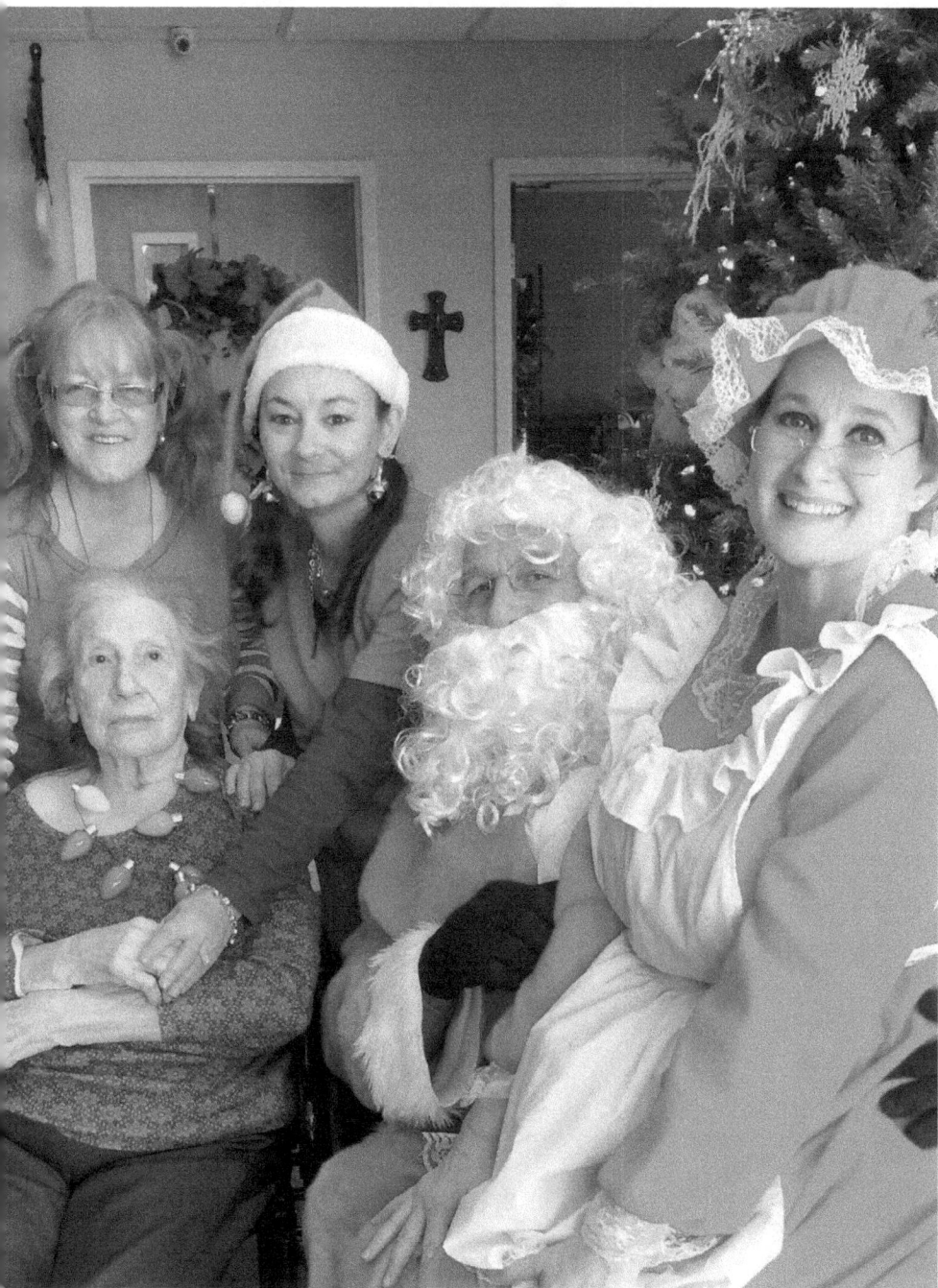

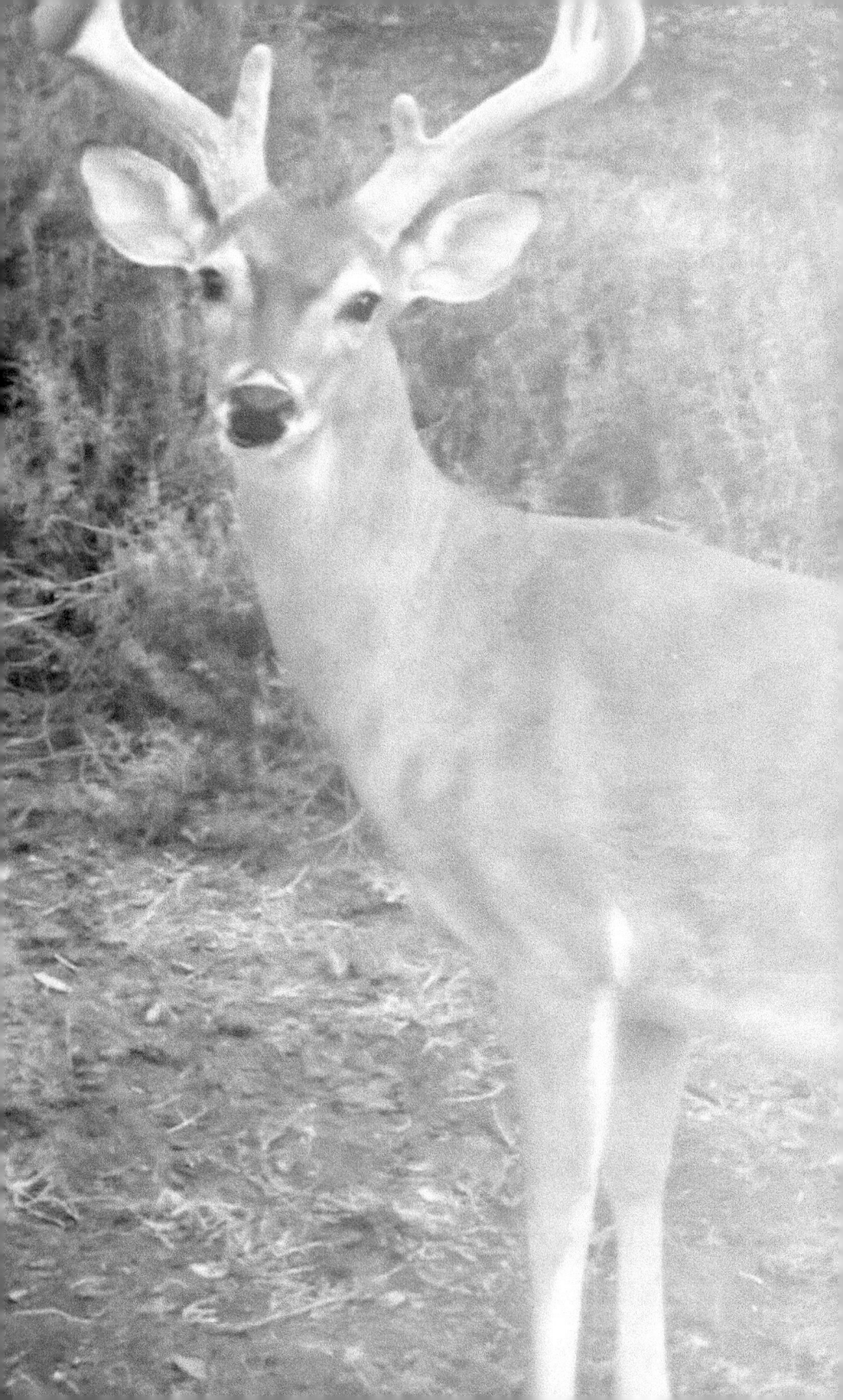

# CHAPTER 56

# MIND YOUR OWN BUSINESS

EACH NIGHT as I approached the back door of the special care unit, I rang the doorbell and then waited (sometimes 15-20 minutes) before one of the aides showed up to unlock the door. There were typically only two aides on the floor at night and they were busy. Since I arrived near 7:00 pm, most of the residents were already in their beds. After a hard day's work, the staff tried to stop for a short break, but some nights were unpredictable.

This particular night, I was approached by the two aides on duty. They began talking to me about how my private sitters were "robbing me of my money." I never left any money in the room, so this puzzled me. They continued by stating my sitters were not doing what they were supposed to be doing. *Hmmm...Mama was sleeping. What did they expect them to be doing?* They surmised my sitters should have been turning her in the bed every two hours. *Really? By themselves?* I had been instructed by hospice that the air mattress on the hospital bed was so no one ever had to turn her. I ended the preposterous conversation. I was floored they even approached me in this manner.

The night shift could be difficult. Granted, some nights were totally sleepless nights and they were hard. Mama relentlessly tried to get out of bed. She talked to imaginary people while she waved her hands in the air. She could not settle down. On those nights, I pushed the recliner beside her bed, spoke to her, and held her hand. Those were difficult. One night Mama called the two aides that put her to bed trolls. TROLLS. Where in the world did a 90-year-old hear that phrase? More comedic material from Norma Jean.

Mama went from 5 PM (noted in the notebook) to 11:30 PM the same night I was approached by these two aides before being checked and changed. She was checked again when I and a daytime aide changed her at 7 AM. *I KNEW THAT WAS NOT THE PROTOCOL* because I have been there on every shift. There was no way I was able to physically change her by myself, believe me I tried. Yes, I could have buzzed for an aide to change her, but this was a test. They failed miserably. Even knowing a family member was in the room, they didn't fulfill their duty. This same set of night shift aides took their smoke breaks outside, leaving no other employee inside the special care unit. In my opinion, they needed someone else on shift to sit at the desk, open the door for visitors, and answer the phone. At night, there was a nurse on shift to hand out medicines but she covered all the residents in the front and the back. There was no way she could be in two places at once.

I was so upset that night. When I was relieved in the morning, I went straight over to the director's office. She had not arrived. I called the office after I got home as soon as 8 o'clock rolled around. I told her I wanted a meeting with her ASAP about two of her employees. I did have a meeting with her. She said she was going to speak to both of them. One, more than the other, led the conversation, and I made her aware of that. I don't know what came of the meeting, but having been in the facility for nine years, I had never before had a conversation with an employee telling me how to run my business or care for my mother. I didn't see them for a while, and the night shifts were a lot better because of it.

In contrast, the other two aides who worked the opposite night shift were completely different. I never saw them outside; they were very quiet and respectful of residents sleeping. They worked independently of each other, covering a lot more ground quickly. I could set my watch knowing every two hours my mother would be checked. The aide caring for Mama was quiet, sweet, and gentle. She didn't even turn the overhead light on. She used the light from the lamp and the bright light streaming from the bathroom. She never had any trouble with Mama fighting her at night.

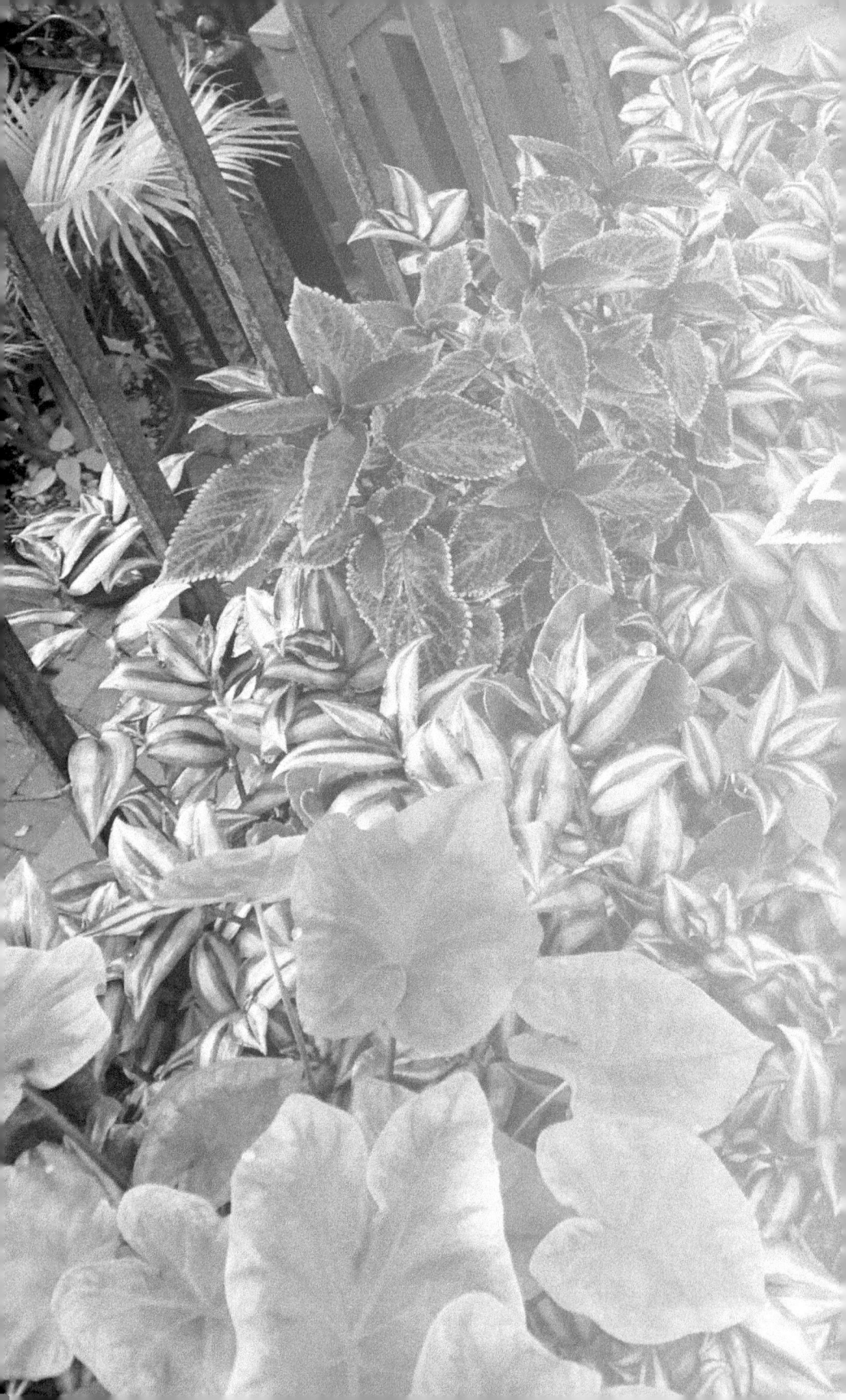

# CHAPTER 57

# BE AN ADVOCATE

Be an advocate for your family member. Watch, listen, and speak up!

DURING THE SUMMER, I noticed Mama's stomach started swelling to the point she looked pregnant. Sometimes, it went back down to normal by nightfall. I watched it for a month before I mentioned it to hospice. I had a photo I took of Mama lying in bed, and she appeared nine months pregnant. I wanted to know the cause of this swelling by perhaps getting a scan or blood work. Her clothes were beginning to get snug, and as the months went on, I had to purchase a bigger size.

After getting nowhere with the hospice nurse, I asked to speak with a hospice doctor. He called me and I shared my query and concern. I requested some imaging to be done to see why she was so swollen. He retorted, "We are not going to go to the expense of testing. Why do you need the results anyway?" *Seriously! Are you kidding me? I wanted to know what was happening to my mother. How hard was this to comprehend? Might this eventually be her cause of death? What if its hereditary? I wanted* to know. The doctor stood firm in his decision, and I was livid. Mama continued to have a substantially swollen, watermelon-sized stomach until she passed.

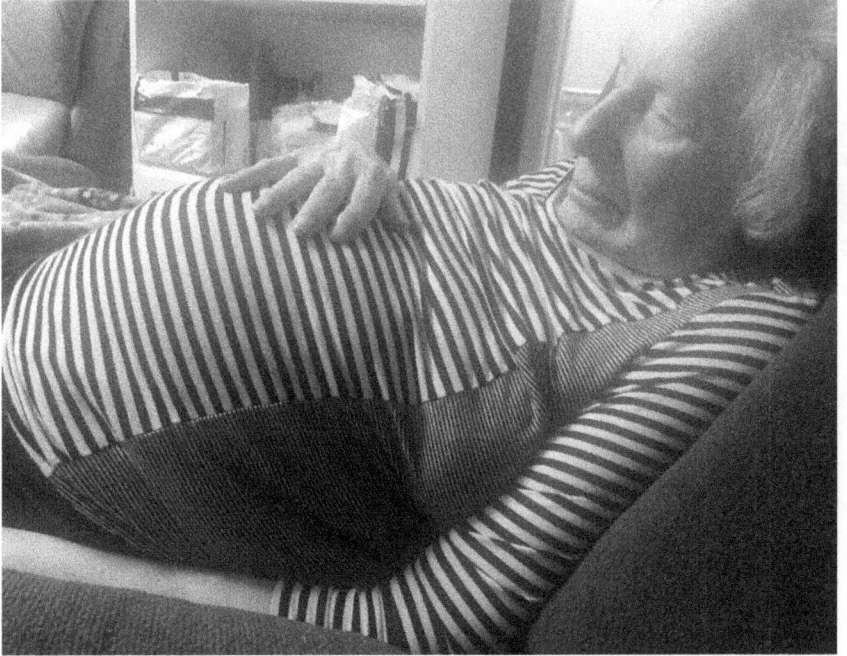

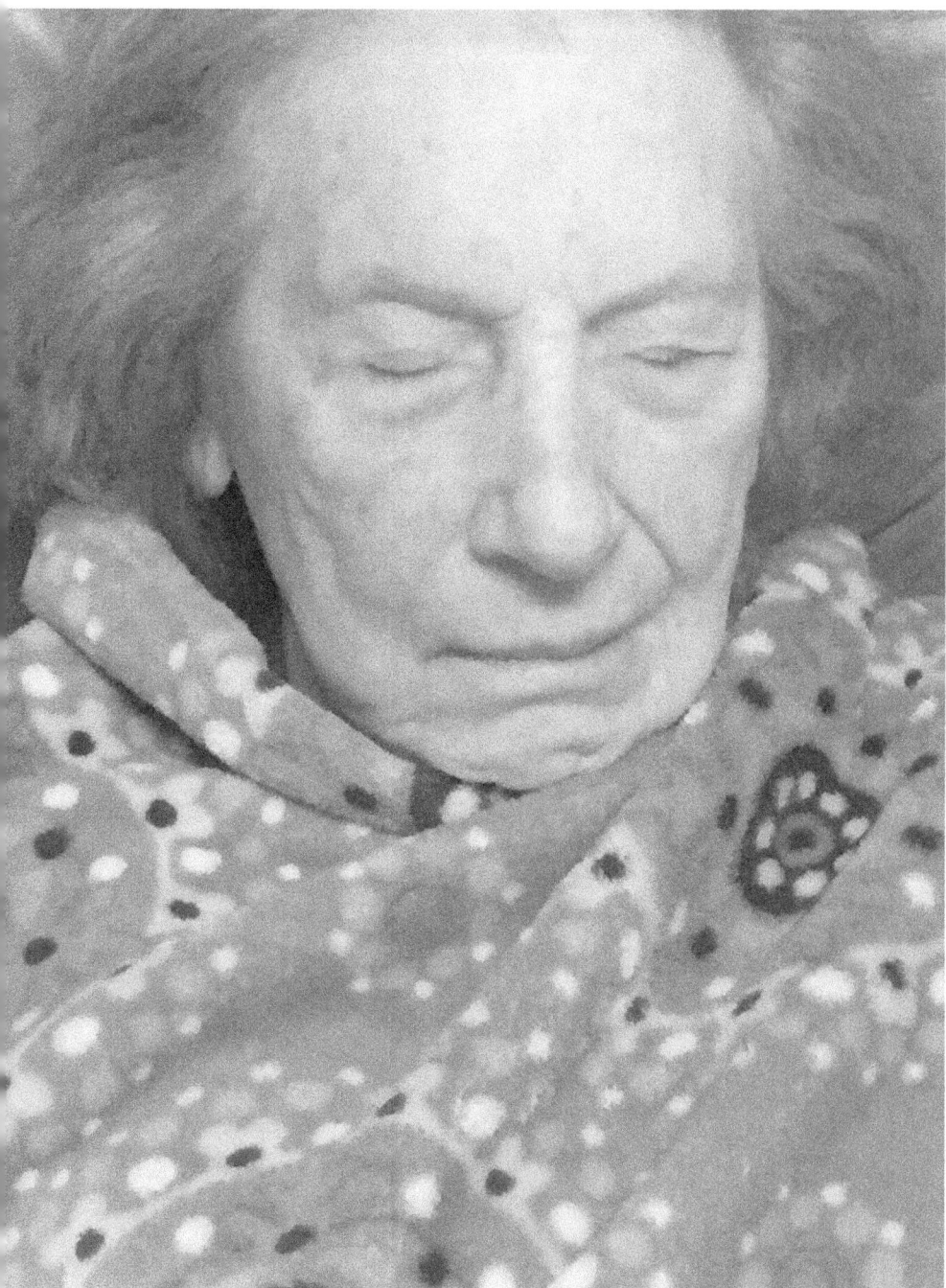

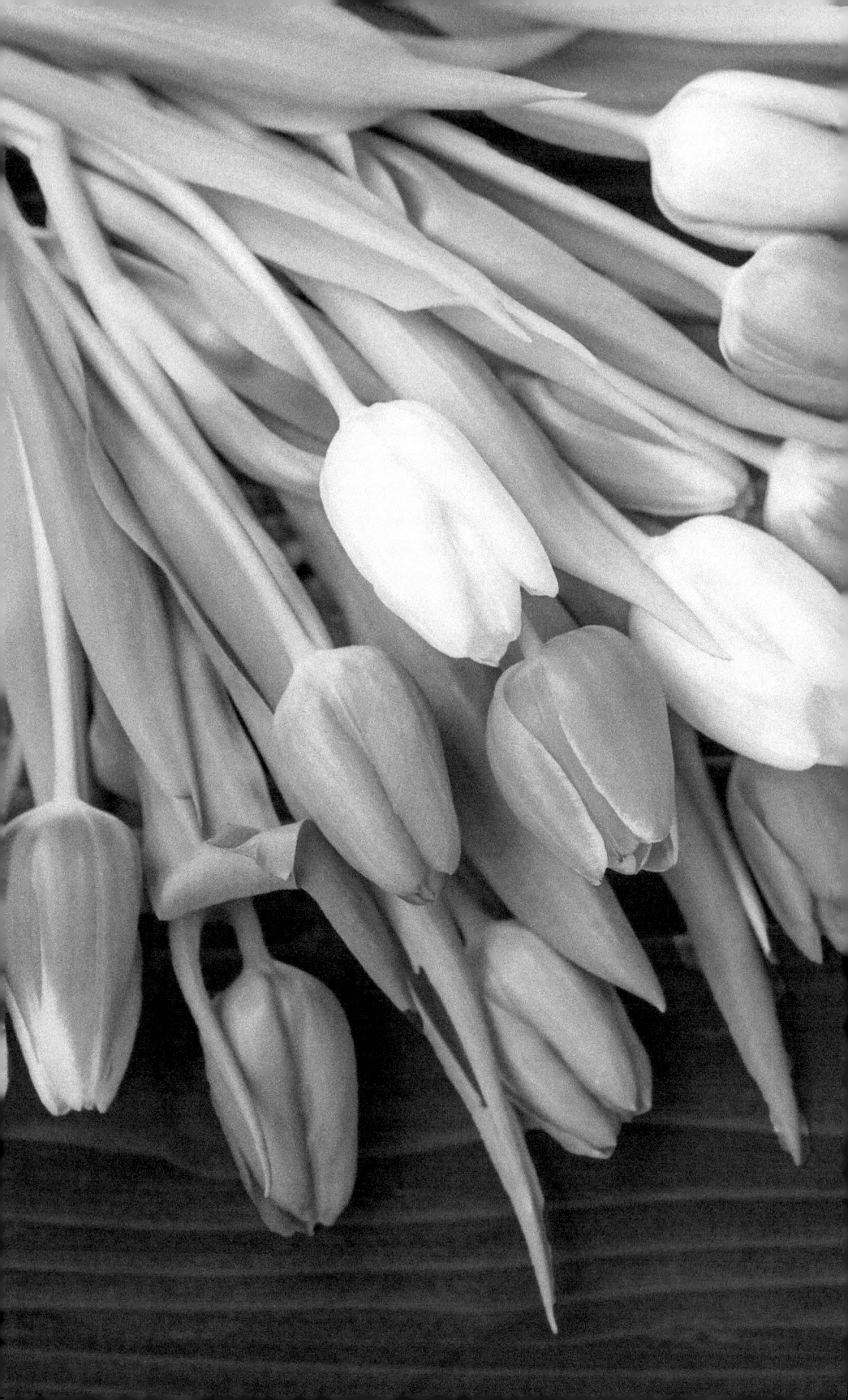

# CHAPTER 58
# WHERE'S MY LITTLE GIRL?

ONE MORNING AT BREAKFAST, I mentioned to Mama it was raining outside. She replied, "I think I've seen that before." Yes, Mama, I'm pretty sure you have. You really never know what Mama will say. I'm not kidding.

<hr/>

I've decided to draw up legal documents to change Mama's name. I think she should be Norma Jean EP (Extended Play). When you thought she was down for the count, this was THE call, Norma Jean proved otherwise. Her song was not over, it still had more verses to sing apparently, and it gave me more opportunity to whisper sweet nothings, which you and I both know were farewells and heart-wrenching whispers of my deepest admiration and love for her.

<hr/>

Mama and I went for her yearly check-up with her internist. Her office was located on the third floor of a hospital. I had the staff call for a wheelchair when we were leaving the office because there was no handicapped parking available when we arrived for the appointment. I parked quite a distance from the entrance.

Gone were the days when I could drop Mama off at the front door and trust her to sit inside and wait for me. Nowadays, she got up and wandered around the hospital.

So, back to the wheelchair. An employee stood with Mama outside and waited on me. I pulled the car around, walked over to Mama, and opened the passenger door. I helped her stand, and all the while, I was talking and using the word "Mama" repetitively so she'll know who I am. I tried to move her to the car, but she stopped. She looked all around.

Front, back, above, and below. I asked what she needed. She said "My little girl. Where is she?" I said, "Mama, I'm your little girl." She cupped her hands around my face and smiled brightly. The aide began wiping tears. I thanked the aide, and Mama turned to the aide and kissed her on the cheek. Another memorable treasure given to me by Norma Jean. I love how she let me know she knew exactly who I was. I also loved how she loved on people, strangers no less, with no effort at all.

People have written and called me throughout the years about how a photo or story I wrote about Mama touched them. Mama loved people, and she was loved by many, spanning several decades. Every time I saw her say or do the perfect thing at the perfect time and witness how it affected a person (myself included), it reminded me God was not finished with her here on the earth.

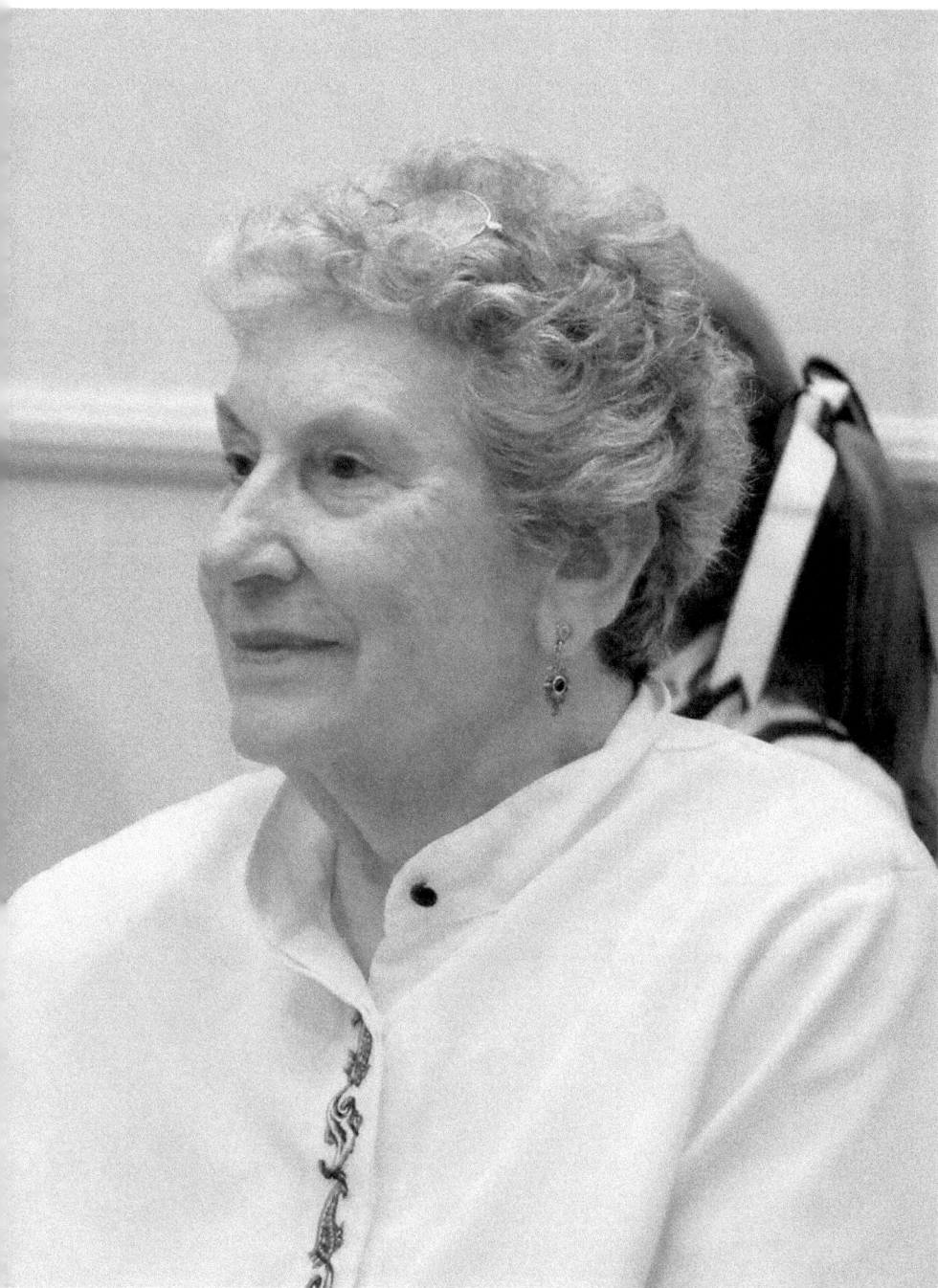

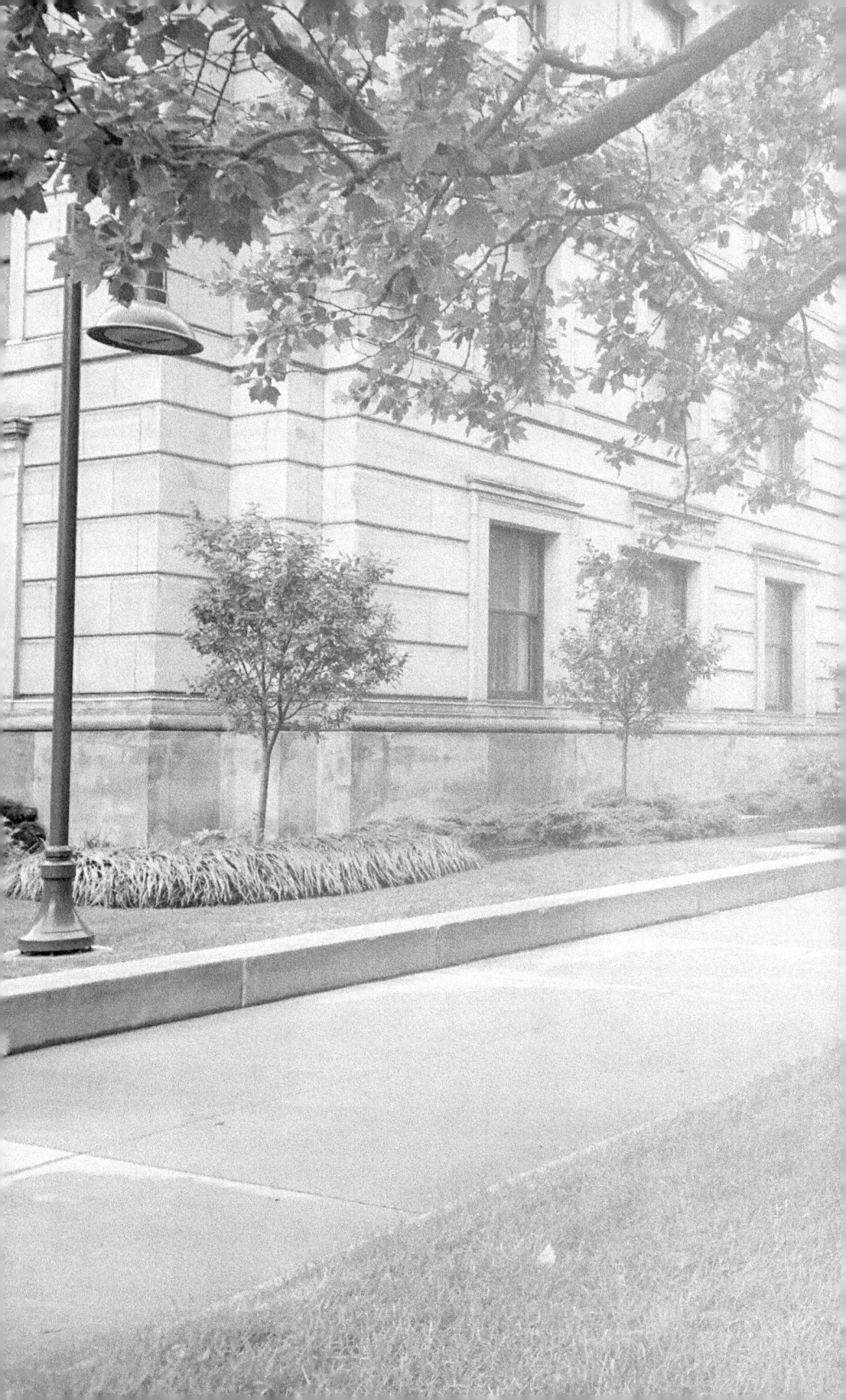

# CHAPTER 59
# SAGE ADVICE

THE MOST DIFFICULT thing for a caregiver to do is to ask for help—especially simple things. Bring them a coffee or soda, bring lunch, or visit them while they sit long hours with their loved one. Bring a meal for their family because it's easy to let things slide at home while keeping their head above water. Their priorities have changed significantly. Their home and their family will likely suffer as a result. Send texts or cards to remind them you are praying for them. Call them, and if they can't talk, be understanding. You have no idea what they are in the middle of on the other end of the phone. Bring them reading material. Be a listening ear. Expect varied emotions (fear, anger, bitterness, loneliness, fatigue), and don't judge them.

When the caregiver has been in place and is very knowledgeable of the patient's needs, please don't come in and try to be the superhero by changing the protocol that has been working. As temperamental as Alzheimer's patients can be, a change you think may be minimal could rock their world. If you were there for only a short time, you may not see the consequence of those changes you implemented. The primary caregiver has to deal with the repercussions long after you have left.

Please heed my warning if you are genuinely interested in being the caregiver for someone because perhaps you have cared for other patients except, they didn't have Alzheimer's. It's not the same; not better or worse, just different. I helped with my aunt, my grandmother, and my father-in-law. My mother was completely different and caring for her had the highest learning curve to date.

If you've volunteered or were hired to sit with a patient, please do not bring a friend, spouse, or child with you. The family expects you to give the patient 100% of your undivided attention. With the paranoia most Alzheimer's patients experience, the presence of too many unfamiliar people could be alarming. Sadly, the more the disease progresses, private needs arise. I'm sorry, but it is just wrong to have someone else in the room when tending to these needs. My mother was still my mother and deserved the same respect she had before Alzheimer's captured her mind. Be mindful and considerate.

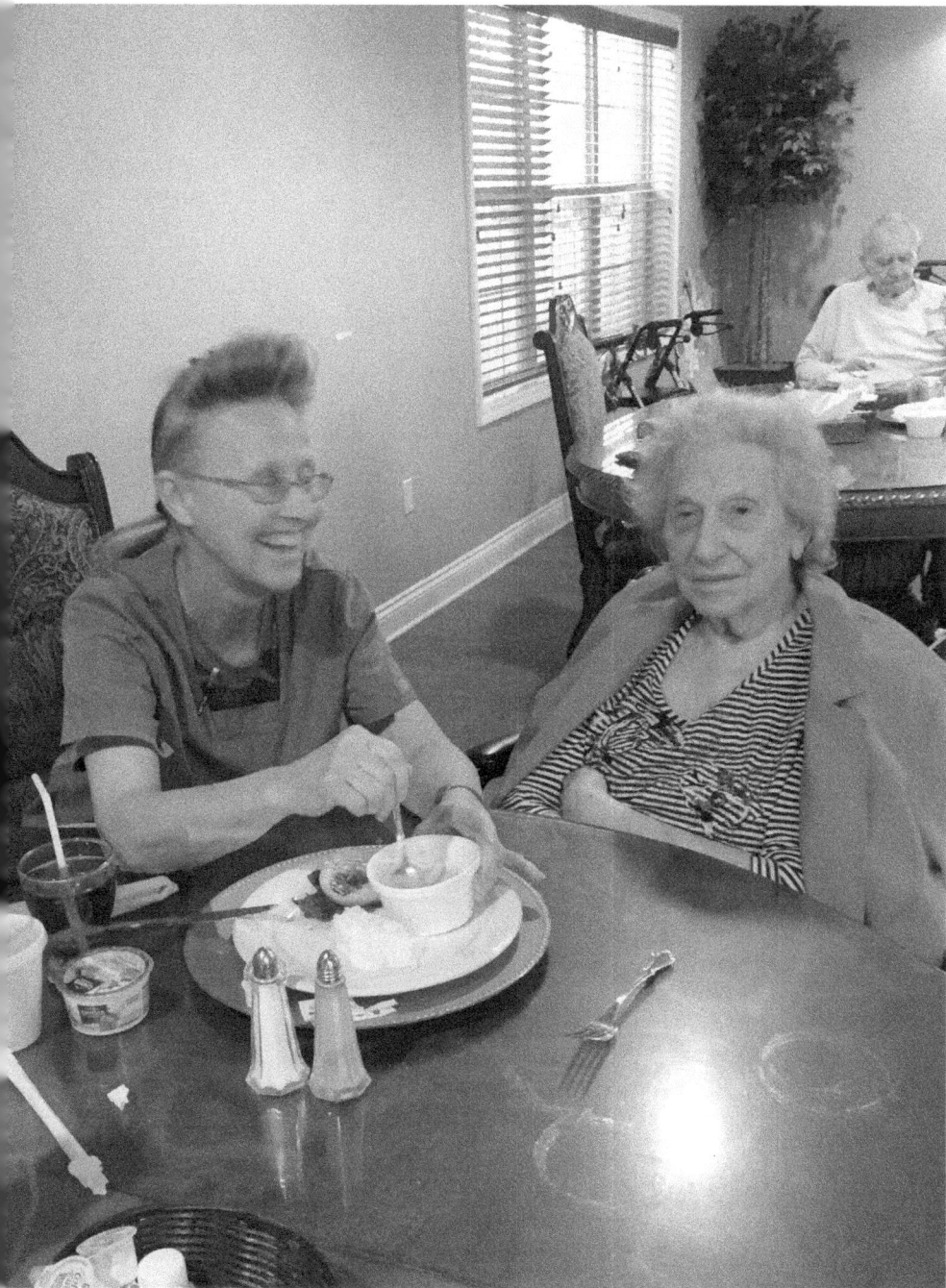

## CHAPTER 60

# LINES OF COMMUNICATION

I WAS OFTEN ASKED why I felt the need to see my Mama in the special care unit every day, twice a day (before and after work). Here is a prime example and one most folks never grasped unless, well, you've been a caregiver for some time.

I typically saw Mama every morning and every evening at shift change in order to keep the lines of communication open between the employees, Mama's sitters, hospice, and myself. The sheer number of things that could change in 24 hours can be astounding; perhaps not life-threatening, but changes nonetheless.

⁓⊶⊰⊱⊷⁓

Lydia and Suzy came into town to visit and noticed Mama did not get her 8 p.m. medicine. No worries. She slept fine that night. They asked the aides about it and were told they were out of the drug, and they had left a note for the nurse to fill. (*Hmmm, I wonder who will do "something" with the note?*) The next morning, my sisters were informed that as a matter of fact, Mama didn't take any medications in the evening.

*Really? That's funny because she has been for months now.* On the second day, the night medicine was not administered yet again. Mama lost an entire night's sleep, slept through almost all of the next day, and finally returned to normal by midday on Monday.

Next, we noticed a line of bruising on the back of her knee and thigh area. We have no idea what happened, but we attribute the challenging task of getting her into the wheelchair when she becomes rigid and unyielding as the root cause. A couple of nights later, while putting on her sock that had slipped off, it was discovered one ankle and foot were twice the size of the other foot. She had no other symptoms, but we monitored the situation closely. Yesterday, she started wheezing in the shower and not again until last night. That's just in the scope of seven days. So much can change in the elderly, and if they are unable to communicate with you, you have to play a Columbo-type detective while caring for your loved one.

Don't be a stranger. Check on your family, often. You'll be happy you did.

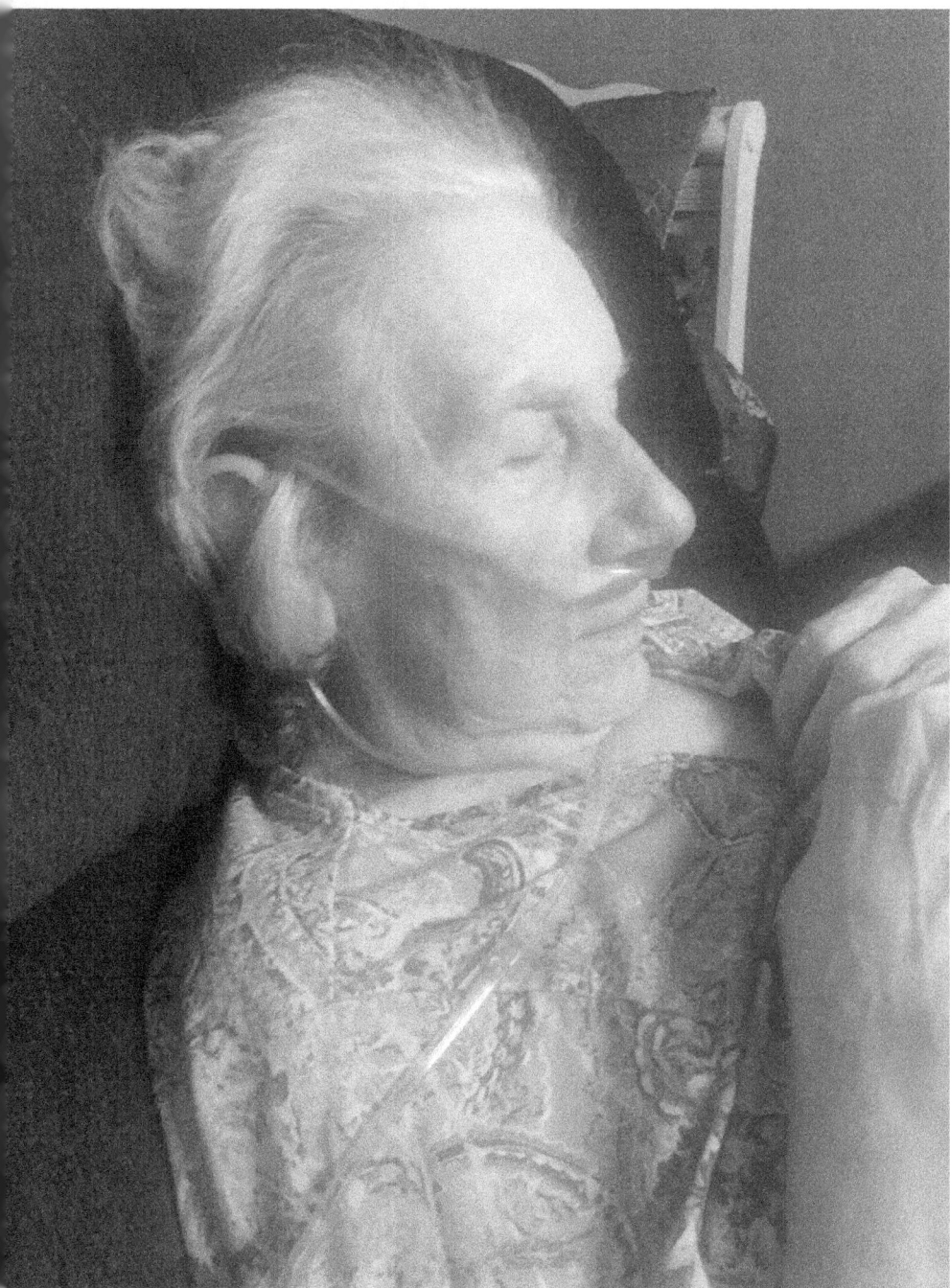

# CHAPTER 61
# ALTERNATIVE MEDICINE

I ADMIT, I drove my family crazy. I have ALWAYS been one of those people who picked up a prescription, and before reading the instructions on the bottle, I read all the literature stapled to the bag. Do you know anyone like that?

⟫⟫⟫⟫⟫

When one of my children ended up with C-diff after taking an antibiotic, I became more serious about reading all the possible side effects of a medication. Honestly, I decided, after a series of hospitalizations with that child, that I would only use antibiotics when it was an absolute necessity. From that day forward, I made it a point to find alternatives to medication. I still read the fine print on everything and researched online with reputable websites as much as possible. I also informed the health professional about my family's situation and why I am adamantly opposed to antibiotics and other medications.

I always sought out other alternatives to Western medicine. My favorite products were essential oils and natural supplements. You can find my list of essential oils I used with Mama, especially her last year, in the **Resource** section of this book.

We have so much information at our fingertips with the internet. Use it. Skip Wikipedia and go to the Mayo Clinic, Cleveland Clinic, or WebMD websites. I have no medical training at all. I am a wife, mother, grandmother, and daughter and the older I get, the more I realize we have a choice. We always have a choice.

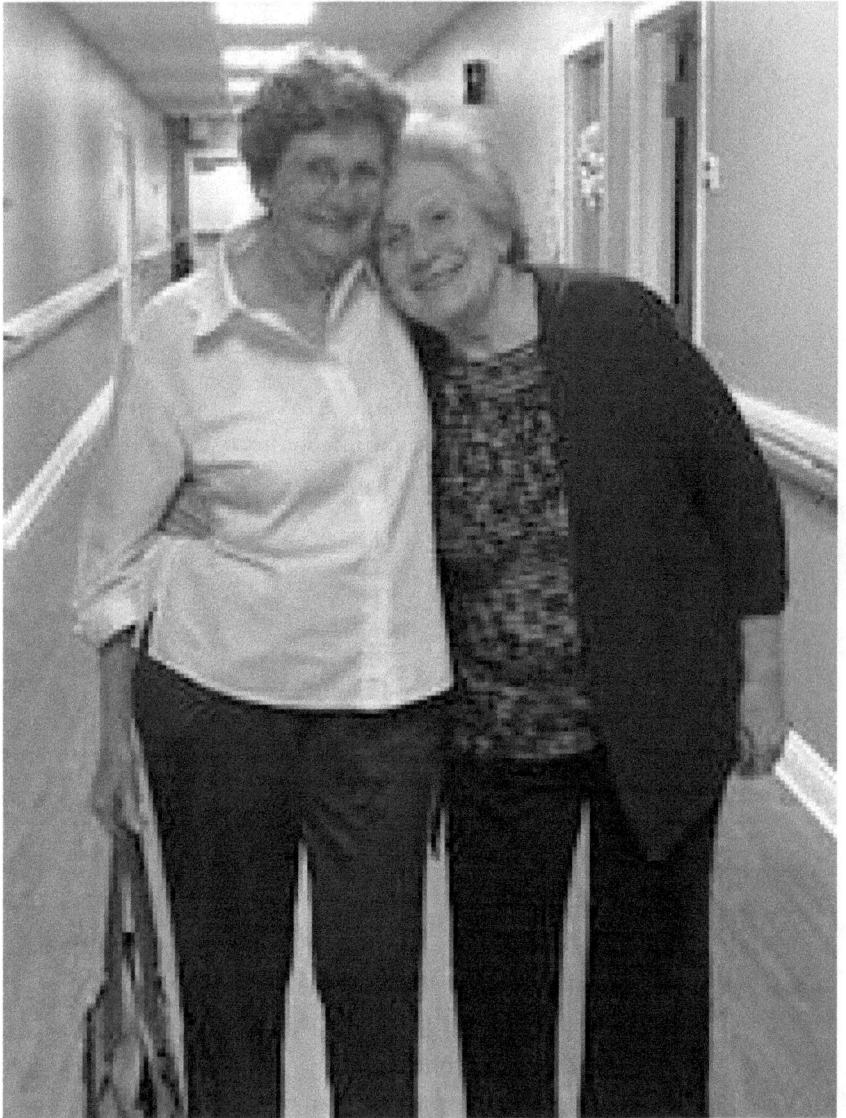

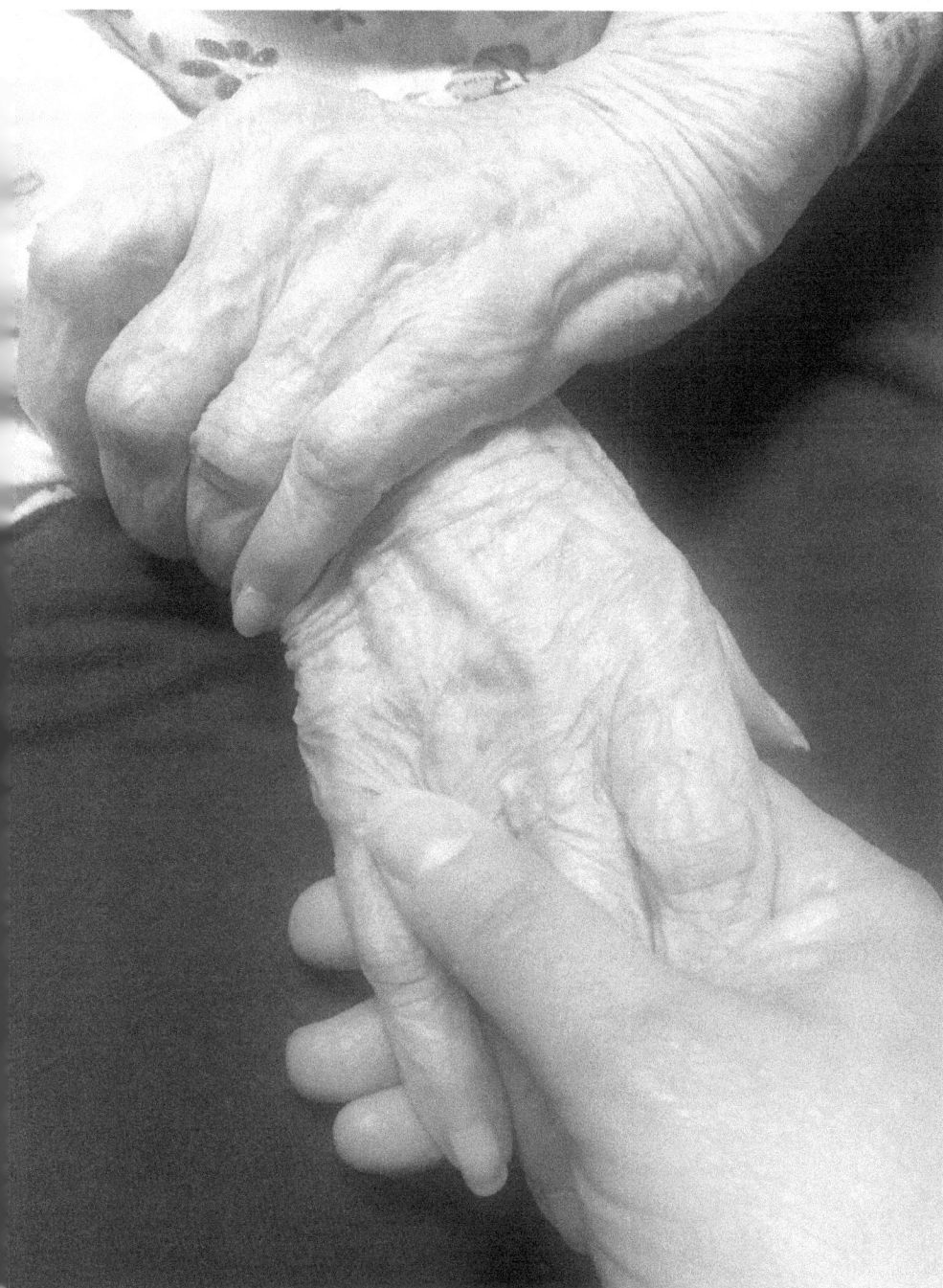

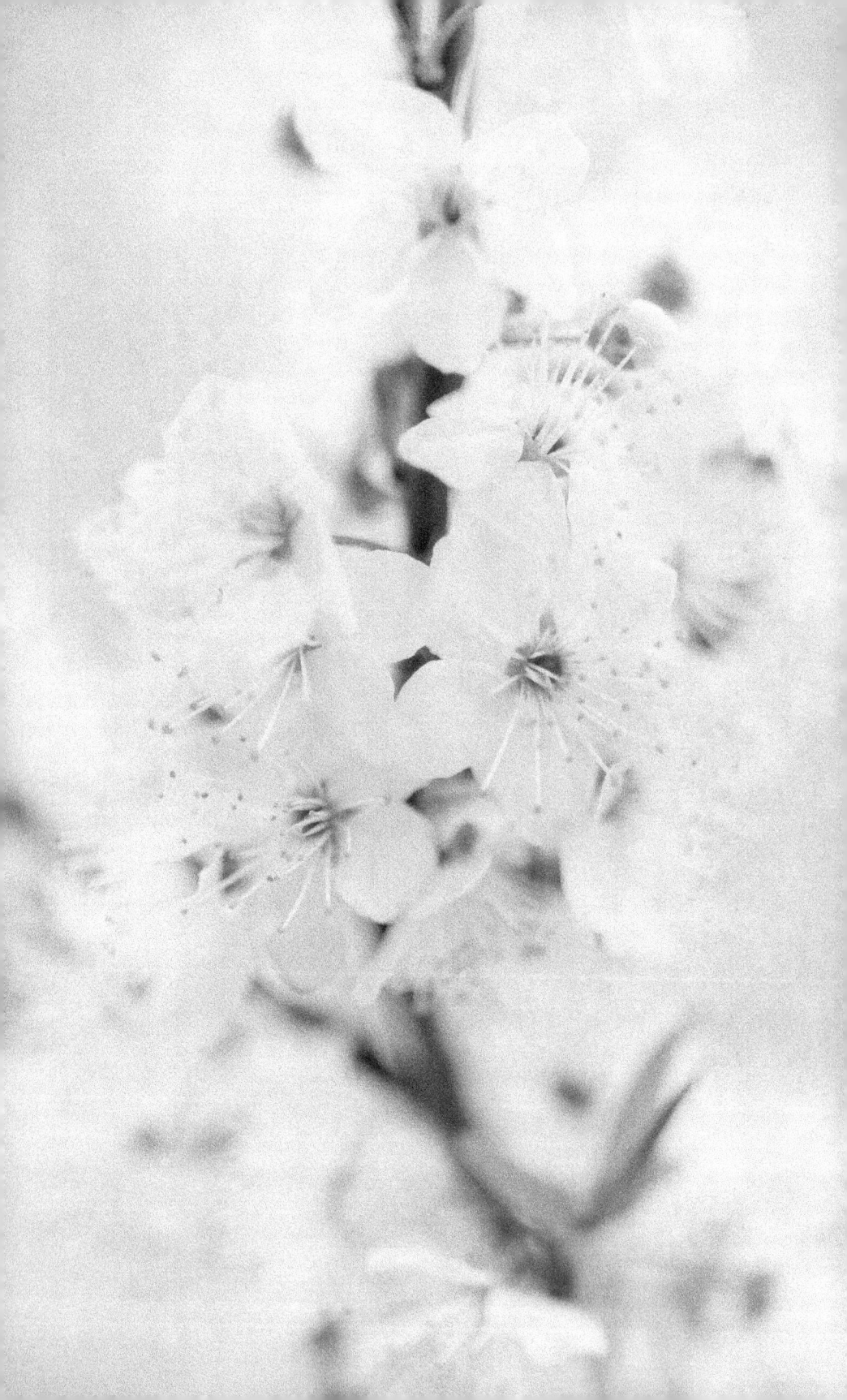

## CHAPTER 62
# DANCE PARTY IN A-130

WE HAD a fun dance party in Mama's room one afternoon. After her little siesta and before supper, I placed her in the wheelchair. She was awake but staring into space, so I turned on some of her favorite church songs. Nothing. Nada.

I tried starting a conversation. Again, Norma Jean wasn't engaging. I resorted to her favorite tunes…in particular Floyd Cramer music, and she immediately started clapping and moving her head from side to side. Mama did the cutest little shoulder action, too. Oh, it brought me so much joy. All six of her children have the same love of music and most love to dance as well.

⤙∞⤚

As Mama listened to her music, in waltzes (no pun intended), Mrs. Brown. Mrs. Brown was another resident down Mama's hall, and she walked nonstop. Often, she stopped in our doorway, surveyed the room, and walked on, but sometimes she walked in, found a seat, and took herself a little nap. Today she heard the music I had playing and came inside the room. I knew Mrs. Brown loved to dance because on a couple of occasions, I helped her walk to her chair in the dining room,

255

and she broke out in the most adorable, playful little dance, and of course, I played along, or should I say, danced along with her. I loved Mrs. Brown. She was very expressive and child-like. As she came one step further into Mama's room, she smiled broadly, then started doing the shoulder motions and some fancy footwork. It was an enjoyable sight to witness these two ladies, completely oblivious of each other's presence within the room, yet finding immense pleasure in the moment. You should have seen the grin plastered across my face.

I hope my children will use music therapy with me when I am older. I saw a substantial difference in Mama's demeanor when I infused music into her daily life. Music runs in our veins. I am grateful Mama gave us a love and deep appreciation for music and dance.

<hr />

My dear friend, Anna Willems, recently shared this post and it resonated with me and reminded me of how profoundly music could not only change my Mama's demeanor but assist a caregiver with all the emotions, frustration, and sadness.

Music has power.[1] Music connects us.

About 25 years ago, I was just a teenager playing the piano for our church's nursing home ministry. We went in and would talk to the residents and wheel them into the big main room so they could join in the service. Many of these residents were not able to communicate verbally with us. Many had problems with their memory and no longer knew the names/faces of their closest relatives. Quite a few of them just sat there staring vacantly into space.

But when I started to play the old, ancient, upright piano and the group started singing... "It is Well with my Soul" ... or "Blessed Assurance" .... or.... "Amazing Grace," **I felt a**

---

1. Anna Willems

**rustling, saw shoulders start shifting, people sat a little taller, lights came on in eyes that only moments before were not focused on anything,** and then I witnessed an actual miracle.

Those voices that struggled to speak and could barely say their own names…rang out clearly and perfectly on key, rose up, and sang with us!

Music has power.

Music connects us.

It has just been so heavy on my mind these last few days…I hope none of my kids ever end up in a nursing home. I pray none of them will ever struggle with a memory or a mind that is failing. But if God forbid that day comes…what songs are my kids learning TODAY that one day they will hear and it will spark joy in their hearts and a flicker in their mind and bring light back into their eyes and comfort their hearts?

We have so many wonderful worship songs our generation sings (and should keep on singing!) but maybe we do need to pause and make sure we are passing on a gift of music to our kids that will root them in truths that connect them to our generations that have passed. For the sake of their future.

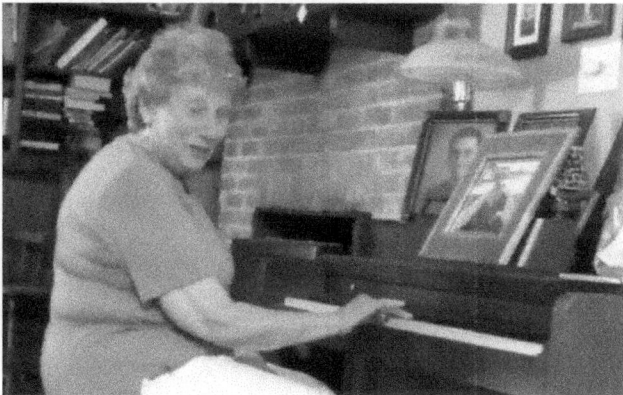

## CHAPTER 63

# NECESSARY LIES

I CHECKED in with the sitter from last night, as I did every morning. I was told Mama had been up since midnight. The sitter checked her frequently to ensure she was comfortable and not hurting or needing to be changed. She was always fine. Turns out Mama had a lot to say last night.

Evidently, in Mama's mind, she was back at work as head of the payroll department at the manufacturing company where she worked. She had some issues with a few men. She fussed at them about getting things right. I mean, *do your job and do it right already!*

Mama ran a tight ship at home and the office, earning the nickname "Workhorse." We often said it was branded on her forehead at birth. I don't know what those men were or were not doing in Mama's mind last night, but boy, they had better get their act together. There was no slacking in Norma Jean's world.

<hr />

The sitters and aides in the Big House were always amazed when Mama was less than cooperative. Sometimes I told her to let me have something (usually something she had a death grip on) so it could be washed. Or, if it was a blanket, I told her I needed to fold it and put it away. Since caring for Mama for the past 11 years, I decided to call these "necessary lies."

I did almost anything to keep Mama happy. When it was hard for me to leave her because she didn't understand and wanted to go with me or she became sad, I decided to start telling her I had a task to do, for example, clean the house, start supper, or something that involved activity and work. When I mentioned those types of things, it became easier for her to let me go. She was glad I was working on something, *anything*. She understood work, even then. She was a hard worker and expected everyone else to work just as hard.

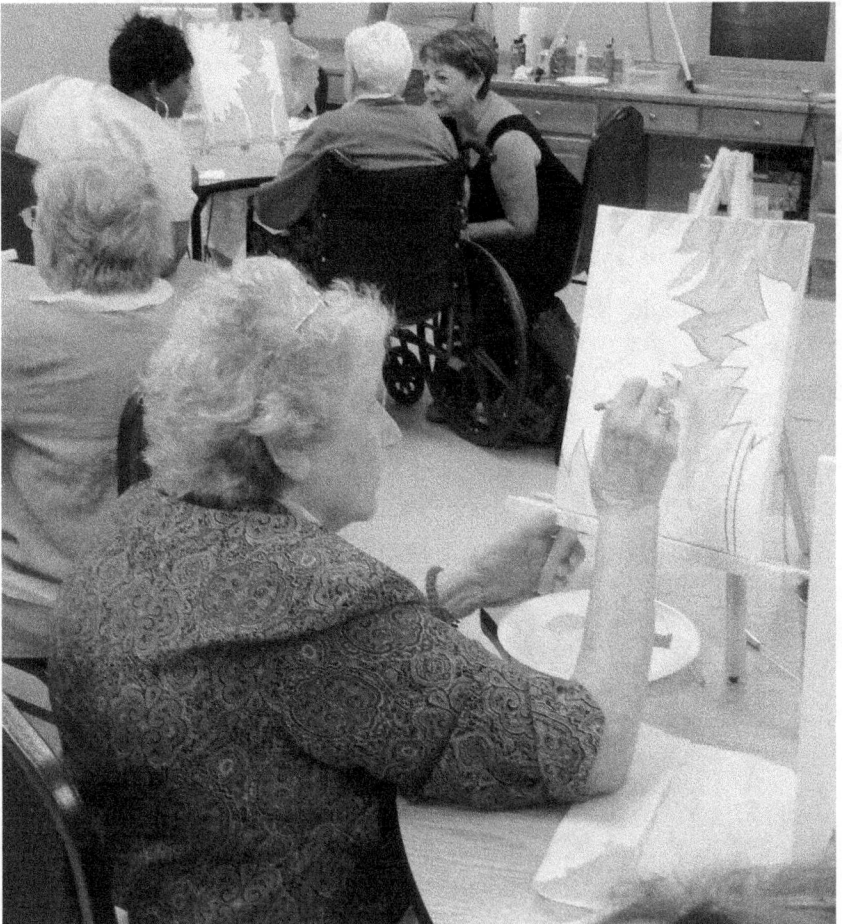

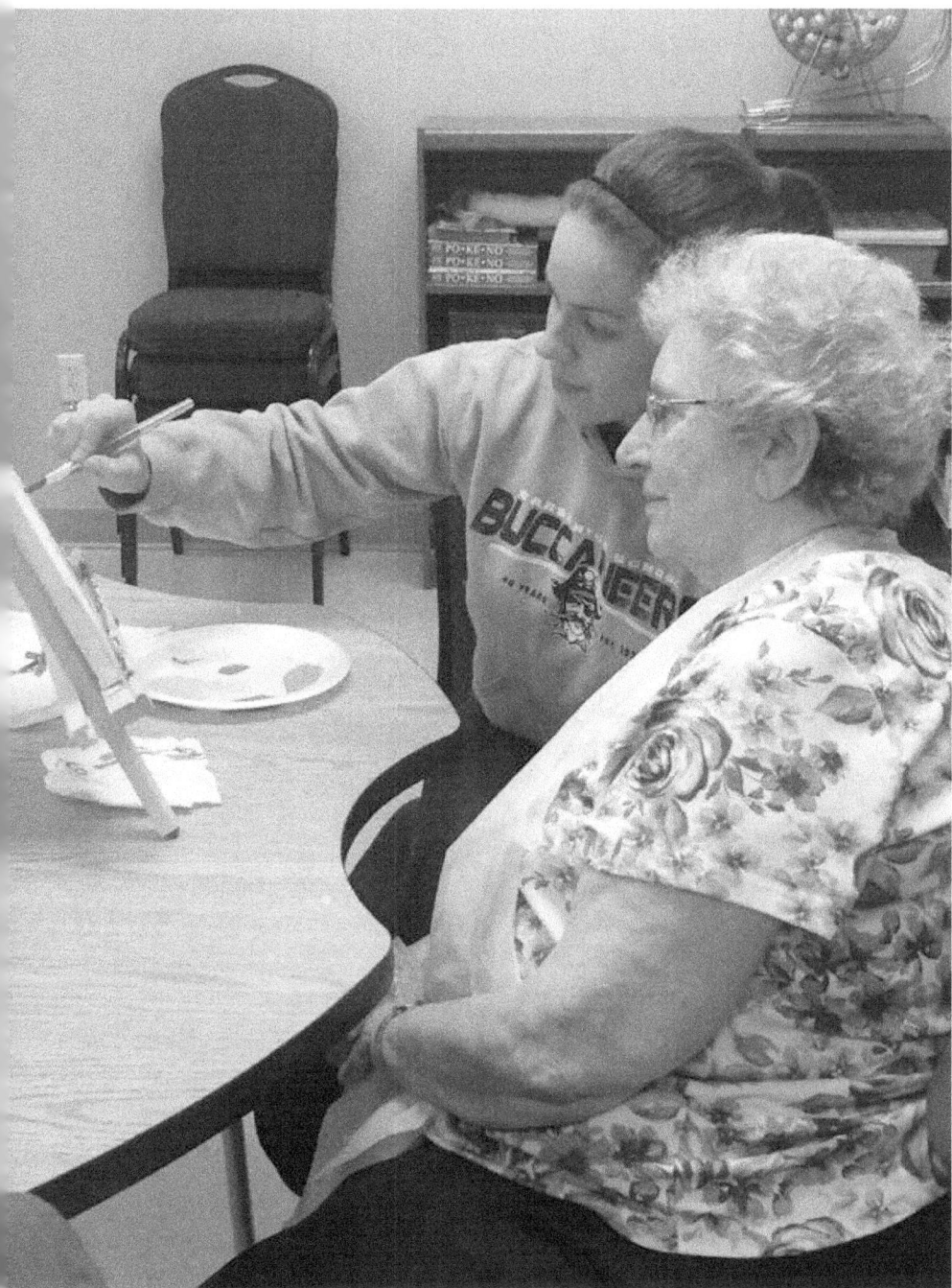

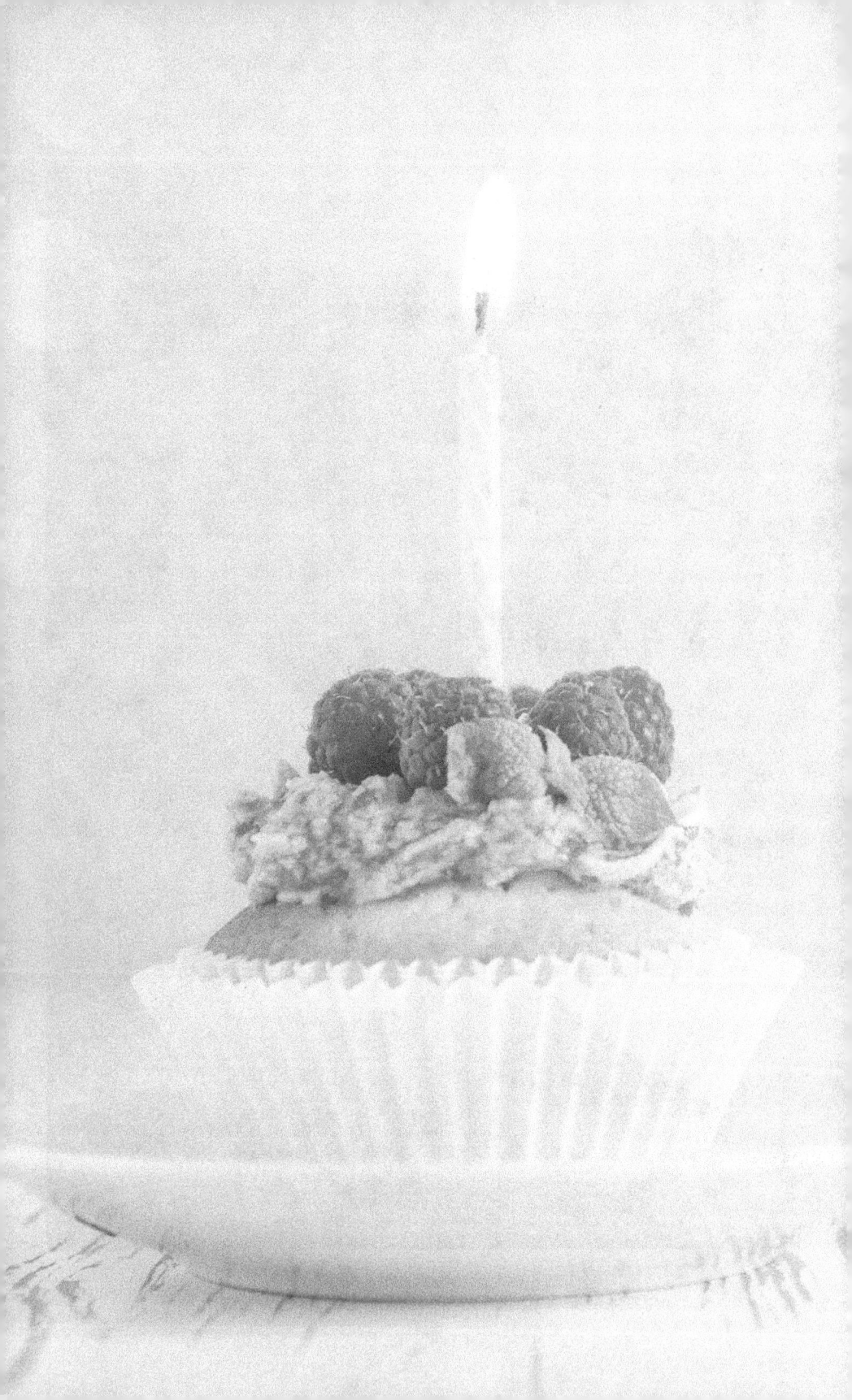

## CHAPTER 64

# THE LAST BIRTHDAY PARTY

IN NOVEMBER, we had a very quiet celebration with Mama at the Big House for her 91$^{st}$ birthday. Her brother and sister, five of her children and one granddaughter came for the celebration. A year ago, I never dreamt another celebration for my precious mother might occur. *Congratulations Mama, you succeeded in living longer than your parents and older brothers and sisters. Your competitive spirit shone through yet again.*

---

I learned valuable life lessons from Mama I don't ever want to forget; how we should treat people kindly, friend or foe, and show gratitude for the tiniest kindness shown to us. Over and over again, I watched Mama make someone else's day better just by taking the time to stop and talk to them. She treated everyone equally, and the best life lesson I learned was we should never act our age, instead stay young at heart. In the past twelve years, I've had a front-row seat to her daily resilience, determination, deep love for people, and uncanny wit.

Mama spoke life into total strangers and didn't even know it. She made me face many fears and grow up faster than planned. I never dreamed I would be caring for her in this capacity or for this length of time. It pained me to know she couldn't remember or see hardly anything; but still, she had joy. Therefore, I had joy. God sustained us.

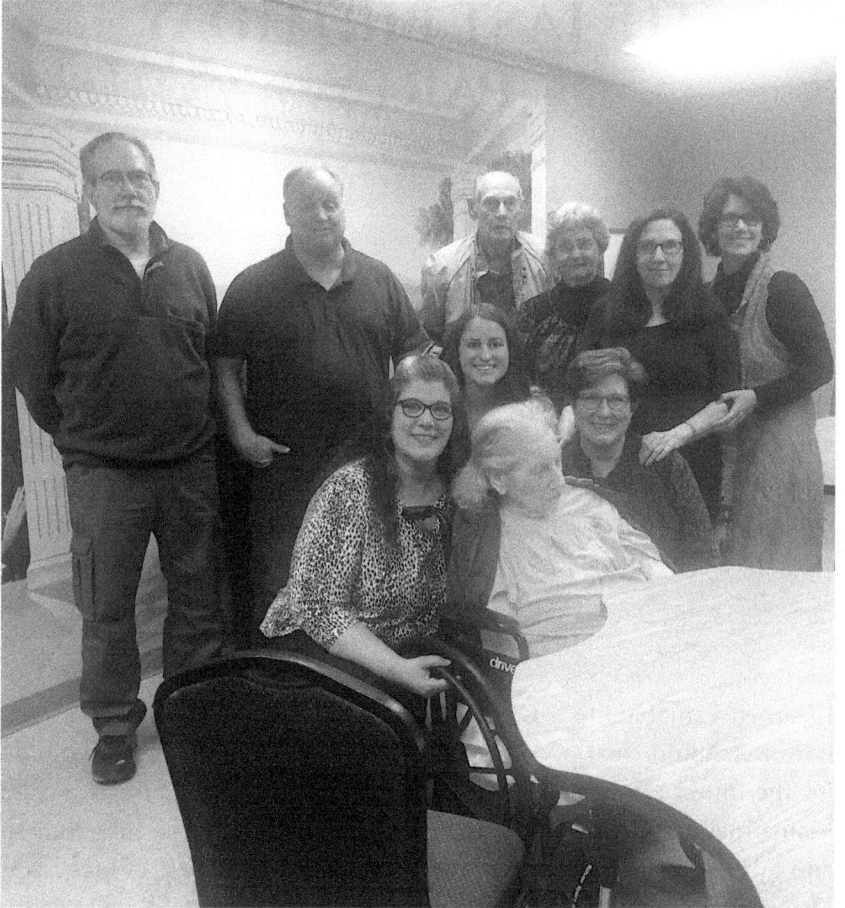

Mama's last birthday party

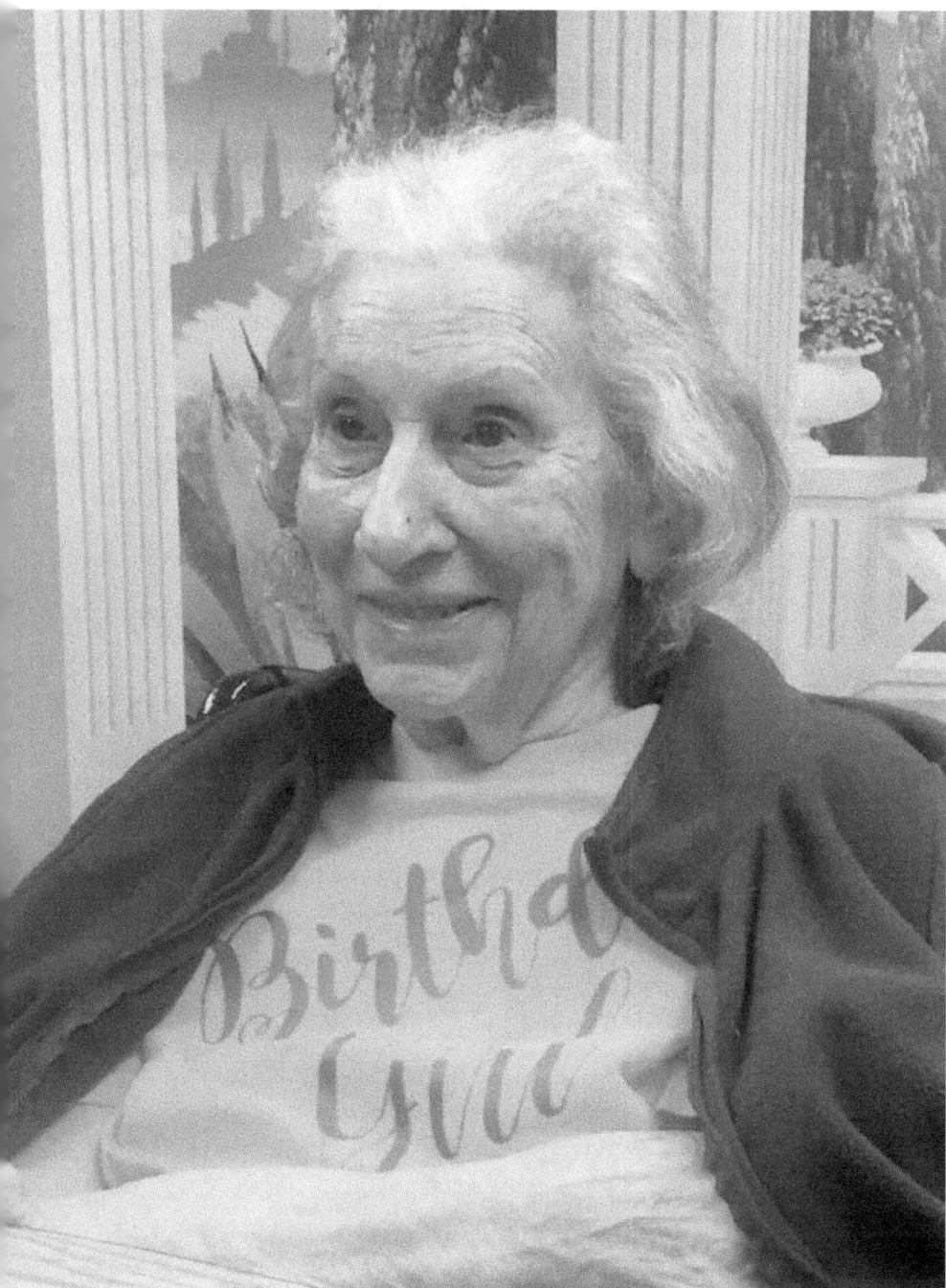

# CHAPTER 65

# THE ANGEL WITH THE WRONG SONG

JACKIE, one of my best friends, called to tell me she had a dream about my Mama. Mama turned 91 on Sunday, remember that as I recount this dream.

Jackie told me she dreamt Mama passed away, arrived in heaven, and was given a white robe. She was then escorted to her new home. Next, she was brought to the choir room to join in singing. *I'm thinking, wow, Mama had to be pleased as punch thus far.* She was in the choir, along with many others, all dressed in their white robes.

The choir director invited her to come to the front and allowed her to lead a song. Much to his dismay, Mama used her limelight opportunity to belt out a Johnny Cash song!

Unbeknownst to my friend, and what made this even more comical to me, Johnny Cash was my dad's favorite musician. Getting back to the performance, the director showed his disapproval but gave Mama another chance because, I mean, it was heaven, right...no better place for second chances. Mama began to sing again and chose to serenade the heavenly choir with Johnny Cash yet again. At this point, the conductor motioned for two angels waiting in the wings, to escort Mama off the stage. The moral of the story was Norma Jean better come up with another song before she can go to heaven.

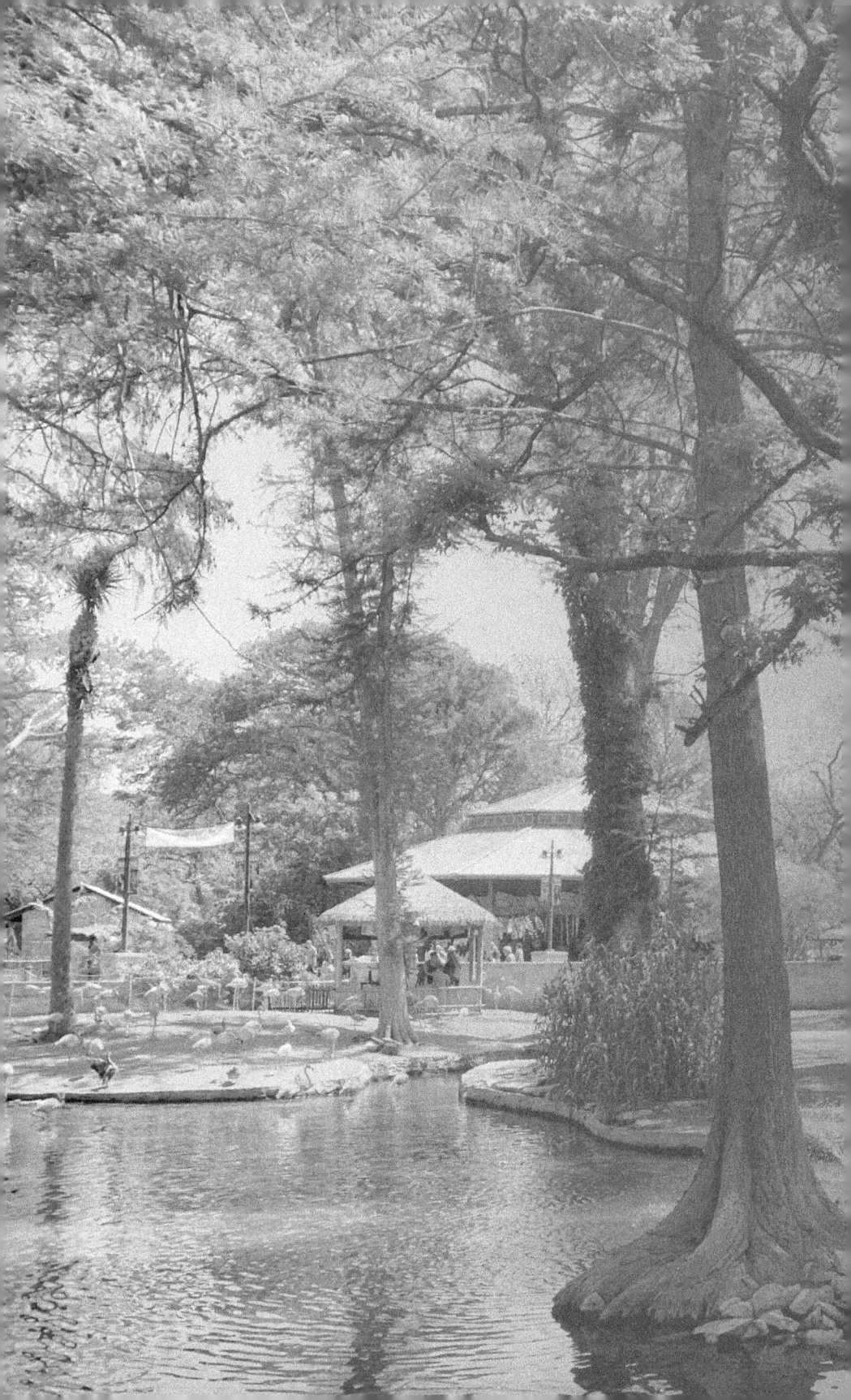

# CHAPTER 66
## THE LIAISON LIFE

As an advocate for someone who could not fully comprehend the scope of endless questions and instructions, I swiftly embraced the role of being a liaison between Mama and her medical team and the assisted living employees.

During the last 16 months of my mother's life, she had several aides, a janitor, the manager of the facility, the nursing director of the facility, the director of the special care unit, the activities director, a hospice nurse, and a shower aide from hospice. As if that wasn't enough, she needed 24-hour care and had a list of eight to ten sitters that each sat with her 12 hours at a time. Let that sink in.

In addition to those fine folks, she also had nurses at the Big House who worked for a contracted company. I paid an extra fee every month since her first day in assisted living to have them dispense her medications. Mama refused to take her medications from me, so I chose that route, which worked very well.

~~~

When we had a doctor's appointment, you had to tell the physician's nurse what company the facility contracted with for prescriptions. If the medications changed, even the dosage, God forbid, it required me to notify the facility director, the nursing director, the special care director, the aides, and the nurses. If you want everyone on the same page, the right page, you better make it your business to make sure everyone knows firsthand.

~~~

During Mama's stint in "the back," there was a nurse who distributed medication while the residents were in the dining room. However, while she stood at her medication cart and administered meds, she was engaged in casual conversations with co-workers, dancing, joking with residents, and so on. This always bothered me. *I'm sorry, no, I'm not really. You were dealing with drugs and these precious residents.* I spoke to the facility's director and the special care unit director about this. They gave me the number to the nurse's boss, who worked for the contracted company. The boss came and saw me at the facility and apologized, and she worked the nurse's shift for several days.

~~~

When Mama required more medications due to her declining health, there was a huge mix-up with the staff, and that was the exact moment I found my voice. I spoke to the contracted nursing company on the phone, while holding a staff member's personal cell phone to my other ear. The facility's director was on that line. I was furious, I was angry, I was scared!

After thirty minutes, we got everything worked out, and Mama got the medicine she desperately needed. These workers were hard workers, but errors happened with so many residents and with the staff spread so thin. When you have too many irons in the fire, orders could be forgotten or mixed up, and you have serious consequences. Because I had a relationship with most of these employees, they knew me. I was there nearly every day of Mama's ten-year residency. I saw how much they loved her, and she returned the sentiment.

The strange thing was even as a mother of four children, I had never been in a position to "fight" for them. When I left the facility that night, I wept. I am a peacekeeper to a fault. I'm not one to openly share my opinion, even amongst family and friends. It was uncharacteristic of me to stand up for her, for anyone for that matter. To demand something be done. I honestly did not know I had that in me. I HAD to speak for her. **I was her voice.**

It is important to note this was the only time I had to fight for Mama in ten years. That says a lot about the facility and the employees. It wasn't a personal attack. It was more of a "Let's solve this problem." Your presence is imperative. Your family needs you to be their voice, their liaison. It does make a significant difference in the care your loved one receives. It is beneficial to build a relationship with everyone involved in their care, from the director to the nurses, aides, kitchen staff, maintenance, and janitors. Everyone matters. The more involved you are, the staff will appreciate you and your involvement.

Just as we always should, be kind and considerate. Aides are the hardest-working, most underpaid people I have ever met. It was a huge blessing when they consistently did their job effectively and sincerely loved their job and the residents they cared for. I am forever grateful for so many workers in the Big House who truly loved Mama in good times and bad. I relied on them in my absence; I relied on them for feedback on changes in Mama's health or demeanor. I relied on them and trusted them. Without siblings nearby, they were my extended family.

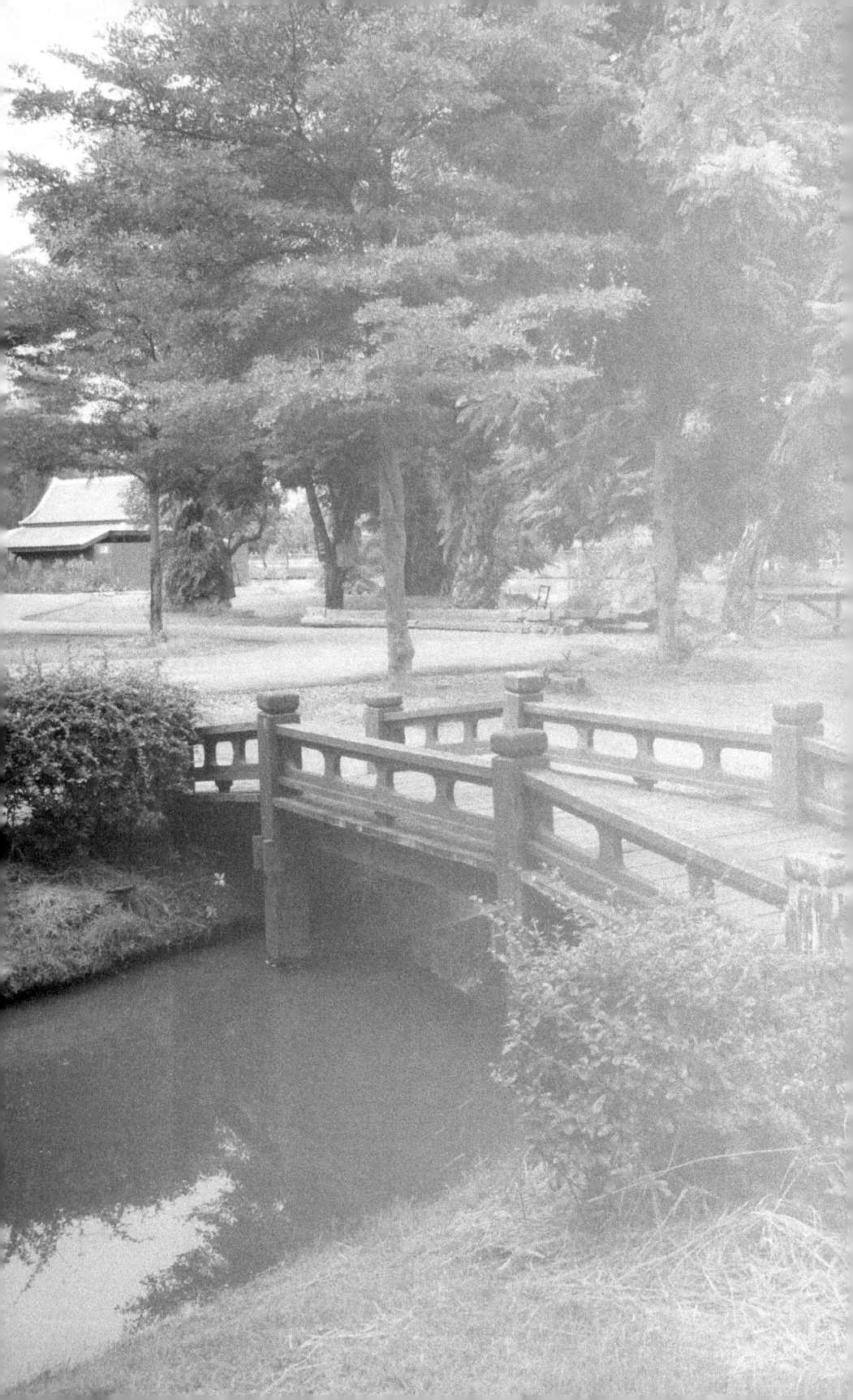

## CHAPTER 67
# CRY, PRAY, REPEAT

ON NEW YEAR'S EVE at 12:30 a.m., Courtney, my daughter-in-law, texted me, letting me know my 34-year-old son, Billy, had been admitted to the hospital due to shortness of breath along with a fever. He was critically ill. He had been on medicine for nearly four days, but he was not responding to the medications. She asked if I could come and help out, and, of course, I said yes. After ensuring I had sitters lined up for my Mama, I informed each of them I would be out-of-town indefinitely and not able to continue with my 7 a.m. and 7 p.m. shift change check-ins. They understood and offered their prayers for my son.

❧

Before I received the text, I had spent Saturday and Sunday sitting with Mama prior to New Year's, which in hindsight, was an extra blessing from God. I noticed she had begun wheezing Sunday, and I decided to make a judgment call and put her on oxygen. I was not alarmed or worried. It wasn't the first time I have had to do that. After receiving Courtney's text, I awoke early from a restless sleep and packed my bags. I arrived at the facility for shift change later at

6:45 a.m. I stopped by Mama's apartment to check on her and the sitter for the day and proceeded to do my usual morning routine with Mama.

Mama was still on oxygen, no better or worse from the previous day and I was confident she was in great hands. I got very close to her, put the back of my hand on her cheek, and said, "Good morning, sweet Mama." She typically then leaned into my hand and put her head on her shoulder, embracing my tender, warm touch. It took me a few times that morning to get her to respond, but I kept trying. I moved to her left side, making the same motion, and added, "I love you, sweet Mama." She quietly whispered, "Thank you. I love you, too." Those turned out to be the last words I ever heard her speak.

I visited with Mama for about thirty minutes. There was no indication Mama's health might decline. After being reassured multiple times by my sitter "Norma Jean would be well taken care of," I gave Mama another kiss and suddenly burst into tears. My emotions were more for my son at this point. I was worried sick about him! However, something in my spirit was different than when I had left Mama for other trips. My friend again reassured me and reminded me, "Mama, your son needs you now."

⚬⚬⚬

I had a five-hour drive ahead of me and this gave me way too much time to think. Billy was young and very healthy. He exercised often and lived an active lifestyle. He had been sick for six days at this point, and this ole girl was very concerned. Half-way through my drive, I called the sitter to check on Mama and her wheezing. Imagine my shock and disbelief when she informed me Mama had started with the infamous "death rattle." I asked her to put the phone to Mama's mouth so I could hear it. I pulled to the shoulder of the road, my head spinning and my heart breaking, and boy, did I wail. I was so torn. My son was critically ill, and now my mother was in the throes of death. In all the times I imagined exactly how Mama's death would play out, this, my friend, was never one I could have dreamt of. I immediately called Suzy and told her to drop everything and get to Mama. I couldn't bear the thought of Mama being without one of her six children by her side. *How could I possibly be in two places at one time?* I felt strongly one of her children should be with her.

Mama had experienced several unresponsive events and serious falls in the previous twelve months. Each time, I called my siblings to let them know. Honestly, I began sounding like the little boy who cried wolf! But this time, I knew. My heart, mind and spirit knew, too. My sister could not get a flight home until the next morning. Mama was in God's hands.

※

When I arrived at the hospital and entered my son's room, I was horrified and ill-prepared for what I saw. The man I had seen only seven days before for an early Christmas gathering was now lying in a hospital bed with no color, droopy eyes, and barely able to put two words together; it was positively devastating. *Oh God, please heal him!*

I am a crier, and I barely held it together for him. I asked Billy if the pneumonia they had previously diagnosed him with was bacterial, and he whispered, "Yes," and then he added, "And sepsis and empyema!" My knees buckled, and I felt faint. I gripped the end of the hospital bed. SEPSIS. *How in the world did this happen?* The wind was knocked out of me. *My son or my Mama. God don't take both of them. I wouldn't survive that loss. Please Father God, NO!*

The next twenty-four hours were categorically the most gutwrenching experience in my life. As I grew more concerned over my son's bizarre condition, I received word my mother was declining rapidly. *How could I be in two places at once?* My precious child and my sweet Mama. I loved them both dearly.

When I entered the hospital room and laid eyes on my son, the gravity of the situation was overwhelming. I quickly reached out to James and our younger son, Ethan, urging them to rush to the hospital immediately. Witnessing my firstborn struggling in the most arduous battle of his entire life, I was terrified! My body was riddled with fear.

※

The doctors were bewildered and unable to comprehend how a young and healthy patient could be in such a horrific and unexplainable predicament. Before I left the hospital with my two grandchildren that evening, Billy began to feel somewhat better due to antibiotics and prayer, lots of prayer! The doctor had decided to try and remove some of the 1,500 cc of excess fluid in his lung the next day.

I stayed the night with my grandchildren at their home while James and Ethan stayed at the hospital with Billy. My daughter-in-law was a trooper and had stayed by her husband's side the days prior to and during this hospitalization and, needless to say, she was exhausted. Their church family rushed to their aid to help in anyway they could.

<hr />

The whole scenario was an impossible dilemma. I had been Mama's caregiver for 12 years. I didn't know how long she had left and my son's prognosis was grim. I prayed like I had never prayed before. I cried out for a complete healing for both of my loved ones; whether in heaven or on earth, I wanted them to be relieved of their misery.

*Full disclosure…I had the audacity to strongly recommend to God to let Mama get her angel wings since she was 91 and begged and pleaded with God to allow Billy to be healed and live a full life well into his nineties.*

When you are crying your eyes out and can hardly breathe, and your precious four-year-old grandson puts his head on your shoulder, hugs you, and says these three things I hope I never forget:

- Grown-ups aren't supposed to cry.
- Angels fly really fast (to minister to his great-grandma).
- We should pray for people when they are dying.

Then he prayed for his Mamaw. This was by far the sweetest moment ever. My grandson now knows grown-ups do indeed cry, and his Meme cries a lot!!

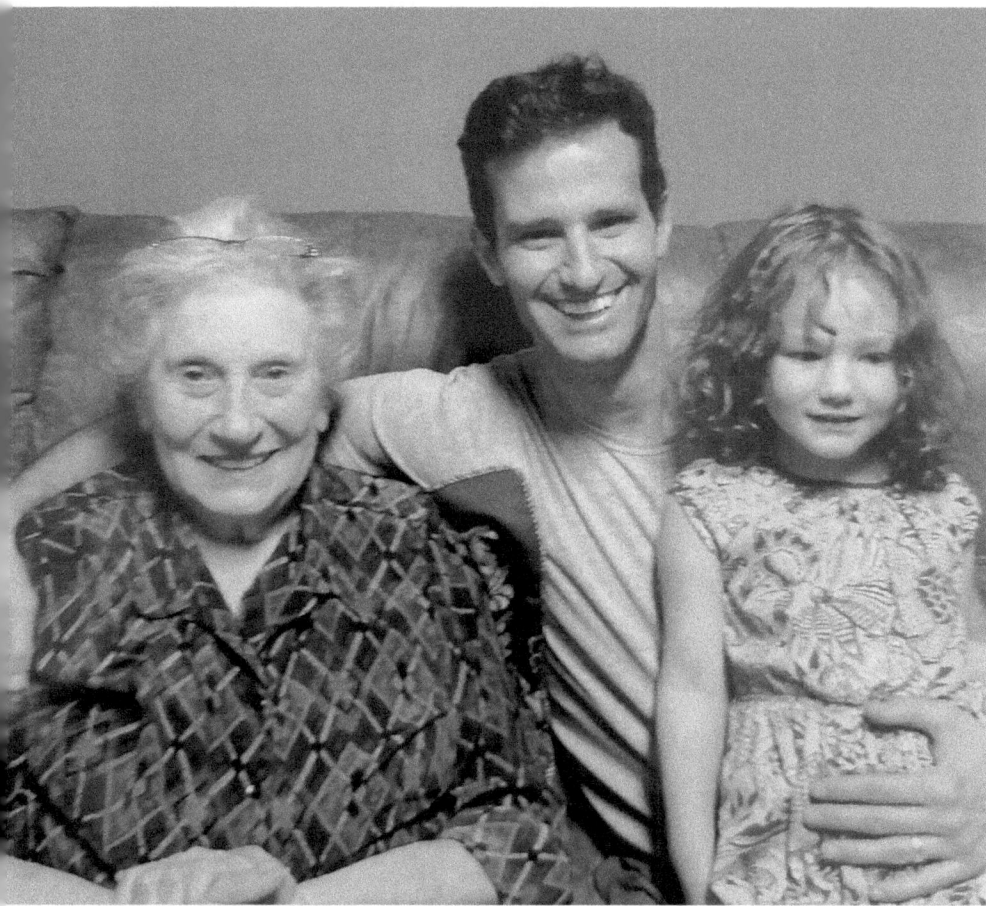

# CHAPTER 68
# TRUSTING GOD

THE LATEST UPDATE on Mama was she refused to drink anything, clamping her lips closed. Suzy was expected to arrive at Mama's soon. I discussed with the sitter and the hospice nurse whether to start morphine with Mama but chose not to at that time. In my conversation with Mama's sitter, she mentioned how bad Mama sounded, the rattling worsening overnight. I was told it sounded like she was drowning. She even recorded it for me so I could hear it for myself. I wanted to clearly understand what was transpiring in the death process. I wanted to be there and couldn't, but that did not keep me from staying in touch.

Suzy arrived midday at the Big House on January 1, and when she walked into Mama's room, she heard the horrific sound coming from our mother. It was indeed the death rattle and our precious Mama was beginning her journey to her eternal home. Morphine was administered to her, and I felt my sister would take excellent care of Mama. Suzy confirmed how quickly Mama was progressing. I was informed my only living aunt and uncle visited Mama to say their sweet, emotional goodbyes to their big sister. Lydia also had driven home to be with Mama.

I was constantly in contact with my sisters, hospice, the facility where Mama lived, and the sitter.

⁓⌀⟨⟩⌀⁓

Back at the hospital, they were not successful with draining the fluid from my son's lung, and they informed us it was the consistency of slush. My anxiety was soaring to new heights! My son's medical team was contemplating putting drain tubes in to help him with his severe back pain and difficulty breathing. This might give him a better chance of getting fluid off of his lungs.

⁓⌀⟨⟩⌀⁓

I do believe with the emotional see-saw I found myself on for well over 48 hours, I was a verifiable "basket case." I couldn't turn off the tears. I was drowning in uncontrollable waves of sorrow. My heart was completely and understandably ripped in two. My husband and sons saw my tormented state; it was a horrific, explosive combination. My husband knew I needed to return home and complete the journey I had begun twelve years earlier with Mama. My sweet son, who could barely talk, looked at me with all sincerity and compassion and told me I needed to finish this chapter with Mamaw to have closure. This was the final chapter. *Oh my gosh, how could I leave? How could I turn my back on my boy?*

I was incapable of making any decision with my state of mind, but my son did. He assured me he was going to be fine. Have you ever had the sensation of a knife stuck in your gut? Magnify that feeling times ten. After much persuasion and assurance by my husband and son, I agreed to head home and am so thankful Ethan decided to drive me. My husband stayed behind with Billy in my absence. Before Ethan and I began our journey home about 5:30 that afternoon, I gave Billy a very emotional farewell, somewhat encouraged by his progress but still extremely concerned about him. All we could do at this point was rest in HIS arms while two people I love more than life itself were battling and fighting hard. God has carried, healed, protected, and blessed me throughout my life. I trusted Him implicitly. Until that moment, I don't think I fully comprehended what 100% trust and faith looked like. I called Suzy while we drove toward home and was told Mama's breathing had worsened. They planned to increase the morphine to make her as comfortable as possible.

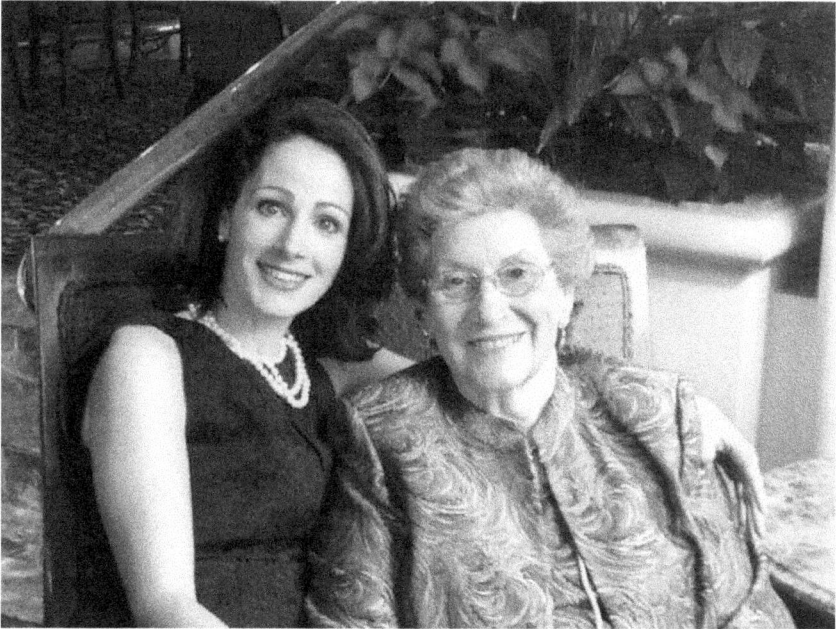

Mama with her granddaughter, Kelly

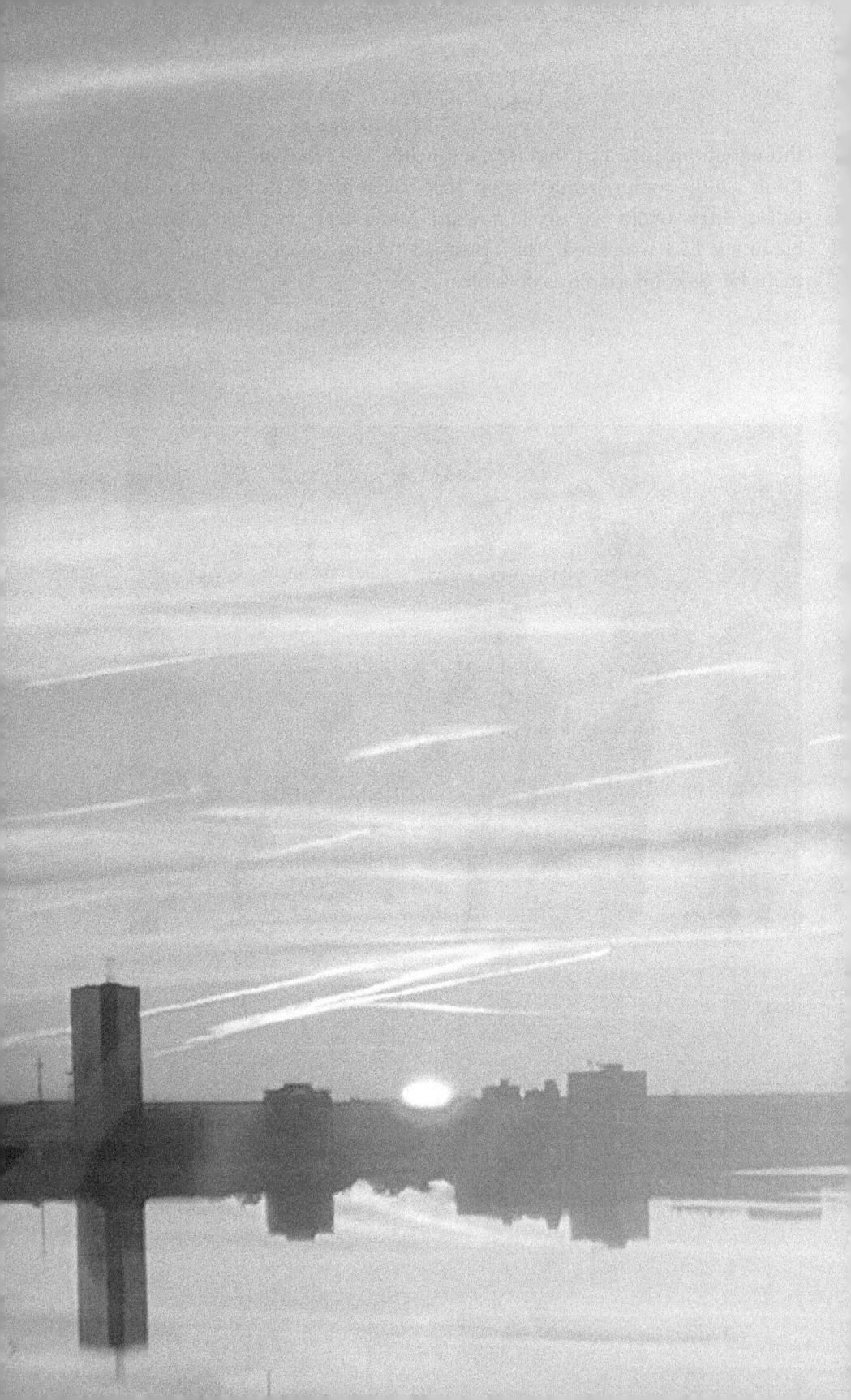

## CHAPTER 69

# ONE LAST LESSON

I ARRIVED at the Big House shortly after 10 p.m. and was greeted by my daughters and raced in to find Mama lying in her bed, struggling to breathe, and I got acquainted with the awful death rattle. I did what I had done thousands of times before. I got on my knees by her bed to get close to her and whisper to her, and the floodgates opened. I was in disbelief this had transpired so quickly and yet so thankful I was able to return and be by her side. Lydia and Suzy came to my side to comfort me. I took in every sound, every breath, and every little movement. The end was near, and I was relieved my husband willingly took my place at the hospital so I could finish my last walk with Mama. I stayed up all night with Mama and my sisters took turns watching her with me.

At one point, things started changing with Mama. The inside of her mouth changed from pink to a dark color. We had to constantly use a sponge to clean the mucus coming from her mouth. Much later that day, her nose began discharging the same dark color and her breathing stopped and then began again. Mama was unusually calm. Dying is a process; just like no two births are identical to another, the same is true for death.

Friends, family, and workers all visited throughout the day and said their goodbyes. Word of Mama's impending death had spread quickly. Norma Jean had always been a favorite at the Big House. We prayed and sang songs around her bedside. We whispered to her she could leave us, and we had each other. We reassured her we loved her and she was a wonderful mother, and then, we waited. Mama would leave this world and enter into the next in her own unique way. I've said this countless times, but it merits repeating it: Mama taught me SO much about various facets of life, and now she was doing it again, except this time it was a lesson in dying.

At that moment, I knew returning to Louisiana was the right thing to do. It was the absolute HARDEST thing to do, but it was necessary. I am thankful for my husband, who stood in the gap for me, and for my son understanding and encouraging me to come home.

Let me pause and tell you what a blessing Mama's sitter, Vicky, was to us that day. I was so discombobulated I had forgotten to update the sitters on the recent developments.

Vicky was scheduled for the day shift with Mama. Having not seen Mama since Friday and not learning of her demise, she was quite surprised to see Mama actively transitioning to her eternal home in heaven. That did not deter Vicky. She could have easily gone home for the day because my sisters were there and hospice and the aides who were on the floor. But she didn't. She stayed her entire 12-hour shift. She washed Mama's face with a warm washcloth. She combed Mama's hair. She cleaned Mama's apartment. She got us anything we needed. What a servant! She even took pictures and videos of us gathered around the bed praying and singing. And, of course, Vicky prayed. I will never forget the kindness and love she showered on our precious Mama that day.

The evening shift change was always at 7 p.m. Imagine my surprise when Mama's night sitter, Cat, walked in the door for her time slot.

Again, I had let the ball drop and had not notified her of Mama's impending death. She was shocked and saddened and wanted to stay with us for a few hours. What a precious soul. Those are the kind of sitters you want for your loved ones. I am thankful for how my sitters cared for Mama while she was living and as she was dying.

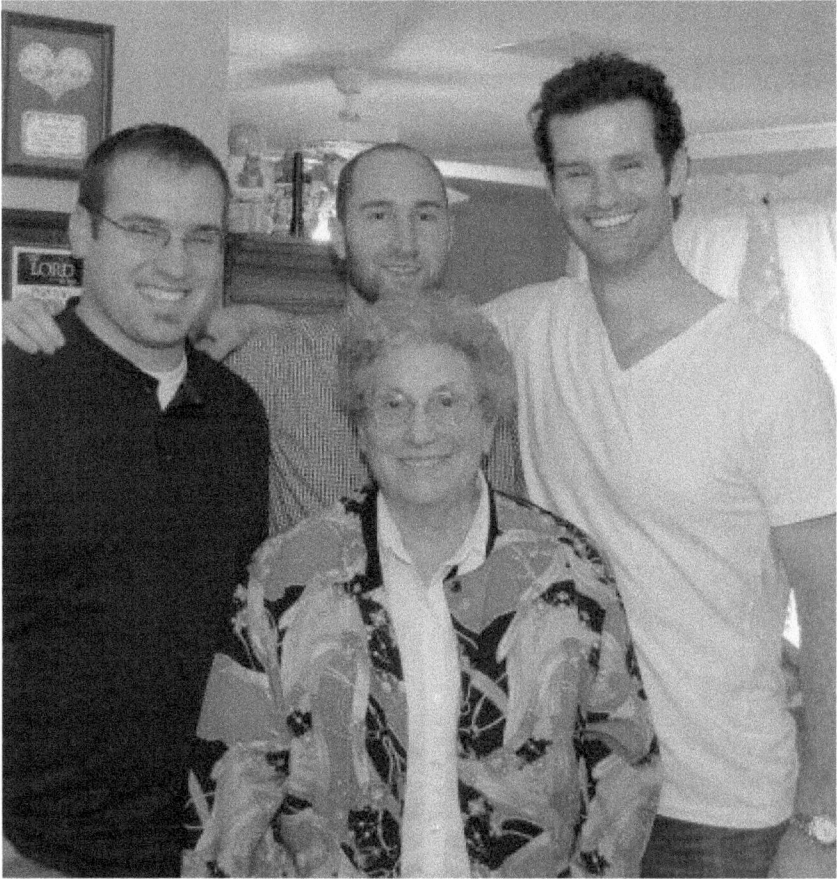

Mama with three grandsons, Billy, Neal, and Ryan

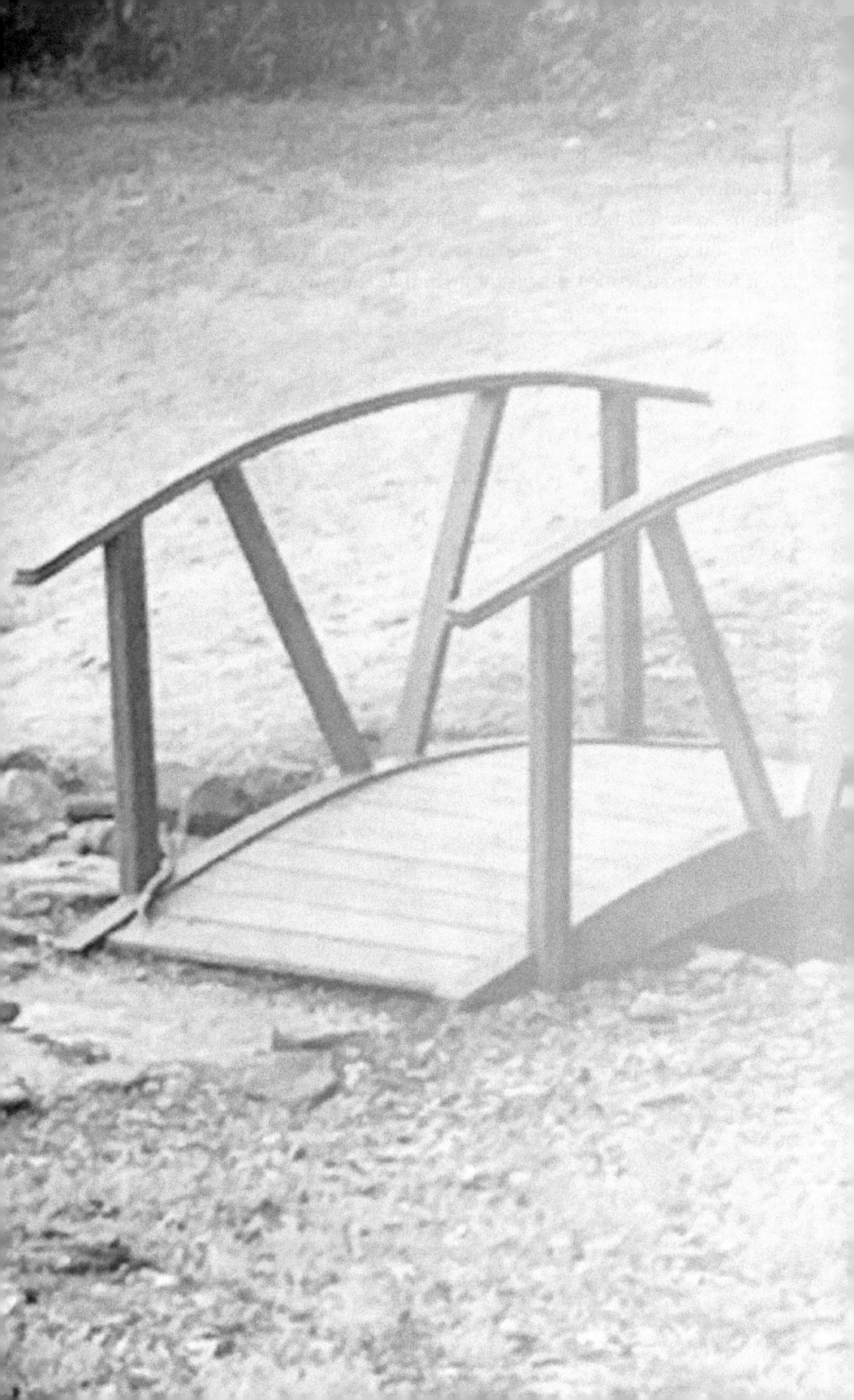

# CHAPTER 70

# THE FINAL CURTAIN

JANUARY 2ND ROLLED AROUND, and the sun peeked out behind the clouds. Reports on my son were encouraging. He seemed to have turned a corner and had procedures scheduled later that day.

That evening as the sun went down, I realized I had been awake for nearly 48 hours, and as I sat by Mama's bedside hour after hour, I was growing weary, very weary. At approximately 9:30 p.m., I looked at my sisters and daughters and told them I was going home for a quick nap. I was utterly exhausted, and we had no idea how long her transition might take. I asked them to call me if anything changed, anything at all. I only lived 10 minutes away, five minutes if I broke the speed limit. Shortly after 10 p.m., Suzy called to tell me "It was happening." I ran through the house, waking the girls up, and we hustled out the door. I confess I did, in fact, break the speed limit in my rush to reach Mama.

~~~~~~~~~~

Upon arriving at the facility, we met people standing in the hallway waiting for us. We ran down the halls until we reached Mama's room. I rushed in and went to her bedside. No more rattling sounds, just weeping in the room. I kissed Mama and asked my sister, "Is she really dead?" I had thought about this moment many times, dreamt about it, and could *not* believe I was standing by her side and she was gone. No more waking her up, holding hands, getting her dressed for the day and then again for bedtime, feeding her, standing in the gap for her, being her advocate. No more songs, silliness, or out-of-the-blue poignant and profound statements. She was gone.

I looked at Mama lying in her bed, completely at peace. Watching Mama die was scary, different, and somewhat bizarre to us. In the end, God answered my prayer. He was merciful. Mama did not suffer.

Realizing the finality of the situation, realizing the prayer I had been praying for two months was answered, I sighed deeply and whispered, "My life has just drastically changed!" Eleven years of seeing her nearly every day and the last year twice daily with much more intense care. It was over. I am very thankful He honored my plea to take her swiftly without prolonged suffering.

After things settled down, I overheard Lydia talking to my daughters, who were standing in the hallway. What she said hit me hard, "Girls, you get to have your Mama back." Just let that sink in. Not only did I make sacrifices while caring for Mama, but my husband and children did as well. On the evening of January 2, my twelve-year journey of caring for my sweet mother ended when she took her last breath. Seeing those words in print as I write them still evokes emotion down to my core. The previous 48 hours of her life wrecked me and, in the same sense, released me from the caregiver position. What a whirlwind of emotions. At 91 years old, she was no longer trapped inside her diseased body, a far cry from the beautiful, brilliant, hard-working, active woman we had known and loved.

It was finished. The battle was over. She was healed and whole, walking and running in heaven, and her mind was beautiful again. She had seen her Savior face to face and would spend eternity in His presence. She had also been reunited with loved ones.

Caring for Mama with this horrible disease came with some of the darkest times, difficult decisions, and an extremely high learning curve that never seemed to end. But God guided my decisions and steps, and Mama, in her own way, encouraged me to keep pushing forward.

I've said this before, but it bears repeating.

---

**Be careful who you marry because one day your spouse may be taking care of your Mama.**

---

Words cannot fully convey how much I love my sweetheart. He was incredibly good to Mama. James Stephens, you were the best, and Mama and I were so fortunate you took and continue to take such incredible care of those you love.

One scenario that had never entered my mind in all these years was my husband, my best friend, my strong man, would not be there with me, holding my hand, when Mama died. I depended on him so much. He had stepped in many times and cared for Mama. He was amazing with her. He was a son to her. She absolutely lit up around him and she did anything he asked her to do. The workers were always happy when my husband sat with Mama. It made their day easier.

I found myself going on two, three, four, then five days without him while the family gathered in town and we prepared for the funeral. I was grateful we had postponed the funeral services a few days and relieved when he arrived for the visitation the night before Mama's funeral. Again, in his absence, God was holding me up, literally.

The morning after Mama passed, Billy began making progress and had one chest tube removed. Everyone was happy with the direction things

ELLEN PETTIJOHN STEPHENS

were going. He remained in the hospital for another week with his wife by his side and unfortunately, but understandably, he had to miss his Mamaw's funeral.

I am happy to report my son made a full recovery, and we were thankful for all the prayers. I am convinced on January 2, God could have taken either one of my loves or both for that matter, but I am eternally grateful He chose Mama. She lived a beautiful, fulfilled ninety-one years. I know her first order of business when she reached those pearly gates was to ask God to heal her grandson and He did.

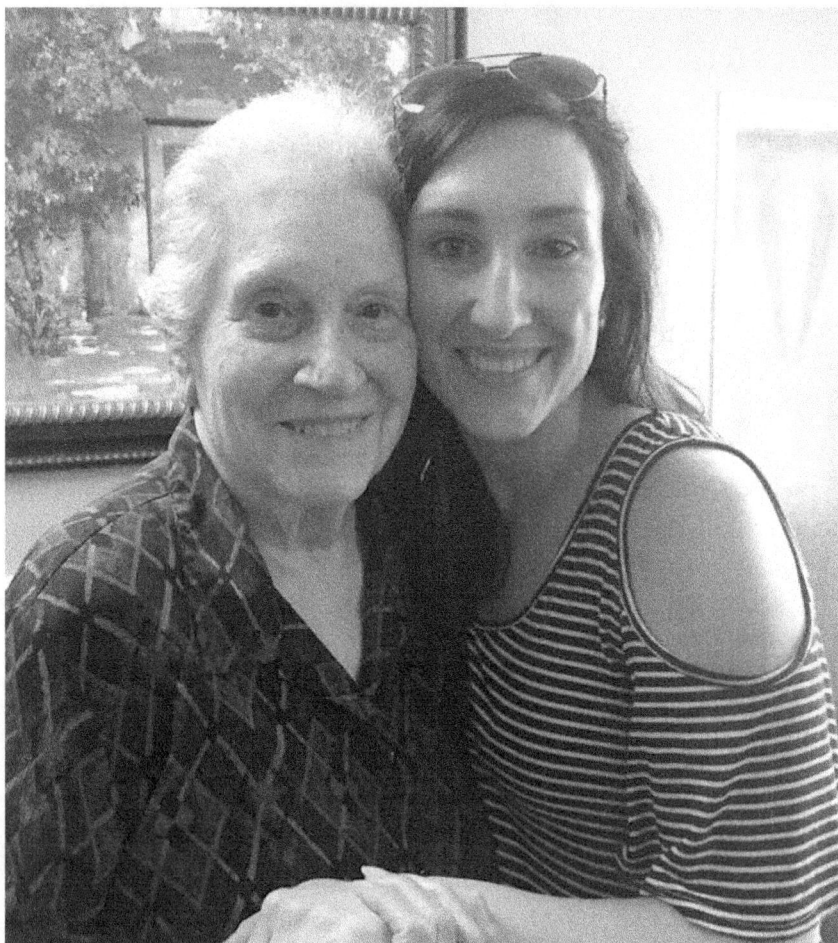

Mama with her granddaughter, Rochelle

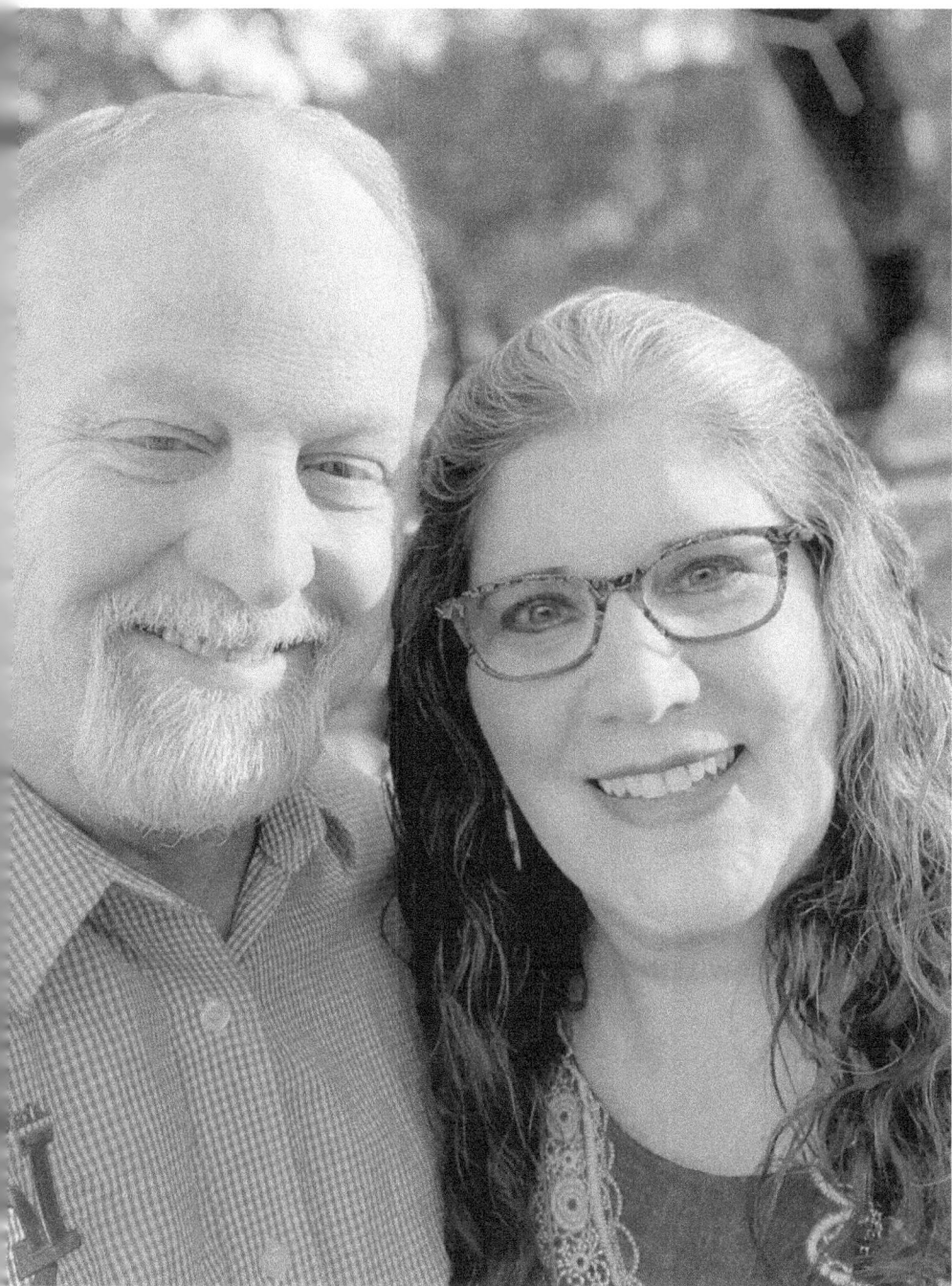

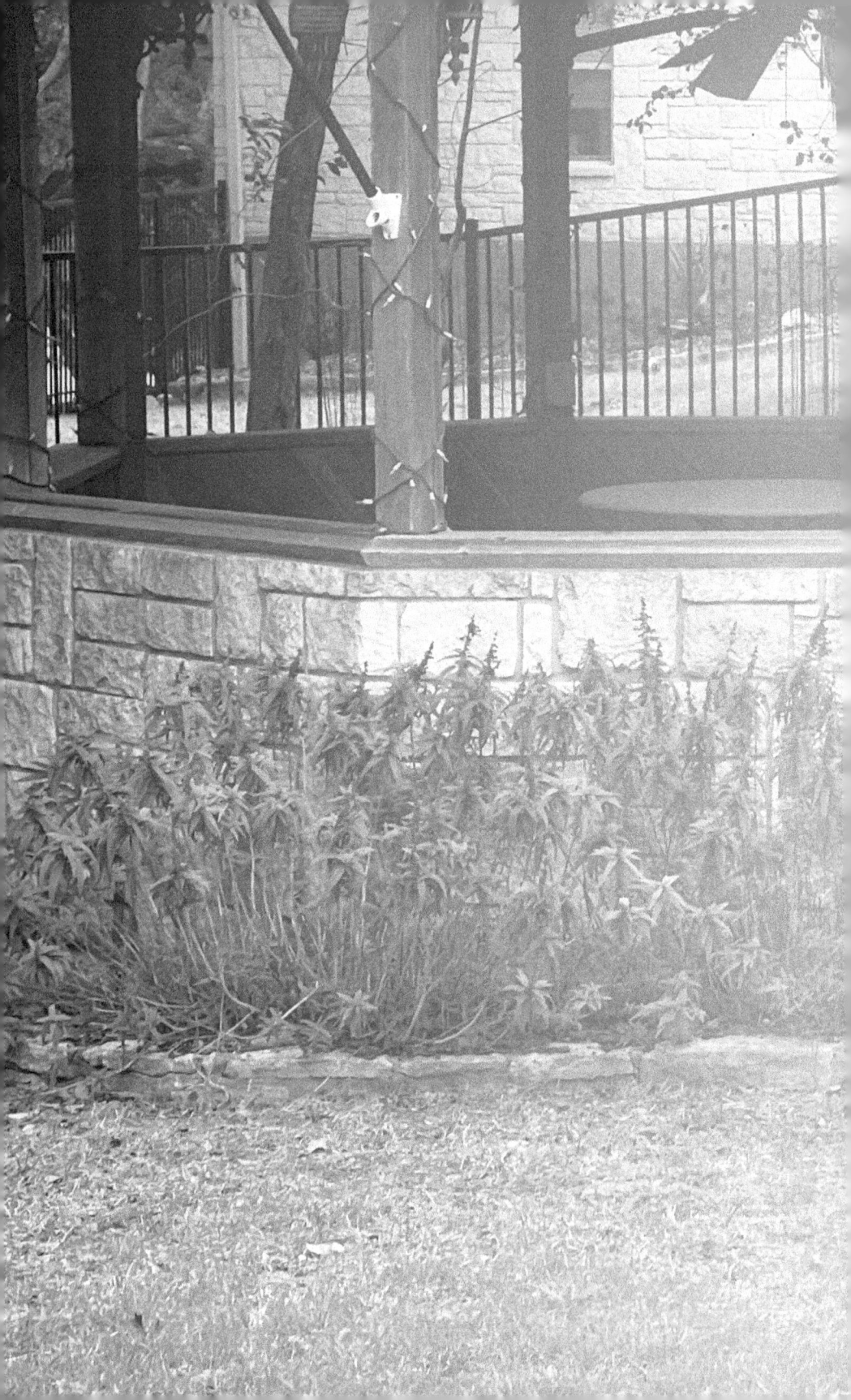

# CHAPTER 71
# A LEGACY OF LOVE

I WANT to believe I was an example to my children of how we should care for our parents and the elderly in general. I hope I was an inspiration to them and others. I trust they learned about respecting and caring for the older generation over the years and how to care for those with memory loss, in particular. I pray I leave my children with a legacy of love for others, even those who may make you feel uncomfortable.

---

Work through it. Everyone needs to feel loved. Stop and take time to talk. Open doors. Sing songs. Hold hands. Push their wheelchairs. Sit at their feet. Who cares if they ramble? Let them ramble. I've learned through all of this not everyone is a caregiver, but everyone can be kind and caring.

---

One of the unique things I wanted to do for Mama's funeral that certainly got the *Norma Jean seal of approval* was to get the whole gang together and go to her favorite place, Dairy Barn. After a hard day working in her flower beds, Mama drove there for a burger and a chocolate shake. After I brought her to Saturday evening Mass, we often went there to eat supper. All the employees knew Mama. We headed to Dairy Barn when I needed to lift her spirits. When friends and family came in from out of town, she brought them to Dairy Barn. When she wanted to treat the grandkids and great-grandkids, you guessed it, Dairy Barn.

Pierre, the owner, and his staff were fantastic. They allowed us to utilize such a special place for our extended family to gather. The restaurant was packed out. There was delicious food, my siblings, grandchildren, great-grandchildren, her brother, many cousins, and some friends.

I surveyed the room filled with laughter and overheard several colorful storytellers and imagined what joy this would have brought Mama. Nothing made her happier than her family. I could feel her spirit there.

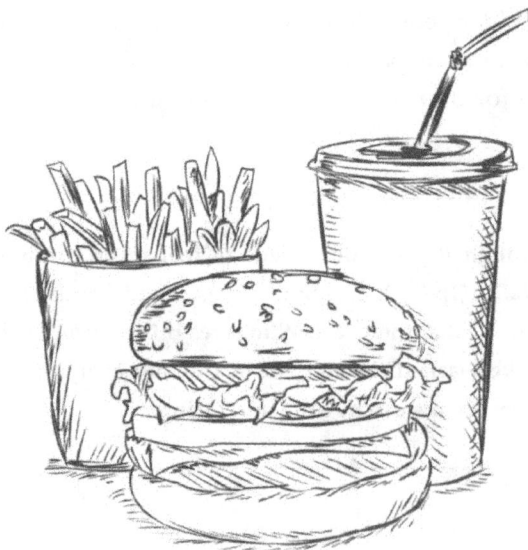

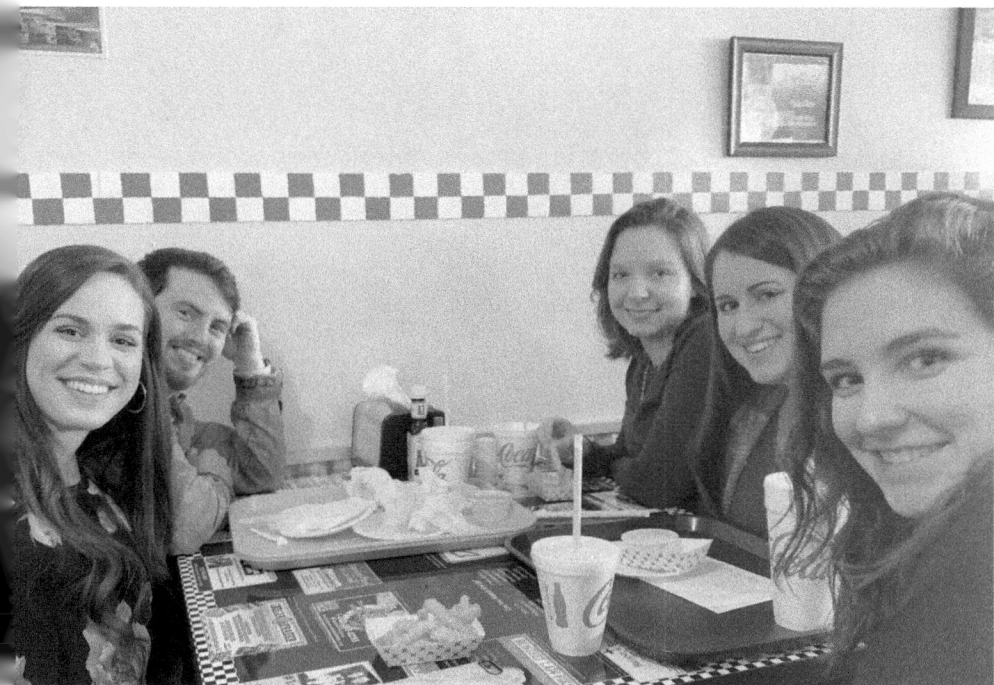

# CHAPTER 72
# A FLOOD OF MEMORIES

IMMEDIATELY AFTER MAMA PASSED AWAY, I was very emotional, which was to be expected. Twenty-four hours later, with my house bursting with my siblings and their families, I slipped away to my bedroom and began to experience a sinking feeling in my chest coming over me. I just had to flee. I needed to get to Mama's apartment immediately. I was running out the door, bawling, when my three sisters asked what was wrong and why I was leaving. I told them I was going to Mama's apartment. They were puzzled and asked for clarification. I responded, "For over a year, I had been there every day to check on Mama. I arrived every morning between 6:45 and 7:00, and every evening between 6:45 and 7:00, I returned." Without further discussion, the three of them jumped in the car with me.

As I got in the car, I looked at the digital clock on the dashboard, and it was 7:00 p.m. My chest was hurting, and I could hardly breathe. I could not get there quickly enough. It was where I was *supposed* to be.

<hr/>

We arrived at the Big House and three of my favorite employees were at the nurse's station. We hugged and cried, and as we began sharing stories of Mama, the tears turned into laughter and continued for over an hour. It was just what I needed. The healing process was beginning for me.

⌑

All of Mama's daughters walked down the hall to Mama's room, and as we strolled quietly, I glanced to and fro and recalled with a deeper meaning, every single place, every chair, every hallway, everywhere I had been with Mama the last five years. I was snapping mental pictures in my mind so I would never forget the journey.

We came to her apartment, which was completely void of furniture except for the lift chair. My siblings had gone earlier and cleared everything out for me. My sister commented, "She's not here anymore," to which I replied, "Oh, but she is." Her presence was everywhere I looked in the room. The place where her couch used to be became a special space where we called my siblings on their birthdays. Mama belted out "Happy Birthday" to them, not knowing if it would be her last time. We sang, and sang, and sang some more. It was the impromptu student's desk for Mama where I continually tested her memory unbeknownst to her.

My eyes caught the dim light coming from the bathroom. The bathroom is where we spent countless hours, and honestly, I learned more lessons in that tiny square footage than anywhere else. Hard lessons, practical lessons, lessons in grace, sweet lessons in forgiveness and gratitude. I know it sounds odd, but anyone in that room with my mother knows what I am speaking of. That bathroom was literally my classroom.

I next turned to look at the place where her beautiful bed was and remembered how she fought us so hard to lie down in her bed. She was much more content just sleeping on the couch or even her recliner. It reminded me how content she was with a simple life. If I did get her to sleep in the bed, she wanted me to lie down next to her, and we engaged in sweet, memorable pillow talk, all the while teaching me, encouraging me, and stretching me.

I looked at the space where her hospice bed had been placed. Oh, my goodness. The pain I felt as I thought of that piece of equipment was immense. Some of the hardest struggles in Mama's life were in or near the bed. Thankfully, it wasn't all painful memories. She passed away peacefully in that bed. During the six or seven months before her death, she had multiple encounters as she slept, we believe, with family members who had already passed or perhaps with angels. During the night shift, she often raised her hands in a slow, graceful movement to the ceiling as if reaching for a hand or praising the Lord.

Other times, she clapped softly. What a sight to behold. Every time this occurred, a hush came over the room to see if Mama uttered anything that might give us a clue as to who she was interacting with. To our delight, the person she spoke of the most was her Mama, our Granny. Oh, those were special, holy encounters.

The last item I recalled as a fixture in the room she inhabited was the wheelchair. Mama, even at 90 years old, had required no assistance with walking. However, after a series of falls, the worst one required us to put her in a wheelchair. My legs were the bruised and battered storyteller regarding my daily battle with that wheelchair, as I transferred Mama from the recliner to the wheelchair multiple times a day. My claim to fame would never be a graceful caregiver. Bruises of all colors, shapes, and sizes were constantly on my lower extremities. Even so, there were good memories, as good as some could be, of the wheelchair, too.

My favorite memory was Mama sitting in the wheelchair in her room, and we turned the music up a little louder than normal, and she maneuvered that chair all over the room, all the while getting in some great rhythmic shoulder action to the beat of the music.

As we left Mama's room that night, her presence was so strong to me. As I walked down the hallways, I looked into the dimly lit dining hall to the table and chair where Mama sat at every meal. I touched the couches and chairs she sat in outside the dining hall. I peered into the TV room...her spirit was there. I felt her presence around every corner particularly her recliner in that room. I had spent hours there, days even.

Thank you, sweet mother of mine, for being such an incredibly inspiring role model even in the darkest years of your life. Rise up, persevere, work hard, be smart, love hard, be innovative, cherish your husband and children, honor your parents, be good stewards, laugh and laugh often, have fun, don't be afraid to get dirty, and go see this beautiful world. Thankful for these and so many more lessons she taught me.

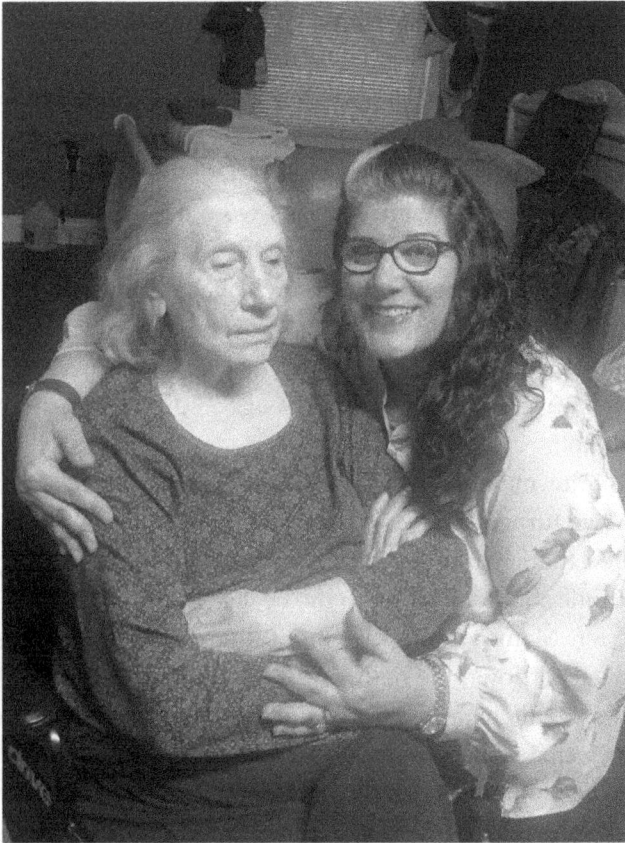

The moment when Mama said her last words to me

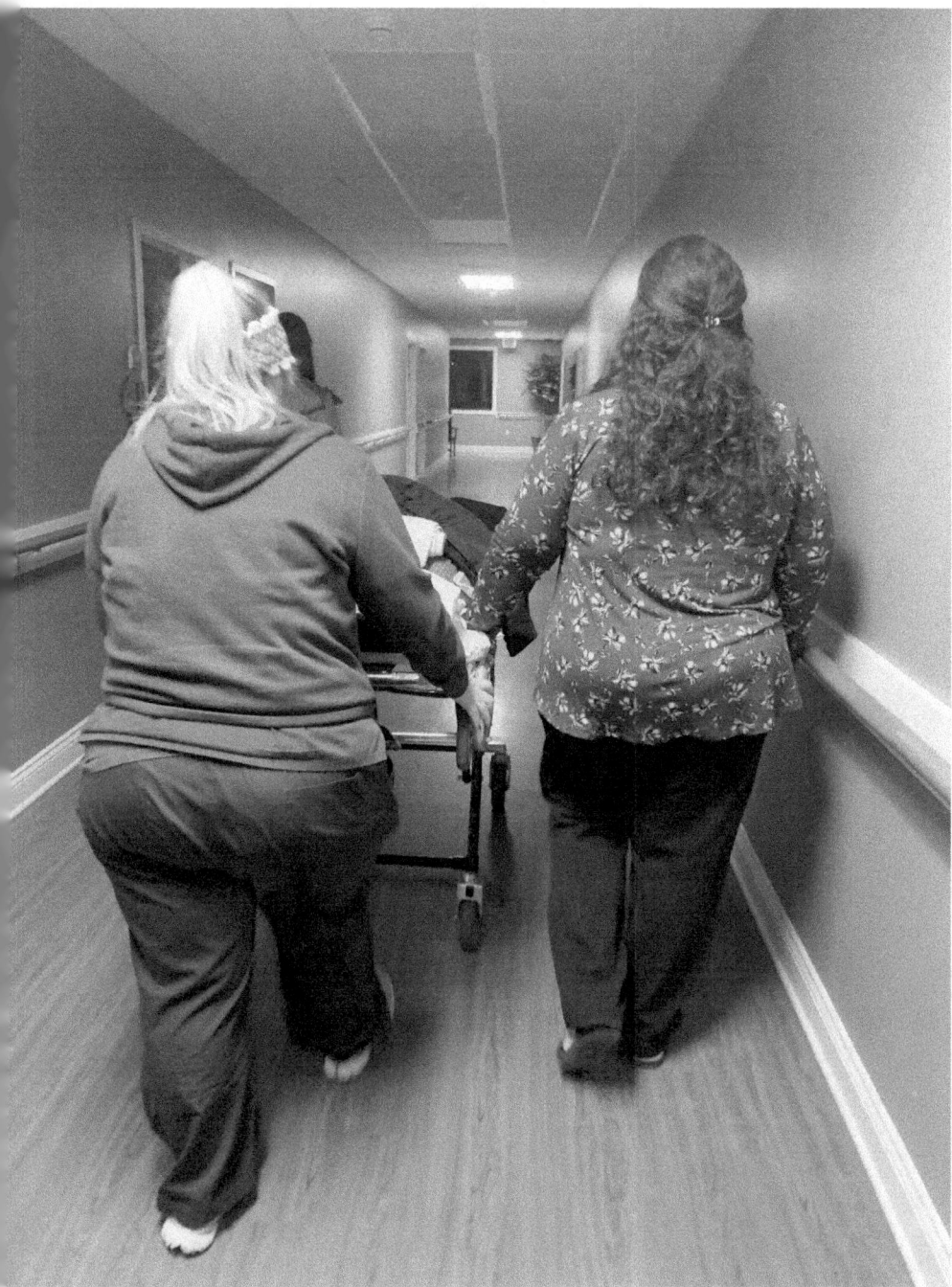

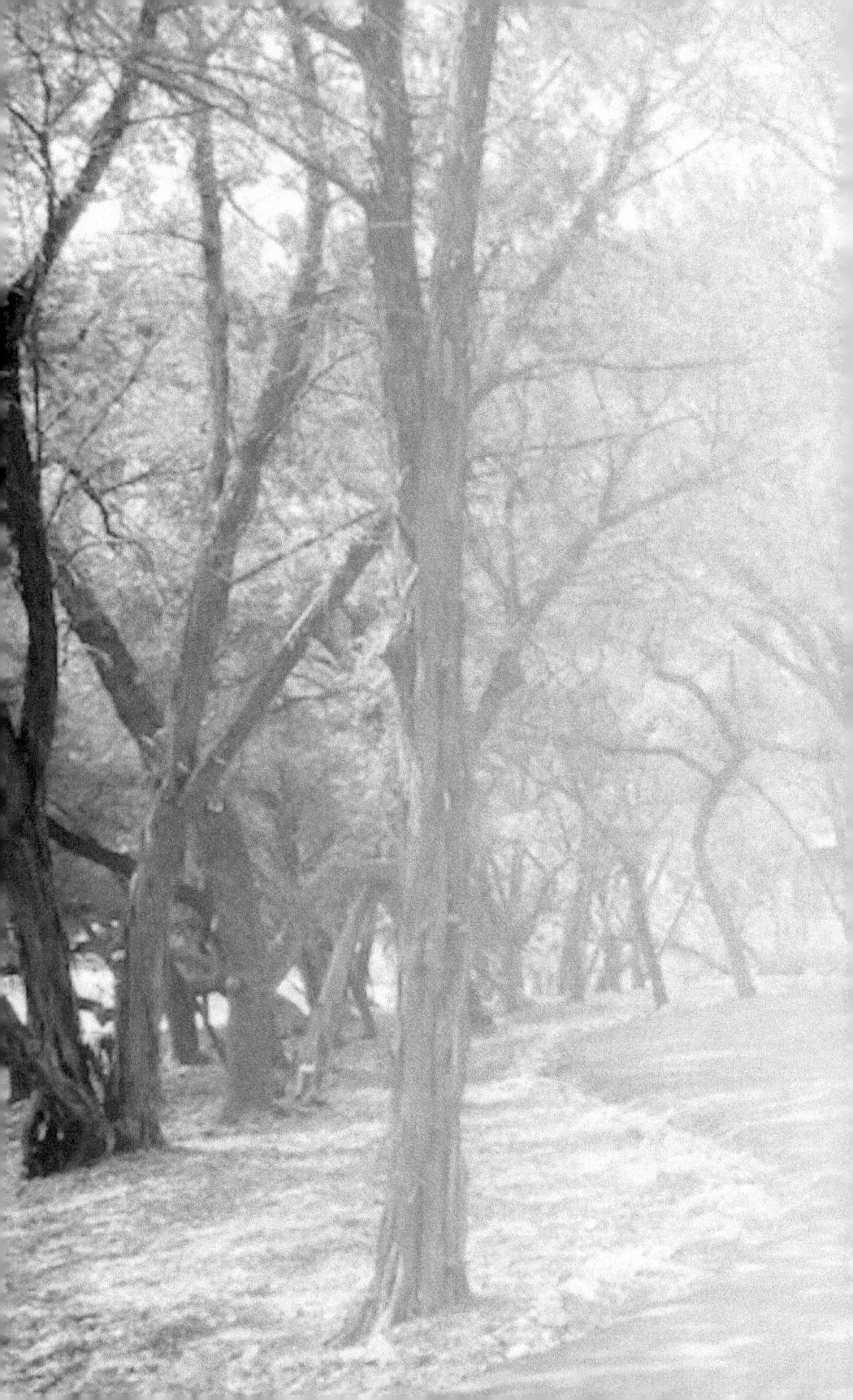

# CHAPTER 73

# THIRTY DAYS LATER

WE WERE APPROACHING the one-month anniversary of my mother's homegoing. This month had been incredible. I had been loved on, cradled, hugged, prayed for, and encouraged, even by strangers. God sends people into your life when you need it most. When the nights were darkest, and the sunrise did not come soon enough, God sent angels to minister to me. I had an extra dose of "angelosity" this month and am forever grateful. Yes, I think I will coin that phrase.

At the end of my first month without my sweet Mama, I had to be content and peaceful and know with full confidence what I did for Mama, be it right, wrong, or indifferent, well, it was enough. *It was enough.* I have zero regrets. I attempted to do everything to the best of my ability. I loved Mama unconditionally and treated her the way I wanted to be treated. That was my daily goal. Was it easy? Oh, my goodness, no, not at all. Would I do it again? I received countless blessings, memories, and lessons and lived out what God's Word tells us to do right in front of my children and grandchildren. I have to say a resounding, "Yes, I would do it again!"

I am pretty shocked, yet delighted to share with you how well I find myself adjusting to such a drastic change in my life, not only losing my sweet Mama but having so much free time every single day, particularly during important family times such as early mornings before my girls left for college and in the evening. My family was enjoying having me home again. It was mutual.

~~~~∞~~~~

I attribute my peaceful transition to God's strong arms carrying me and the love and encouragement of many people. That, my friends, was living water to my soul. I have an unspeakable peace knowing one day I will see her again in Glory. I bet I'll find her in the choir room. Lastly, I believe one of the reasons I am not an emotional wreck, which would be my usual MO (mode of operation), was because, during the past decade, I gave Mama my time and attention and tried to the best of my ability to meet her ever-changing needs. I prayed God would never make me place her in a nursing home and He didn't. I prayed He would not let her suffer, and He didn't. I prayed most of the children and grandchildren were able to come to the funeral, and all but one came, and he was in the hospital. He literally had a doctor's excuse.

~~~~∞~~~~

Reflecting on my journey as a caregiver and the financial responsibilities that came with it, I have come to truly appreciate the foresight and planning of my beloved Mama. In sharing my experiences, I feel compelled to emphasize the importance of financial preparedness for the later stages of life, particularly when it comes to long-term care such as assisted living, memory care, or private sitters. It is my sincere hope that by taking the time to discuss and establish a solid financial plan with your spouse and children, you can avoid the burden of financial strain on your loved ones in the future. In the last year of Mama's life, I paid for memory care and 24-hour sitters and spent $200,000.

---

**Now is the time to have that talk and plan ahead.**

---

I returned to the Big House one day and I met the head maintenance man, Ricky, and we hugged, tears in his eyes, and went on our separate ways. No words were required. I entered Mama's apartment, and evidently, Ricky had been working there, covering up all the holes in the walls and prepping the walls for paint. It was empty without her furniture and pictures, void of Mama's things. As I left the room, Ricky returned with a fresh can of paint, stopped me, hugged me again, and said how hard it was for him to be in her room. He started crying and telling me what a difference Mama made in his life. She was ALWAYS happy to see him, ALWAYS had open arms for him, ALWAYS smiling at him, and ALWAYS made him feel loved. He said it was their job (the employees) to make the residents feel good and keep them happy, but Norma Jean flipped it and made the workers feel loved and important, making their day more joyful. That was her gift.

Wesley walked up, too. You may recall he and Mama shared the same birthdate. He LOVED her and held my hand while the three of us talked. These two men, the way they looked after my mother and they looked out for me, they were also considered my family. I hope they knew what their friendship meant to both of us.

305

# CHAPTER 74
# LOVELY LETTERS

My COUSIN, Tesa, wrote me a letter that summed up Norma Jean so well.

*When Aunt Norma first went to live in assisted living, I visited her often, and it was never hard to find her. Every morning, she got up early, got dressed, and went downstairs to sit in her favorite seat across from the front door. She said she sat in that spot so "she would not miss anything." It was ground zero to her. She was the Queen of Hospitality and never met a stranger.*

*She had a way of seeing the humor in every situation and could make you laugh with her silly songs. The fact that the child inside her stayed active and engaged is why everyone flocked around her, especially actual children. They found their buddy, their partner in crime, and their Mary Poppins in her. She was always up for an adventure.*

This thank you card from my aunt and uncle is one I will always cherish.

> *Elle,*
>
> *Thank you for the lovely card. It is not you who should be thanking us, but Uncle Leonard and I want to say "thank you" from the bottom of our hearts for the unbelievable care you gave our sister, without a complaint, for 10 long years. It will never be forgotten.*
>
> *Aunt Bobbie and Uncle Leonard*

Mel gave me several floral envelopes and dated them according to the day I could read each one. You never know who is watching you.

> *From you, I learned the importance of being selfless and forgiving of others. Watching you take care of not only your mother for twelve years but also Pawpaw and Mawmaw, is the epitome of being selfless. You could have easily said I don't have time for this because you were still raising me and Chrissy, but instead, you said, "Yes." You did what you needed to, and you did it with grace. You stepped up to the plate when no one else would and didn't expect anything in return. From you, especially recently, I've learned forgiveness is extremely important. Forgiving people lifts a weight off your shoulders.*
>
> *So, thank you, Mama, for showing me at a young age that you do what you have to in order to take care of your family, even if you sometimes want to pull your hair out.*
>
> *Mel*

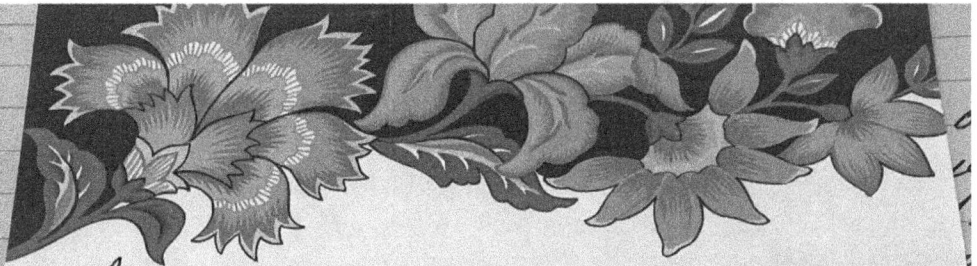

Dear Elle,
    Thank you for the nice card.
Its not you who should be thanking
us, but Leonard and I want to say
"thank you" from the bottom of our
hearts for the unbelievable care you
gave our sister, without a complaint,
for 10 long years. It will never
be forgotten.

# CHAPTER 75
# MAMA'S FIRST BIRTHDAY IN HEAVEN

TODAY MARKS the first birthday my mother was not here, touchable, tangible, huggable. But, oh, she was here in spirit. Even without her physical presence, that absolutely could not stop me from honoring and celebrating her life and legacy.

I woke up several times last night, smiled, and whispered out loud, "Happy birthday, Mama." I dreamed I was feeding her at the facility where she had lived for the past ten years. I've never had a dream like that. She looked great and was wearing a red mock turtleneck.

Yesterday, my daughter, Mel, told me she planned to drive to the gravesite with me this morning. Her gesture and thoughtfulness touched me. Within a few minutes, I received the sweetest text from my niece, Kelly. Cue the tears!

Thirty minutes passed by, and in my door walked Chrissy bearing gifts. She had the day off teaching school (Veterans Day). She brought me a slice of Mama's favorite cake, an Italian Cream Cake, and a flower arrangement with some of Mama's flowers she had incorporated in her recent wedding. She crawled into my lap, and I cried.

My two daughters were there to support their ole Mama, and all this transpired before 7:30 a.m.

311

We spent time at Mama's grave and I recounted stories to the girls of my "first rodeo" in the arena of grief when my father had died. I was 17, and it was in the spring of my high school senior year. Daddy was only a few blocks away from my office visiting his fishing buddy. From my office, I heard a siren that afternoon and like I had always been taught, I stopped and said a prayer for the patient. Little did I know, I was praying for my own father. My dad had suffered his fourth and final heart attack. He was given CPR at the scene and brought to the ICU where he stayed for one month before he succumbed to his fate. We went for visits, but Dad was uncommunicative. I was so torn up. Our relationship was never great. Dad was very serious and stern and had a bit of a short temper. I loved hearing him talk on the phone to his fishing buddies. He laughed and cut up with them and I loved hearing that side of him. He adored Mama. What lovebirds those two were. We dared not upset Mama or the wrath of Daddy would be upon our heads. With Daddy gone, I became painfully aware I had no opportunity to build a better relationship with him or introduce him to my future husband or his future grandchildren. I wanted him to be proud of me, to smile when he looked at me. In high school, I even took guitar lessons and learned his favorite artist's song to suck up to him. The artist was Johnny Cash.

After Dad's death, I was given his white Ford pick-up truck to drive until Mama could muddle through more important issues. That's where my love for trucks began. I felt Daddy was still with me. I played his beloved country music station just as he had always done and waved my hand to other drivers with the same little shake I had seen him do a thousand times, the pointer finger slightly higher than the other fingers. Silly, I know.

Several months later, my Mama decided to sell the truck, bringing my second wave of grief. Mama was occupied with many typical post-mortuary details and also my high school graduation followed by beginning college. Add to that mix, my sister's divorce. She and her four small children moved back home.

<hr/>

I felt awful for the new owner of my father's truck because this wrecked girl was stalking him. Everywhere I saw the truck, I left a note on the windshield or the driver's window. It was pathetic. In a small town, I saw Daddy's truck often. The pitiful notes read something like this:

Please take good care of my daddy's truck. He died this year and loved this truck.

OR

This is a great truck. My dad took excellent care of it. He's dead now.

OR

After my daddy died, I drove this truck. My Mama sold it, and now I have nothing of my dad's.

It's pathetic, right? That went on for six months, and I don't know if he painted the truck, sold it, or moved, but I never saw it again—poor guy.

During the same time, I was entering my first year of college. My Creative Writing class proved to be invaluable. I used the opportunity to research heart health, the left ventricle of the heart, ICU, and morticians. Sounds exciting, right? What every 17-year-old was interested in. They were all things involved in my father's passing. I dealt with this heavy heart as best I knew how, and writing was the perfect outlet.

I made straight A's in the class, but after my fourth paper, the professor asked me to stay after class. His conversation alluded to the fact I was freaking him out with all the death topics, and he wanted to hear, from my voice, about my father. Who he was, his hobbies, our relationship, and how he died. He cared. He knew I was fighting some demons. I am forever grateful to him for giving me a powerful outlet and also expressing his concern for me.

<hr/>

My first year after losing my Daddy I was a hot mess. I began drinking more, visiting the graveside more, and incessantly crying. Mama had returned to work and was occupied with her personal grief and new role as the primary breadwinner of the home. Looking back, I think she handled it very well. Her sister, Aunt Verda, had been a widow for a long time and held her hand through the entire process. I believe that made the transition to becoming a widow easier. Not easy, but easier.

⁂

When I met my future husband and realized he was the one, one of our dates was going to the gravesite and "introducing" him to my father. Weird, I know, but it was the last place I saw my father. My boyfriend was very understanding and compassionate. He didn't think less of me.

He didn't ditch me. He didn't think I was a freak show. This guy was a keeper. I never read about this tactic in the book "Dating for Success," but it worked for me. We didn't stay for long, but the fact he knew visiting the grave brightened my day, well, I knew he was something special. I married that guy the following year, and we recently celebrated 42 years together.

I continued this oddity with all four of my children. I brought them to the gravesite as infants and told Daddy all about them. My firstborn was named after my dad, and it turned out he resembled him, too. I'm happy to report, I am older now and have an ounce or two of maturity under my belt. I only visit the cemetery to replace the flowers and pay my respects on birthdays, anniversaries, and holidays.

⁂

I always encourage friends not to forget the family, especially the first year when they are going through major events like the first birthday, the first Christmas and Thanksgiving, the first anniversary, the first Mother's Day or Father's Day without their loved one. I don't even need to mention the anniversary of their death. It means so much not to feel forgotten. The pain doesn't go away as you drive away from the graveside. Actually, the reality begins to set in. Cards, letters, and phone calls are appreciated.

---

**A brief visit accompanied by a heartfelt hug might be even better. If you get nothing else from this book, please remember the families.**

---

⊷∞⊶

After my girls and I left the cemetery, we returned home, shared one slice of cake, and talked. I thoroughly enjoyed this much-needed time with my girls. Chrissy told me she planned to take me to lunch at Mama's favorite restaurant, Dairy Barn. I think they thought of everything. It made for a much better day all the way around. Lastly, Suzy called me to make sure I was okay. I was glad to report I was and I am. One day at a time, sweet Jesus.

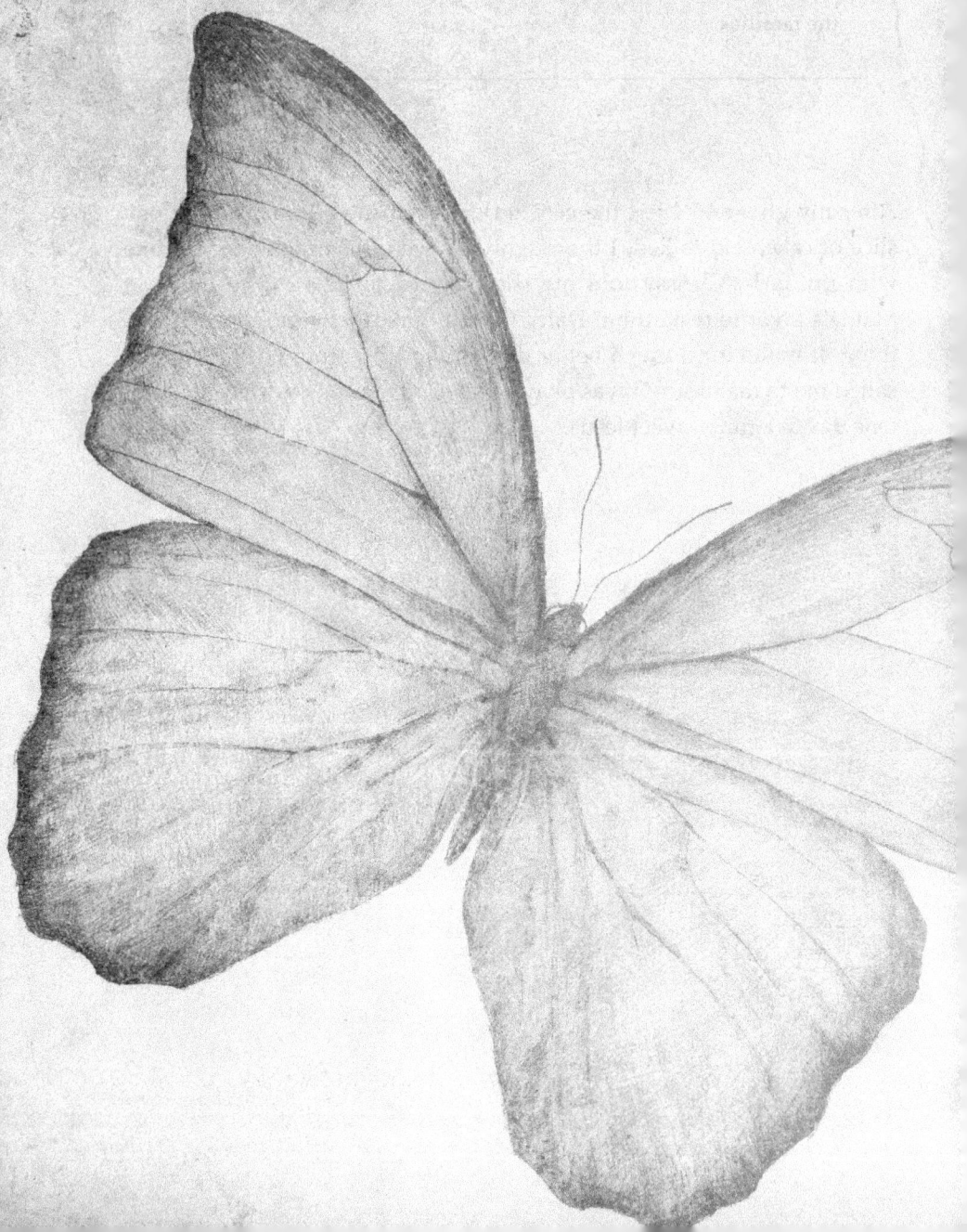

## CHAPTER 76

# THE FIRST ANNIVERSARY OF MAMA'S DEATH

A YEAR later we have walked through all the firsts and survived. My sisters and I filled the first couple of months with group calls on Marco Polo almost daily. (I highly recommend this app). It was very therapeutic. We *were* going to make it.

As I was walking out my door this morning, my daughter, Chrissy, and her husband, Austin, pulled up in the driveway. I thought, *these kids are GOLD! So thoughtful to remember Mama's anniversary.* About that time, the back door slides open, and out steps Suzy from Alabama. She was here for the first anniversary of Mama's death. I was so touched. Many, many hugs and tears all around. What a welcomed surprise.

Suzy joined me for my usual walk around the neighborhood and we enjoyed a beautiful time together. After we returned to my house, I got dressed to go to the cemetery. The two of us drove out to the country graveyard where several of our family members were laid to rest, including our father, our grandparents, and now our precious Mama. It was Suzy's first time to see the headstone with Mama's name engraved on it. After only seeing Daddy's name etched on the granite

317

headstone for forty years, it brought us some comfort to see our mother's name, too.

They were together again and it made our hearts happy. Thankfully, the grass had finally begun to cover the dirt that made it look barren for so long. We picked weeds around the headstone, wiped it off, and reminisced about the life of our mother. I was grateful to have my sister there with me.

⤙⟋⟍⤚

After my mama passed away, and still five years later, as I write this memoir, I noticed the most wonderful occurrence. In the past five years, more often than not, her birthdate, 11- 11, appeared on my phone as 11:11. In our bedroom, we have a red digital reflection of our clock that cast the time onto the ceiling. Again, it was not unusual to see 11:11 on our ceiling. It was a good night sign from her. When I get a text from someone with a sweet or poignant message and the time stamp is 11:11, I pause and am reminded she's not suffering anymore. Other times, as I play my music in the car and the perfect song comes on to remind me of my mother or to encourage me, the time stamp is, you guessed it, 11:11. Before Mama's passing, I don't remember ever noticing that happening. I've never had that happen with my father's or father-in-law's birthdates, either. It carried on Mama's tradition of making her birthdate a special one.

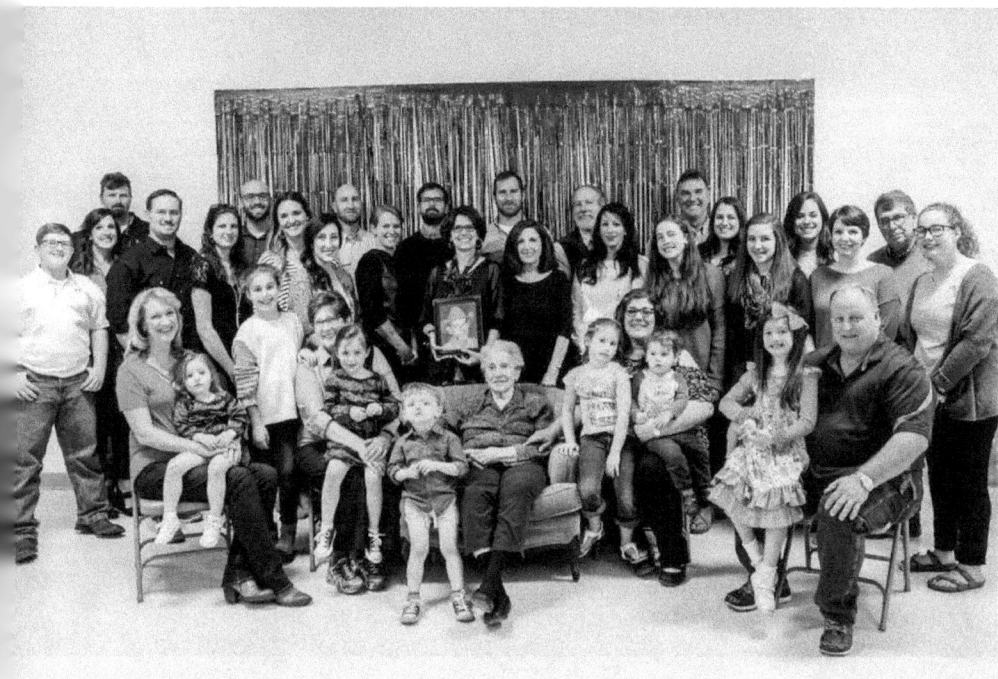

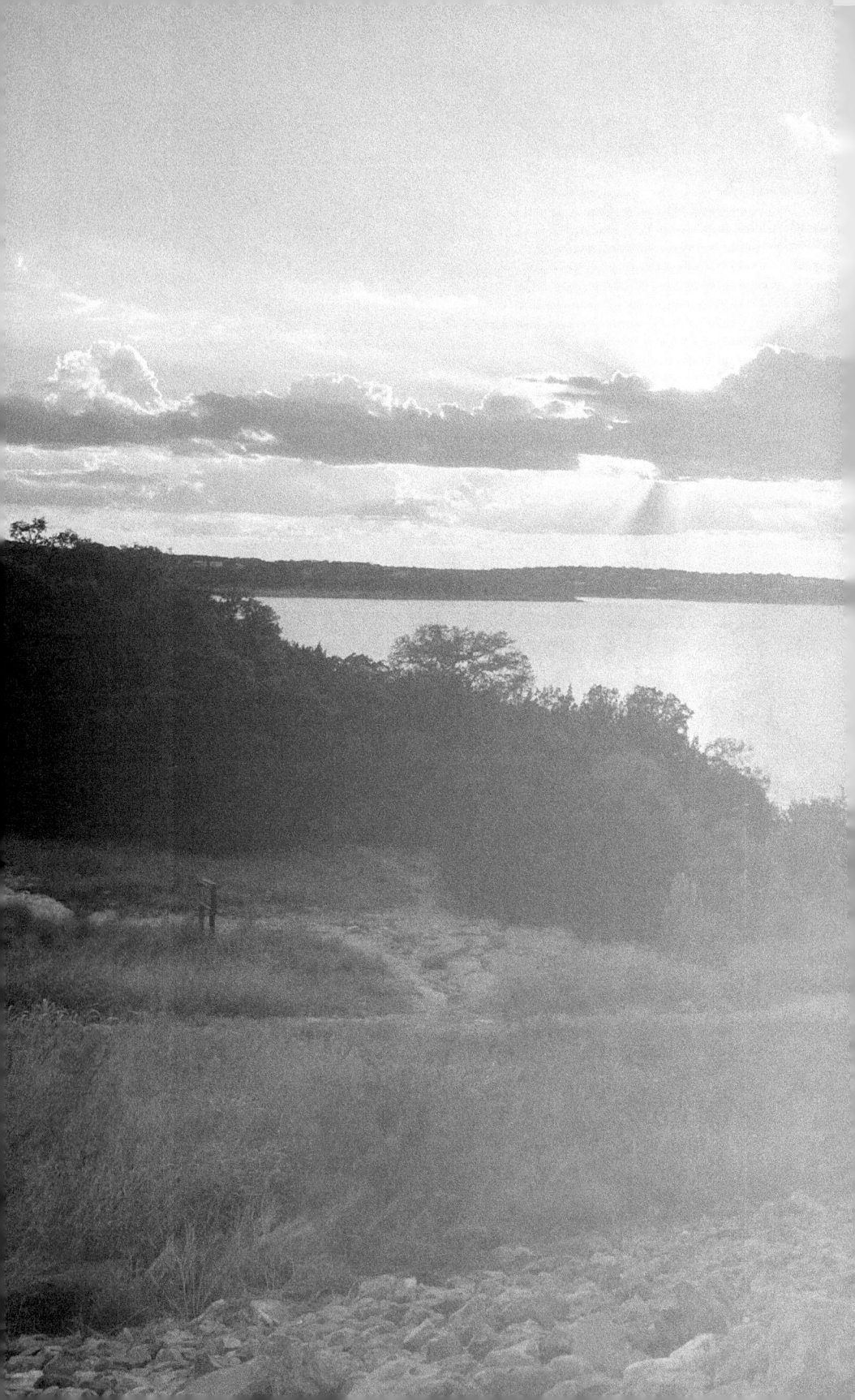

# CHAPTER 77
# MY PRAYER FOR YOU

MY PRAYER for everyone reading this memoir, is you find help, hope, a resolve to do your absolute best no matter what, and remember, the person you are caring for needs you. I can't say for how long, or at what level of care, but they need you.

---

Be present, be willing to learn the necessary skills, be flexible, love them as they are, don't try to change them and please don't correct them. Do everything you can so you do not have a single regret when they pass.

---

Be patient (yes, I said the "P" word), ask for help, and, as always, remember to take as many photos and videos as possible.

There is so much peace and healing in those two words...no regrets. You fight hard, you do your level best and you usher them down this treacherous path. I believe in you and I personally thank you for not turning a blind eye to someone in need.

~~~

Please, please, please be their advocate in all things. Find a support system. Lean heavily on the Lord. He will be your saving grace.

I wish you a burdenless journey. I pray you can look back on your journey and see how much you've grown and see you are a stronger and better person in every area of your life as a result of it. You can't be a caregiver and not be changed in some way, shape, or form.

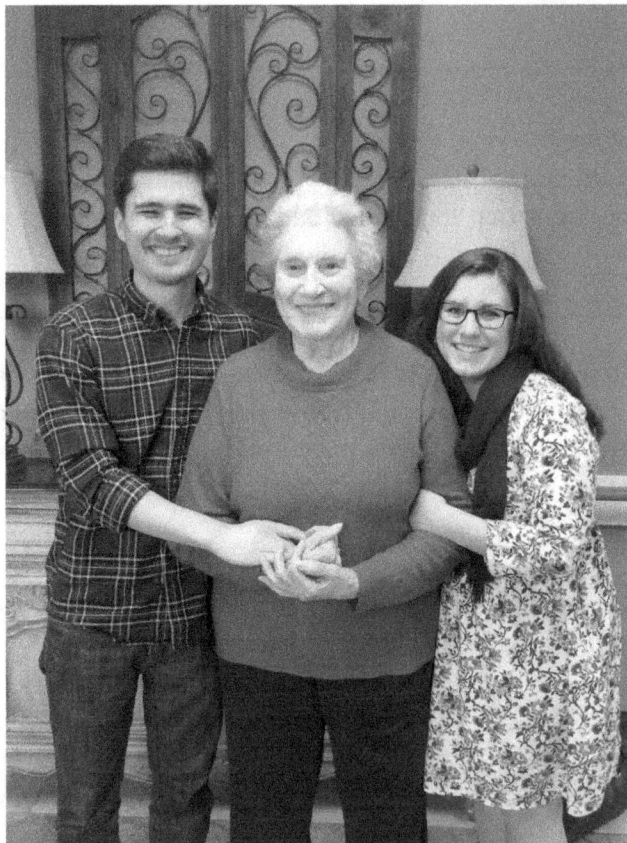

Mama with her granddaughter, Maddie, and her husband, Nick

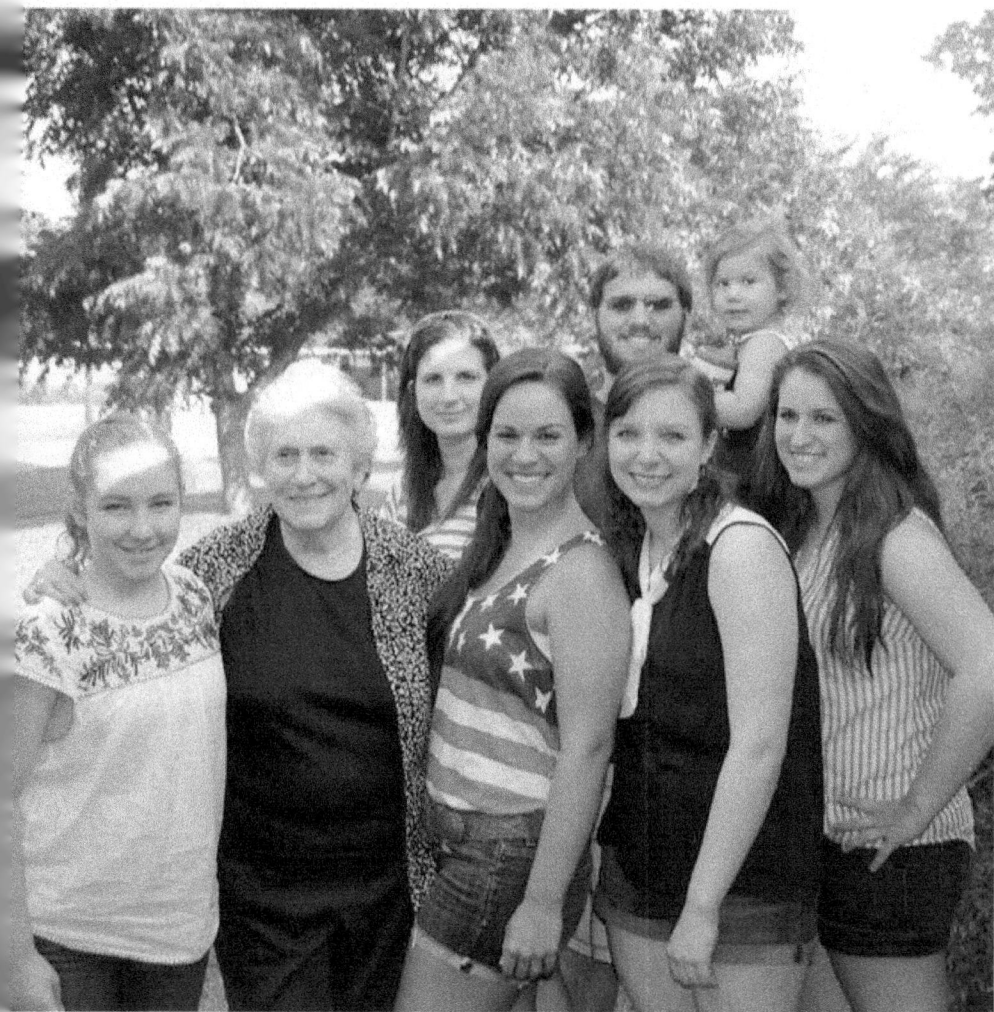

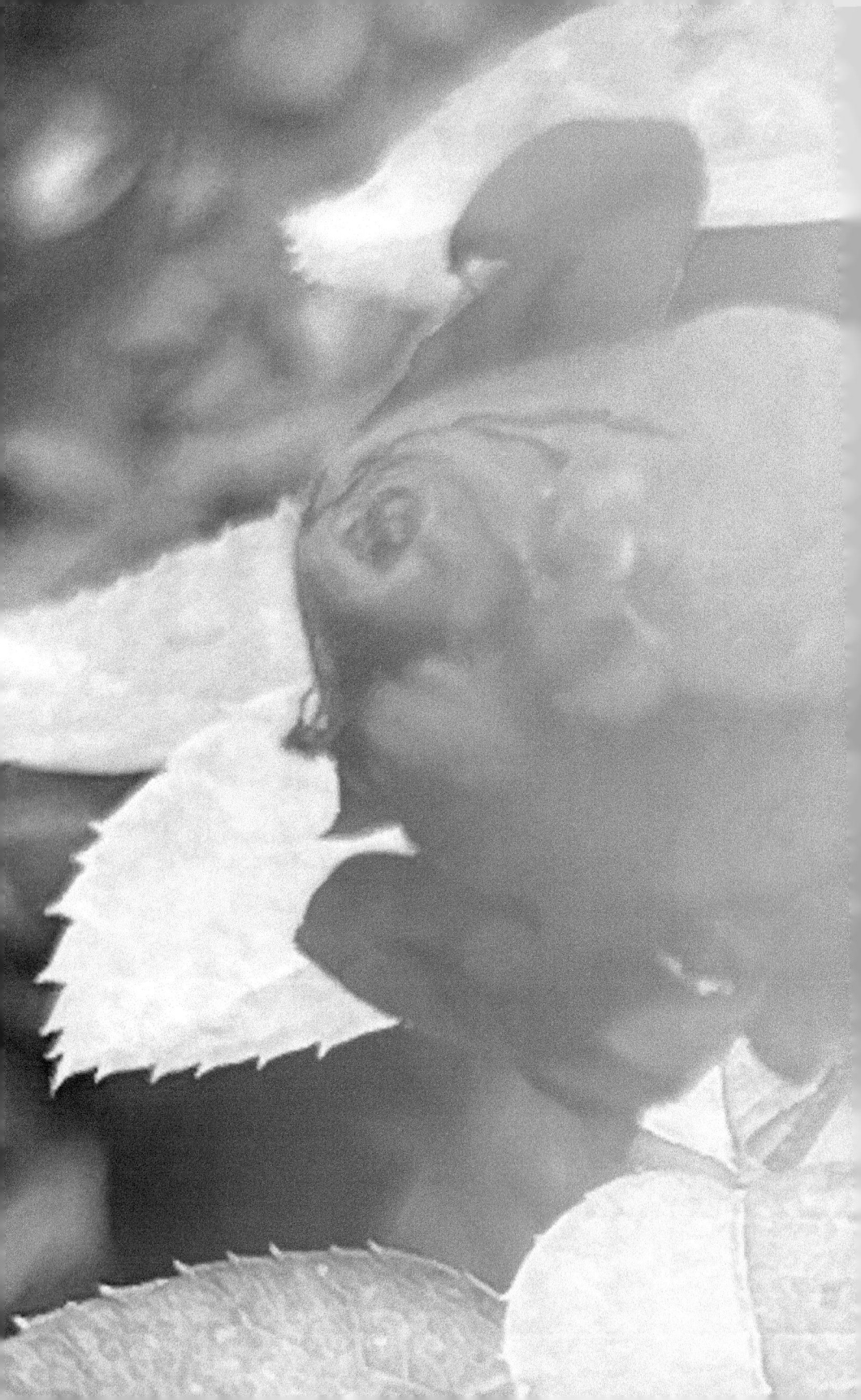

# EPILOGUE

Mama, I am deeply grateful for our newfound closeness when it wasn't always so. I was extremely honored God put me and my family in a position to be your caregivers, even when it was the most challenging thing to do most days. I am thankful for the long car rides, looking at landscaping and beautiful homes; thankful for Dairy Queen Blizzards; thankful you taught me NOT to act my age but turn up the music and dance until you couldn't anymore.

I'm grateful for your undying love for Daddy, even though he was only a vague memory to you for the past decade. I am grateful for your pride in your children, grandchildren, and great-grandchildren – and your love of our country and Jesus, our Savior. He was your rock, your fortress, and nothing comforted you like those old hymns and daily prayers.

I love you, Norma Jean. You are one of a kind, and I am blessed beyond measure to call you Mama, Mother, Crazy Woman, whatever. I wish more people in this world could have a Mama like you. Over the last few years, I have learned what an irreplaceable treasure you are. I pray I have inherited your best traits and pass those onto my children, grandchildren, and great-grandchildren. I love you, sweet Mama.

# NORMA PETTIJOHN

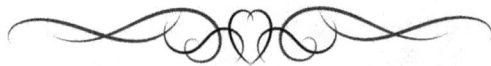

## REST IN PEACE

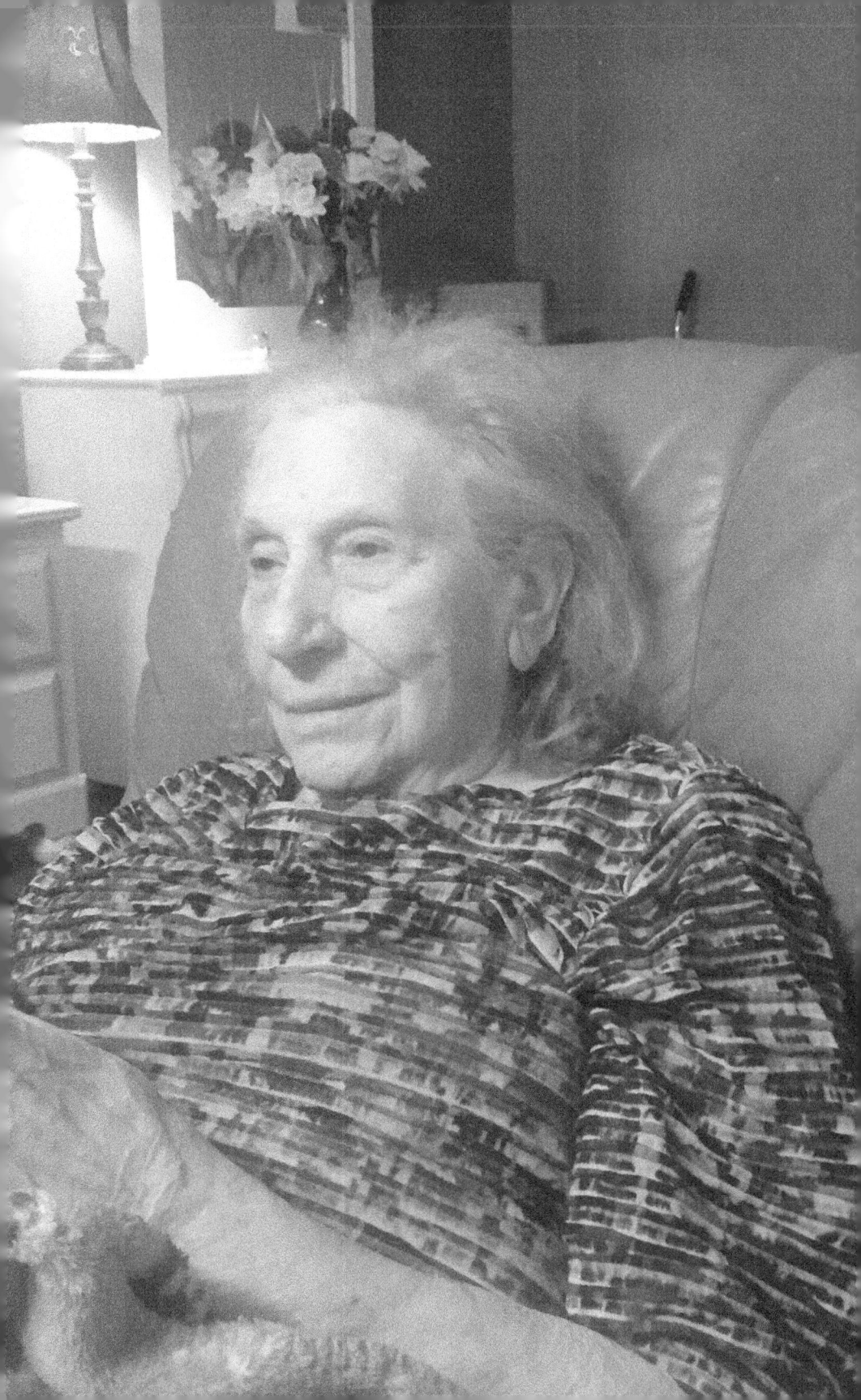

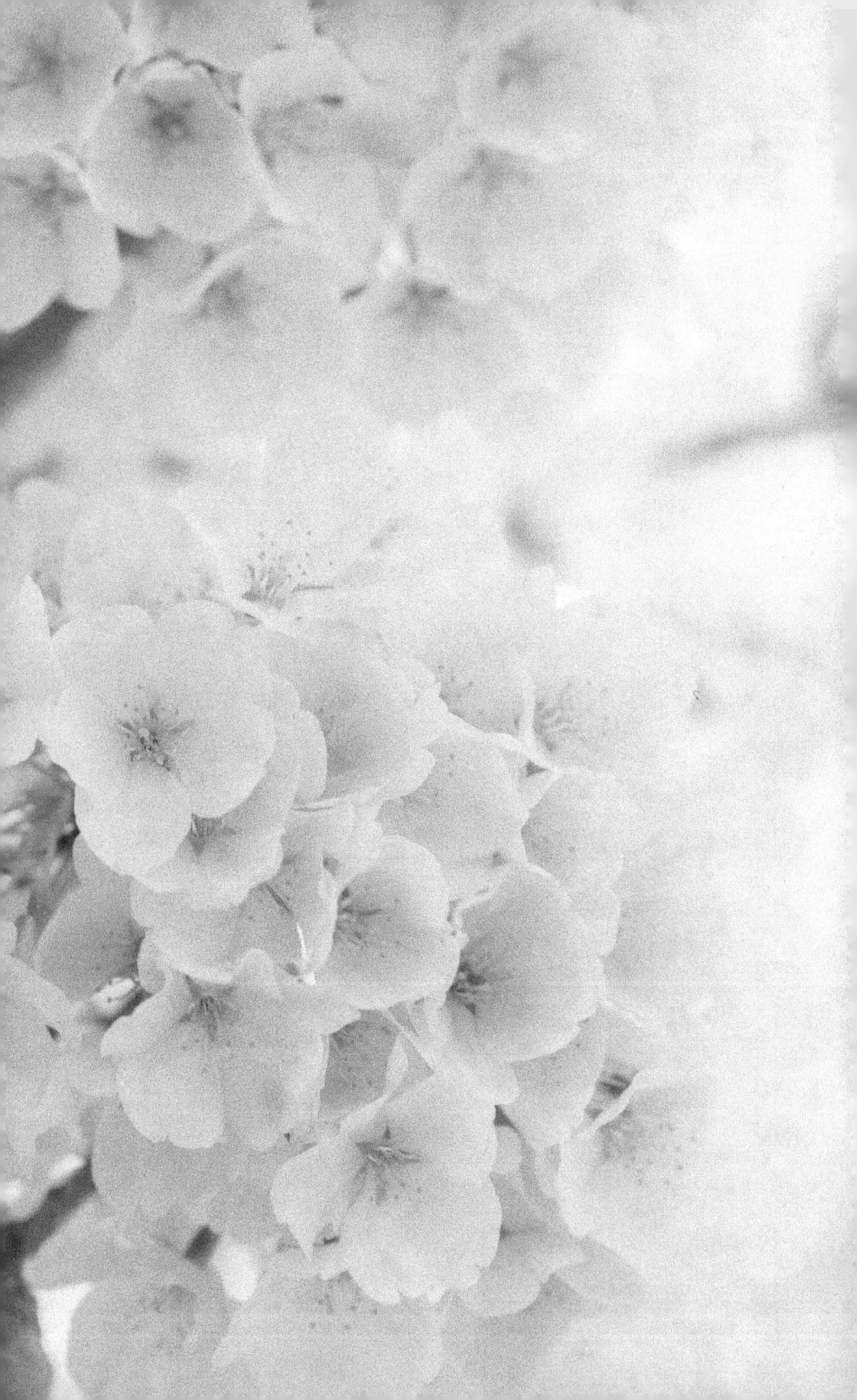

# CAREGIVERS TESTIMONIALS

The stories on the following pages are for you, the reader. I trust you will take the time to read them. I promise you will be moved, inspired, and educated. Each caregiver has a different journey. Some care for their person entirely at home, others are living in nursing homes, assisted living, or memory units. Diagnoses and disabilities differ.

In an attempt to give my readers a broader scope of experiences, I asked friends of mine to write about their journey. Some of them refused, apologizing, stating it was just too painful to go back there. They couldn't do it. I respect each of them immensely. Several called me, needing encouragement and clarification. I told each one, "I just want to hear your voice because your experience matters to me and to those who will read it."

When they understood it was for the purpose of helping others, they allowed themselves to be vulnerable. I know all too well when you try to put an emotionally and physically difficult experience on paper, it is tough! I'm so proud of each of them for pushing through their tears and memories and allowing me to share their stories.

I am forever grateful.

# THE CAREGIVER'S TRIBUTE

## BY ELLEN PETTIJOHN STEPHENS

YOU MAY NOT HAVE HAD a choice when the need arose, but you answered the call without regard to the cost.

It is daunting, time-consuming, emotionally draining, back-breaking, and lonely. You navigate through unnatural, undesirable, and awkward emotions as you decipher your new lead role in your loved one's life.

It may not have been in your wheelhouse of Fortune 500 companies, and your name will never be on letterhead or an office door, but the impact you have made on this individual has dividends that far outweigh most all occupations.

It's complicated, gut-wrenching, ever-changing, and downright scary. But with all the burden, you get the blessings, too. The thank you's, "I appreciate you," the chant of "love you, love you, love you," the kisses on your hands, their head on your shoulder showing you their love and appreciation, and hand holding. Thousands of times, you've held their hand to guide them, but a thousand more, they've clutched yours because you are their rock, their strong tower.

You are the unsung hero.

You are the escort in their final walk.

You are the Caregiver.

# THE FROZEN MOMENTS

## BY ITASCA CASTILLE BROUSSARD

My friend, Itasca Castille Broussard, beautifully penned this, and allowed me to use it here as a reminder of "The Frozen Moments." I am so thankful, Itasca.

"TODAY, if you are sitting with a loved one or if you are in the waiting, I lift a prayer for you and remind you that YOU ARE NOT ALONE. God sees, God knows, and God cares.

※

"There are moments in our lives that seem to be frozen in time. Not always events that we are happy to recall or desire to live again, but moments that seem to capture the true meaning of our existence. Being there with anticipation as those we love make their last exhale. Knowing that God is the giver of life and death and partaking in an event that only He can orchestrate gives richer meaning to those frozen moments. For the believer to exhale on earth means to inhale an eternity of the perfect breath of life.

"I'm grateful God allowed me precious moments at the bedside of my mother-in-law. There were many through the years but none so life-changing as the last one. It's a moment that is frozen in time."

# TAKE THE TIME TO BE PRESENT

## BY DENISE BROUSSARD FREY

AT THE AGE OF 78, my mother, *Jolene Broussard*, found herself alone for the first time since my dad died. In 2013, Mom unfortunately had to have her left leg amputated below the knee, leaving her with a prothesis.

At that time, I, along with a couple of my siblings, alternated staying with Mom. In 2015, I moved in with Mom. My younger brother lived there as well. Together, we cared for Mom until I remarried and moved from Louisiana to Texas in December of that year. Fast forward two years.

My brother moved out of Mom's house, leaving a couple of us to care for her during the weekdays and him on most weekends. I traveled to Louisiana from Texas once a month, staying five to six days, 24 hours a day. As time went on, the frequency of my visits changed to as often as every other week. That was my life for the next five years until Mom passed away on March 20, 2022. It was so hard, emotionally, to see the physical decline of my mother. Separating my time between Mom and my husband was very stressful. I felt so guilty no matter where I was.

I'm thankful for all the special one-on-one time I was blessed to have with Mom. She told me so many stories and I was able to see

Mom for not only the wonderful person she was to me, but also the girl and young woman she was long ago. She shared stories about growing up, her family, and the early years of her and my dad's marriage. I loved going through old picture albums with Mom as she described each one.

My mom was such a strong woman until the end. During this time, I learned that I could do **anything** that I **had** to do because with God, *everything is possible!* (Matthew 19:26) God was definitely with me through all those trying years. *"Come to me, all you who are weary and carry heavy burdens, and I will give you rest."* (Matthew 11:28-30)

"To care for those who once cared for us is one of the highest honors."[1]

---

1. Tia Walker, The Inspired Caregiver: Finding Joy While Caring For Those You Love.

# KEEP THEM ACTIVE

## BY CHERYL REDMOND

MY DAD, *Wilbert Bourgeois*, was diagnosed with an early stage of Alzheimer's at the age of 62. One thing I learned to be very beneficial was to obtain a proper diagnosis from a medical professional proficient with treatment options for Alzheimer's patients and to get the patient on medicine right away. I attribute the early admission of medicine to the enhanced quality of life and the prolonged life he was able to live for the next 12 years.

As my father became more forgetful, we noticed the family dynamics changing. It was hard for my mother to accept that her soul mate for 50+ years was no longer the person she so heavily relied upon for daily activities. As time progressed and my father's condition deteriorated, we had to separate our parents to give both him and my mother a break. As his condition further progressed and our mother passed away, my sister and I became his primary caregivers for eight years. My other siblings chipped in whenever possible.

It was very sad and frustrating to accept times when your own father didn't recognize you nor had the basic abilities to accomplish simple tasks like feeding himself, but we never tried to make him remember something or someone – it only irritated him more.

It was very helpful to do activities with my dad that stimulated the brain. We had him do easy puzzles, elementary math sheets, play catch with the dog, or swing outside and sing songs from his time. He even read the newspaper to us orally every day. After hearing the front page several times, one of us yelled, "Turn the page." To lighten the mood of a really bad day, we turned on something like "Golden Girls"- you couldn't help but laugh at them. My dad belly laughed through several episodes. We tried to avoid telling him what to do as a command. Instead, we said, "It's your turn" (to bathe), or "Let's try this" (and let him think all along that it was his idea).

My dad was an electrician, so some days we turned off the breaker to a certain outlet on the counter and told him it needed to be repaired. Trying to fix the wires literally kept him busy for hours. They have no concept of time so he thought he was repairing it by taking wires apart and putting them back together over and over and never became frustrated. My dad followed my husband around the barn, or as he worked on rent houses. We took him everywhere including numerous camping and boating trips. He always enjoyed being with family, even if he didn't recall our names at times.

The hardest part of being a caregiver was the mental awareness of what he was doing at all times. For safety, we installed alarms on all of the doors. Some of the best advice I could give to others in this situation is to always REDIRECT!

If something was not working or frustrating the loved one, change direction. Having a routine keeps you mentally in check. If physically possible for the loved one, take them everywhere, for instance, church, grocery shopping, and restaurant dining. Our kids played tournament ball, so we took my dad camping out of town every weekend to ball games.

More great advice is to have a backup to give yourself a break once in a while. I utilized my husband, my teenage kids, or their friends to play cards or games with my dad while I was gone.

I mentioned that my sister shared the responsibility of caregiver with us. However, we lived three hours away from each other. So, at the beginning, we each kept him a month at a time. As the Alzheimer's worsened, we met in the middle and relieved each other every 3 weeks, then 2 weeks, then every other week. This was a great mental relief for myself and my sister. Neither my sister nor I could have kept him home for so many years without each other. It did get to the point of placing him in a facility for the last nine months of his life.

The entire experience was a great lesson for our children to learn respect for the elderly. They shared in the load on a daily basis. We relied on God and His Word to get us through. We stood on Phil 4:13: *"For I can do everything through Christ who gives me strength,"* and Isaiah 41:10: *"Don't be afraid, for I am with you. Don't be discouraged, for I am your God. I will strengthen you and help you. I will hold you up with my victorious right hand."*

# THE GIFT OF TIME

## BY KATE CHRISTIAN

My name is Kate, and I was Jason, my husband's caregiver for 14 months. On January 21, 2021, at the age of 43, he was diagnosed with stage 4 pancreatic cancer. From that moment, our lives changed drastically and to some extent, for the better. When you get a terminal diagnosis, it shifts your perspective to what really matters: for us that was focusing on God and making sure our children knew Jesus. Thankfully we both already knew Jesus and three of our four children had already been saved and baptized. Knowing that gave Jason a great level of peace.

I had already quit my job six months prior, and I remained off work to be home with him throughout his chemo treatments. He owned his own business and made the decision to give the business over to the employees running it. He didn't want to spend whatever time he had left working or negotiating the sale of it. After a few months, he worked very little. His first treatment was Folfirinox, which was the standard of care for advanced pancreatic cancer. It was administered through his port once every two weeks. He came home with a bag to be administered through the port for 48 hours afterward. The most noticeable side effect initially was neuropathy in his hands and feet.

He tried to stay active at first, but as time progressed, the side effects worsened and it eventually affected his vision.

One of the most difficult parts of caring for him was not being able to manage his pain, especially in the last couple of months. Morphine was the medicine prescribed for pain. At first, lower doses morning and night were given; then every four hours in between.

For the last six weeks, liquid morphine could be given every hour in addition to the other doses of morphine.

I remember quietly crying in bed next to him when he was trying to sleep yet unable to because of the pain. One of the side effects of morphine was constipation, which was very painful. On top of the cancer spreading, we tried to manage the pain of constipation. It was heartbreaking to watch, but I tried not to let him see me upset because that just made it worse for him.

During the first 10 months after Jason's diagnosis, I stayed active and walked a lot to manage my stress. I had lunch with friends and talked about my fears that I didn't want to burden Jason with. I napped when he napped. Even when we traveled, we did our best to come home for Sunday church. Our family and church family were huge support systems through his illness. We also played golf which allowed us to be outside and spend time together.

Six weeks before he died, he became anxious, which I know now was part of the disease/ dying process, but at the time we didn't know what it was and thought he was very near death. We called everyone to come visit and it was an emotional day.

He never really felt better after that. For the last six weeks of his life, he was in an extreme amount of pain. I had to write all his medications down because he was taking so many that I could not remember the time and dosages of them.

A huge benefit, especially in the last couple of months, was allowing people to help us. They offered to bring food and pick up his medicine. I permitted them to because I knew that was their way of loving us and at that point, I didn't feel safe leaving Jason to go run errands. Before he got sick, Jason never needed anything, so he was a little hesitant to receive help, but I reminded him how much we loved helping others, so we needed to allow others to help us in our time of need.

He remained at home until four days before he died. He became scared to take his medicine orally because he had a hard time keeping anything down at that point. He asked me to take him to a nearby medical facility. We found a beautiful, hospice retreat where He died peacefully. With the family surrounding us, and while I held his hand, he passed away.

Along with the physical pain, obviously, the emotional toll was high for both of us. There were moments toward the end when he knew he was dying, and he just cried out for his children because he would be leaving them. This was our second marriage, so the three younger children were his from his first marriage. He only had limited time with them and that made it so much worse.

I tried to be strong and let him know that he had done his job here on earth and that God would take care of us. There were many times as I was caring for him that I told him how much I loved him because I never knew, towards the end, when God was going to take him. One time, in the middle of the night after I said that, he said, "I know you do or you would not be doing all this for me."

Although it was the most difficult time in our lives, it gave me the opportunity to show him how much I loved him and that truly was a gift from God. We had 14 months to talk about many things. He got a chance to tell me all the things he wanted for me in the event he died, and I know many wives don't get that. I got to see him draw closer to the Lord more than ever before and have immense gratitude for the life he had been given. He often wept at God's grace and mercy for him. It was so beautiful. We got to know each other and love each other in the most beautiful ways. We spent a lot of time talking and reading our Bibles. When he could not read anymore, I read to him, or we listened to sermons online. In the end, he just wanted to sit in silence, and I knelt next to him and just held his hand. I truly believe he was in that thin space between heaven and earth during those last two weeks. If we could keep his physical pain managed, he was filled with peace. A peace that was only from the Lord.

It was an honor to be able to care for my husband. Looking back, I know the Lord gave us both strength to get through the most difficult days, and he still gives me strength today to walk through my grief with hope.

# THE VALUE OF SITTERS

## BY CATHY WATTS

MY DAD PASSED into the arms of Jesus on August 30, 2022. He had dementia for about four years, the last two years were the worst.

We were blessed to be able to keep him in his home with the help of 24-hour care. My dear friend, Ellen, was able to pass on her knowledge and list of caregivers that was a lifesaver for us.

My dad had lost his ability to speak and eat towards the end, but his caregivers were able to guide us in ways to help ease his discomfort. Everyone's journey with this horrible disease is different and having a strong support system is necessary.

My best advice to anyone going through this with a loved one is don't be afraid to ask for help because it truly takes a village! Ellen, you were the best part of my village!

# A DEATH DOULA

## BY FAITH HARRISON

In January 2018, my 67-year-old veteran husband was officially diagnosed with ALS, Amyotrophic Lateral Sclerosis. All we knew about it at the time was that it was surely terminal and a baseball player named Lou Gehrig died from it. We learned all too soon that it results in progressive loss of motor neurons that control voluntary muscles, progressing to the point of rendering its chosen vessel completely frozen, trapped in a body that couldn't move, speak, swallow, and in worse case scenarios, couldn't even move the eyeballs. We were told the mind stays intact. That's not always true. They lie when they say it is not painful.

I affectionately and privately called my husband, Mr. Plumb Bob, after the builder's tool. A plumb bob establishes a straight vertical line. It never lies and it lasts forever. He kept our life going in a straight direction, and never lied, but did not last forever.

Now you would think upon receiving a death sentence, such a man would be devastated, angry, and bitter at God, not Mr. Plumb Bob. In military terms, he told himself he was being rescued from the enemy's camp. Life to him was a prison of tenacious nightmares from childhood abuse and family tragedies, from gruesome combat and subsequent PTSD. However, through all of his life's heartbreaks, his heart's song was, "I love you, Lord, I love you." My heart's prayer was for a miracle.

The first non-medical person I asked about the disease was a man whose wife had recently passed away from ALS. Over the phone, he told me, "You have a rough road ahead of you and you will know what it was like for Mary to watch her Son die on His cross."

My daughter, who is a nurse, told me, "Mama, you are Papa's death doula now." "Doula? What's a doula?" I asked. "A midwife, Mama. Birth and death are both transitions. You have been chosen to help him. It's a sacred rite. This is probably the most significant thing you will ever do in your life."

The living room of our little condo became his hospital room. The VA provided his bed, Hoyer lift, shower transfer chair, power wheelchair and wheelchair van, bi-pap machine, and cough assist. *All the stuff*. Then came Covid. My world became very small.

As the ALS progressed, he developed frontal lobe dementia, leaving him both mentally and physically handicapped. A VA-assigned psychologist put him through a few tests and told me, "You are the brain for both of you now."

He couldn't understand why when he dialed 411 the operator wouldn't put him through to the President of the United States so he could get his combat orders. He escaped out the door in his power chair with his shaving kit and his Bible, wearing only his underwear, a T-shirt, and his Vietnam Veteran cap heading for the airport to go to Desert Storm.

Sometimes, he didn't know who I was and demanded that I take him to his house. He watched the same movies over and over again, *Shrek* and *King of Kings*, (an old Jesus movie).

One day, while watching *King of Kings* for the 100th plus time, he ordered me to help him "walk" to the TV believing if he touched Jesus on the screen, he would be healed. By then, attempting to get out of bed resulted in the need to call the paramedics who most likely would not come, plus I had given up on the idea of a miracle. I stopped him. That moment of conflict haunted me more than any other along the journey.

Initially, I had a very romantic idea of my beloved dying in my arms, gazing up at me and with his last breath telling me, I was the best thing that ever happened to him. The end was not like that. I felt like a failure.

Several months after he died, I was still exhausted, alone, and very, very hard on myself. I worked up the courage to seek help from a Pastor in my area who had a very eventful healing ministry. I knew of him, but he didn't know me. We met in his office and I poured out my heart of self-doubt saying, "I could have done better." Thinking maybe he would say something cliche like, "No, I'm sure you did everything you could."

Instead, he said, "We all could do better than we do, but that is not what I'm thinking when I see you. I see a broken heart. Do you know what a geode is? It is a rock that looks very ordinary on the outside, but when broken open it is extraordinary. There is a unique surprise in each one of the beautiful crystals. That's what I see when I look at you. That's what this experience formed in your heart."

I drove home pondering his words and reflecting on my caregiver journey. I was so very inadequate to the task, completely dependent upon the mercy of God and others, and not accustomed to asking for help. Yet at every challenging juncture, in every moment of panic, in every need for comfort and encouragement, serendipitously help was there. My faith in humankind grew from cynicism to gratitude because of my vulnerability. I never knew there were so many kind-hearted, selfless, generous people in the world until I needed them. People in the care industry were angels in disguise. I am still in touch with two of my husband's caregivers. This year, on Memorial Day, both of them visited his grave at Tahoma National Cemetery. One left flowers; the other popped a chilled Corona beer and toasted him.

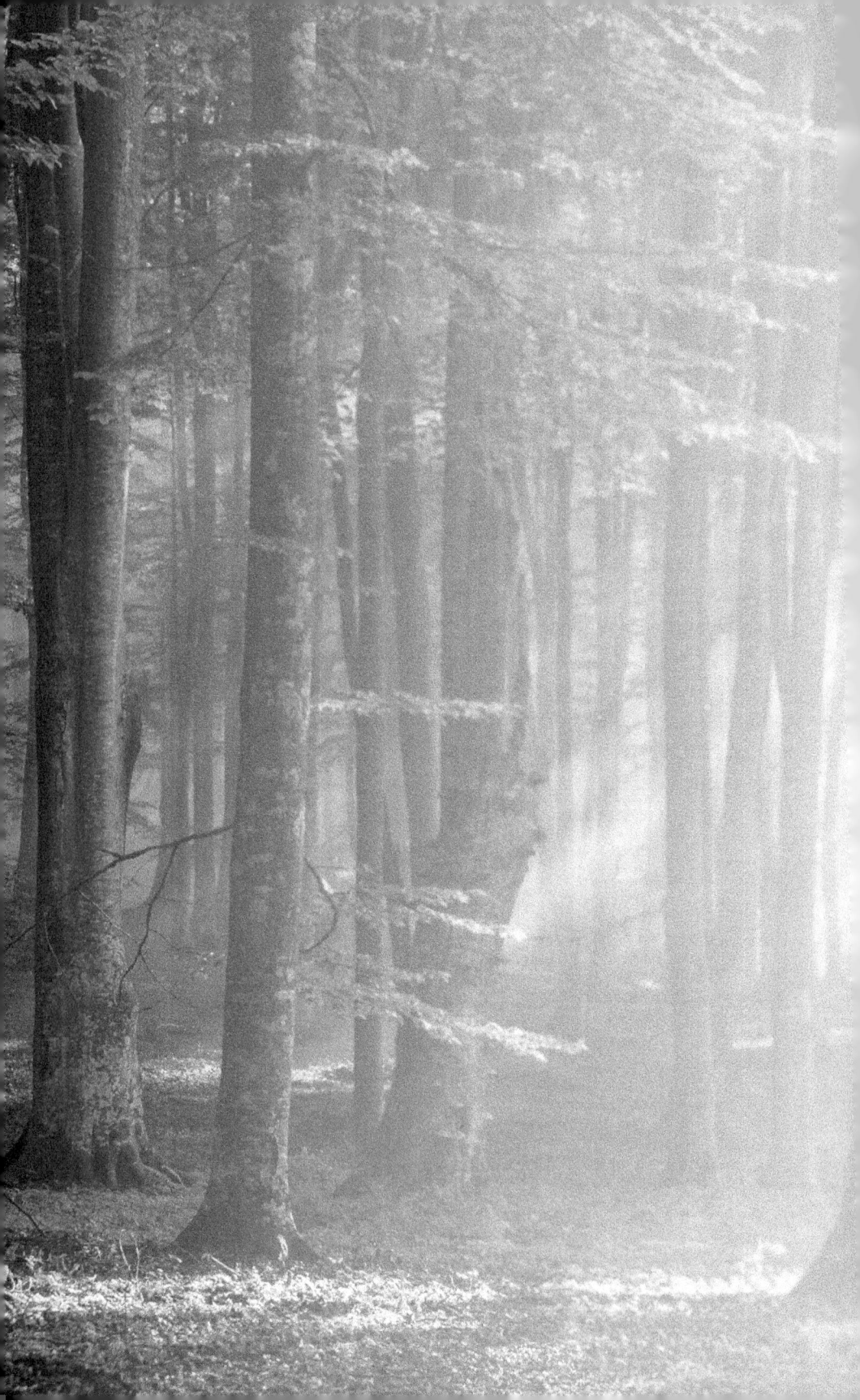

# IN SICKNESS AND IN HEALTH

## BY DONALD M.

I'M CURRENTLY the caregiver for my wife whom I have been married to for 45 years. She has been diagnosed with VCP (Valosin-containing Protein associated multisystem proteinopathy, Inclusion body myopathy associated with Paget Disease of the bone). She came to this diagnosis when she began to have trouble walking, and it progressed to the point where she could no longer walk in 2015. I retired at that time and became her sole caregiver. I was blessed to have worked for a company that enabled me to be able to retire early, as I couldn't imagine anyone at this point that could do a better job of helping her than me, and I see it as a PRIVILEGE to be able to do it!

The hardest part for me was watching this mean and unrelenting disease steal away her ability to do the physical things she loved such as gardening, crafting, sewing and I think most of all, our ability to travel. Fortunately, we were blessed to be able to do extensive travel earlier in our lives, and have been able to reflect on those travels with fond memories. It's also hard to see that our children and our grandchildren don't engage with her like we see them do with other family members because of the limitations she has with traveling and getting out.

Through all of this, again, I am blessed! This woman, while dealing with the daily struggles of just performing normal activities, was very faithful to her God. Rarely, if ever, does she have any 'pity parties.' It amazes me to see her have a positive outlook on life with what she was faced with. I'm very fortunate, as a husband and a caregiver.

I think caregivers are a special group of people, and bring tremendous quality of life to those we are supporting. I think it's important for folks doing this full-time to have some hobbies that can be done while allowing them to provide the support needed. Take up gardening, build an animated, Christmas light show, and learn some new programs that facilitate you to be able to do things you never imagined. Always look for things you can do that you enjoy with the responsibilities you have in mind.

Again, in my case, I see what I do for my wife as a caregiver a privilege. I know that if the tables were turned, she would be there 110 percent for me! Our love for each other is strong! A saying that I think of every day is "Be kind! Everyone you meet is fighting a battle you know nothing about." To all the caregivers out there, God bless you, and thank you! You are making a difference in someone's life today.

# NOTHING MORE DIFFICULT THAN CAREGIVING

## BY TAMARA MONSOUR

MY CAREGIVER'S journey began after recognizing pronounced behavioral and mental changes in my husband. After making multiple visits to various medical specialists, the last thing my husband expected to hear from a neurologist on his 57th birthday was, "I'm sorry to tell you that you have advancing moderate-stage Alzheimer's disease." Both of our lives changed drastically that day - he became the patient and I became the caregiver.

The job of caregiving is every bit as difficult as it sounds. I was working full-time in a stressful position in addition to navigating this uncharted territory. I felt terribly unprepared, unqualified, ill-equipped, and incapable of fulfilling my new role. The caregiving role is something I had to learn; caregiving, at least for me, was on-the-job training as I did not have a nurturing temperament nor the patience necessary for this very important job. Learning how to be a caretaker took much prayer and practice. From the beginning, I had the mindset to treat and make the right decisions for my husband, as I would like for someone to care for me if I were the one with the disease. That mindset proved important as many critical decisions had to be made through our Alzheimer's journey.

Prayer was absolutely essential and was the most valuable tool for me. Supernatural help was needed. My personal testimony is that prayer works! Topics prayed about included the following:

- To find the best physicians and medications
- To keep my husband safe while I was at work
- To let me know when it was time to put him in a memory care facility, not being too early nor too late in making this decision
- To direct me to the right memory care facility
- For financial help
- For strength and patience
- To be merciful to my husband, as this incurable disease turned him into someone no longer recognizable

Answers to prayer flowed continually; sometimes the answers were simply overwhelming to me. Knowing that God was listening and responding in such clear and miraculous ways was the primary factor that got me through this extremely difficult time.

In addition to learning as much as possible about the disease, I also did a great deal of research on how to be an effective caretaker. Talking with doctors, psychologists, and other caretakers was extremely informational as was reading recommended books. *The 36-Hour Day: A Family Guide to Caring for People Who Have Alzheimer's Disease, Related Dementias, and Memory Loss* by Nancy L. Mace, M.A. and Peter V. Rabins, M.D., M.P.H. is one of the best comprehensive books I found on the subject. The book contains valuable information including helpful tips on legal and financial matters that should be discussed with your loved one now rather than later.

While statistics indicate that Alzheimer's can be a slowly progressing disease, don't put complete faith in that statistic. Our journey from diagnosis until the end of life was 5 1/2 years, as my husband was later diagnosed with Frontotemporal Dementia along with Alzheimer's - a double whammy, which significantly shortened his life.

Everything his physician recommended we did. We saw a memory care specialist in Houston, TX. We researched and found a clinical trial for an Alzheimer's drug that was being conducted in our hometown. This clinical trial was found at www.clinicaltrials.gov.

You will quickly learn as a caregiver, safety is paramount. Alzheimer's patients quickly forget basic household routines such as how long to heat something in a microwave. Mowing and using other motorized tools suddenly become extreme hazards. Even very simple tasks like watering the flowerbeds quickly became complicated in a way I could not understand as my husband believed the front door needed to be watered which flooded the foyer. Putting out fires, cleaning up water, and being a watchdog over every movement suddenly became part of everyday life. The Alzheimer's patient becomes angry and frustrated, even combative, as they work to define a "new normal." My husband could not grasp that while he was still physically capable of completing these tasks, he no longer exercised good judgment and could have suffered serious injury had he been allowed to do the things he had always enjoyed.

One helpful caregiving technique employed to reduce his degree of frustration was to name the disease, in this case - "Big Al." When he became angry because he was forbidden to do something like drive, take a walk alone, mow, or use the microwave, I said, "I am not going to argue with 'Big Al' today." This statement was designed to remind him that the disease, not the restrictions, was causing his anger.

Early on as a caregiver, I had the idea that I could do it all and be in control over everything. I could not have been more wrong. My advice is to learn to say "yes" to offers of help from friends and family. Currently, as a 63-year-old, I have plenty of life experiences and challenges upon which to reflect. None of these have been more difficult, both physically and mentally, than my role as a caregiver. Nothing has given me more gratitude than the people who gave of themselves unselfishly during that time. Friends took my husband on short outdoor outings, which he greatly enjoyed. His daughter routinely took him to Sunday School and church on Sundays. This 3-hour weekly outing was so essential for me to have a stress-free break which was a much- needed refreshment for my mind and soul. As a caretaker, you need and deserve a break!

My daughters and I visited all of the area nursing homes with memory care units long before one was needed. We were all in total agreement on the facility that was best for him, as well as for our family. Once it was very clear that it was no longer safe for him to be at home, the transition was much easier, since we had made the facility selection when we were not under the pressure of a time restraint. The staff at the facility was absolutely wonderful to my husband as well as to our family. Visiting frequently and establishing good communication with the staff from the onset is important for all to have the best experience during this difficult time in life.

Having no prior experience with Alzheimer's, I was not prepared to hire feeders and then later, full-time sitters. Family and friends helped when they could, but with nearly everyone working full-time, outside help was essential. My husband stayed at one facility until the last three weeks of his life when advanced care was needed. In hindsight, I should have moved him sooner to the advanced care facility as they had the equipment and resources to keep him more comfortable at the end of his life.

Our family had nothing but great respect for the staff at both facilities. Trust them to care for your loved one. Trust the reports they give you. Be prepared for reports of loss of modesty and boundaries as well as uncharacteristic behaviors including cursing, threats, stealing, and even violence.

Watching your loved one decline mentally and physically is emotionally and physically exhausting for caretakers and families as you feel completely incapable of "fixing" anything anymore. Take care of yourself during this time. If you need a break, take one. You don't need to visit every day when it becomes too emotionally or physically difficult. My experience was that even if you had visited an hour before, your loved one might tell the next visitor he hasn't seen you in months. Don't feel guilty!

You may be criticized by friends that you should have kept him home longer. A quote by author Michelle Bryan, "*Don't let anybody who hasn't been in your shoes tell you how to tie the laces,*" certainly applies. Unless someone lives in the home with you, he or she is not in a position to make such an assessment or judgment about your decisions.

Brush off negative questions and statements. Find a trusted friend that you can talk to. Don't feel guilty!

In closing, I want to share what I learned by God's providence, as I totally believe this was an answered prayer. While having a conversation with an acquaintance, she asked how my husband was doing. After hearing of his current status, she explained she had previously been a hospice nurse and had patients in better shape than my husband. She recommended we call hospice immediately and request an evaluation.

I always thought hospice was a service that was called in at the very end of life. Not so! My husband was quickly approved for hospice care and received the most wonderful treatment for nearly the last year of his life. Hospice provided nursing care at his facility with oversight from a physician. In addition, the cost of his medications and adult diapers were covered by hospice. This was a tremendous financial help during this time.

My prayers go out to all caregivers, who have the most difficult job. Talk to others who have made this journey and ask what lessons were learned. Take care of your legal and financial business as soon as possible. Read as many books and articles as you can, arm yourself with knowledge and coping tools, and join an Alzheimer's Support Group. Accept help from others and don't let others make you feel guilty. Find a close friend willing to talk to you about your feelings. Love and take care of yourself during this time. Trust that you have made the best decisions for your loved one. Most of all...pray...the answers will come and you will pass the test!

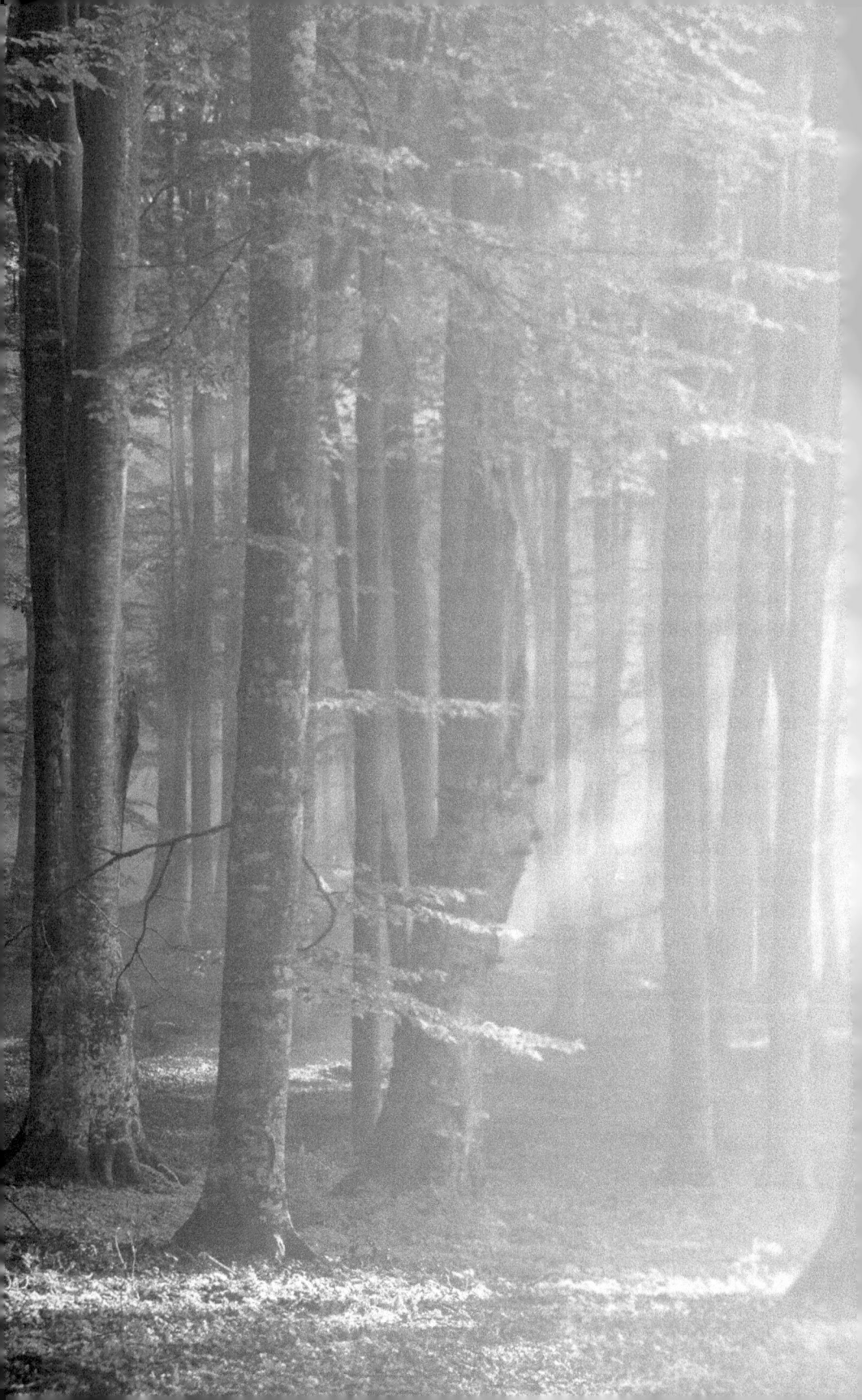

# BE WELL PREPARED

## ANONYMOUS

FIRST, I don't consider myself a caregiver in a traditional sense where day-to-day, hour-to-hour care is needed for long spans of time. I'm fortunate in my situation that we are able to have help through hospice, sitters, etc. There are a lot of people in far worse situations than I. Mom and Dad prepared better than most for their end of life and that has taken much of the physical and financial burden away that others may face.

It's been mentally and emotionally trying for the past 8-10 years or so, and even more constant in the past four to five years. It is sometimes unbelievable how quickly things can take a turn for the worse. Those times can be quite challenging to juggle everything, but like I said, they prepared well, and that helps.

There's a point when I realized the true frailty of the situation and that's when it really became apparent that I was no longer the kid and that it was necessary to look after Mom and Dad's well-being in a very proactive way. That was hard to come to terms with because I didn't want to overstep my bounds in their eyes. I think in a similar fashion, there was a reluctance on their part to ask for help because as a parent, that's not natural. It is hard to see them as fragile, but that's just how it is.

I'm sure that will be the case with my kids at some point and I hope they're able to take care of themselves mentally and emotionally when that time does come. I didn't really have a lot of experience in that area, but maybe in seeing the things I did/do wrong and the things I did right, my kids would be better off for it. I hope we can prepare as well as Mom and Dad to take some of the burden off of the kids.

# ALZHEIMER'S, ALS, AND AN ANEURYSM

## BY MARY TURNER

My sister, Nancy was my best friend. She was funny, energetic, and extremely intelligent. She was a chemistry and biology teacher at a local high school. She loved the kids and they loved her. We were always together sharing our lives with each other. We always said when we got old and it was just the two of us, we would move in together. God had other plans for Nancy.

In 2014, at the age of 50, she was diagnosed with Alzheimer's. This was devastating to her and really, both of us. We cried and prayed together and through the tears, I assured her I would be right there with her. It wasn't long before she had to take a disability retirement because she was misplacing things and forgetting what to do next while working a chemistry problem for the class. That was heartbreaking seeing the disappointment in her that she wouldn't be able to do the thing she loved. She was still able to take care of herself and drive for a few years after she was diagnosed. I dreaded the day she wouldn't be able to drive because that would take her independence away. That day finally happened when I received a phone call from her but there was a man on the other end of the line. He told me she was at a gas station, confused, and didn't know where she was. I panicked because she was an hour away in a different state with someone I didn't know. The man was very nice and said he would stay with her until my husband and I could get there. I prayed all the way over for God to protect her and keep her calm.

It was a long ride home talking about how she wouldn't be able to drive anymore. She kept saying she wouldn't do it again. She was like a child telling her Mama, "I'm sorry. I won't do it again." That was so heartbreaking to see she had to go through that. We cried and I told her it wasn't her fault that it was the disease. Early on the doctor told me right now, it would be harder on Nancy, but later on, it would be harder on the family. This was one of those moments.

Nancy was needing more help, so in 2018, I knew it was time for me to retire after 29 years of teaching in Special Ed. My plan was to retire and take care of Nancy, but God had another plan.

At the end of 2018, my husband, Alan, was having some issues with his muscles in his legs. In February 2019, he started seeing a neurologist in Houston. He was being treated for a neuromuscular disease but nothing seemed to help.

I was still taking care of Nancy and now Alan. Nancy needed more help, so she had a sitter come in for a few hours a day so I could help Alan. He kept getting worse, and by March he could no longer walk. He was still having infusions, but they didn't seem to help. In May, I had to call an ambulance because he was having difficulty breathing. While he was in the hospital, the doctor from Houston called and told me Alan had ALS (also known as Lou Gehrig disease) and there was no cure.

By this time Alan had figured that's what he had. Before he could go home, he was put on a bi-pap machine to help his breathing and a feeding tube. He left the hospital on hospice. We cried, but Alan said, "God is in control." He was more concerned about me and having to take care of him and Nancy. He said he wasn't afraid of dying, because he knew he would be with Jesus in heaven.

When he got home, I knew things had to change with Nancy and she had to go live at an assisted living facility. This was something Nancy and I had talked about early on. She had long-term insurance and she wanted to go to the facility where our dad had gone before he died. I always prayed for God to show me when it was time, and that Nancy would be all right with it.

Nancy could see Alan was hooked up to machines and couldn't get out of bed, so she understood. Nancy loved Alan like a brother and she was sad about him dying, and having to move. The adjustment was very hard on her. She fell and broke her kneecap and had to have surgery that first week. This pulled me in two different directions. I needed to take care of my husband, but also had to take care of Nancy. Nancy had to have a 24-hour sitter because she couldn't stand on her leg for six weeks. Even though it was expensive, that helped her adjust to her new place for a while.

Three months after Alan was diagnosed, he went to meet Jesus on August 24th. By this time, Nancy was getting worse. She was getting upset and I had to go sit with her and calm her down. It seemed I was the only one that could do it. Eventually, Nancy had to be put in the memory care part of the facility.

In March 2020, Covid hit and we couldn't go in to see Nancy. That was really hard on all of us. We were able to FaceTime with her once a week. In August 2020, Hurricane Laura hit and Nancy was evacuated to Mississippi. I went to Texas with my children.

After a few months, Nancy was moved to Mandeville, which was about three hours from me. I still couldn't go and see her because of Covid. The facility was damaged and she didn't come back to our area until November. We could finally start meeting through the glass doors. It was heartbreaking to see how much she had declined. She couldn't hold a conversation and we couldn't keep her attention. After several months, we could finally go in to see her and hug her.

One day while I was with Nancy, I got a call from a friend saying my son, Caleb wouldn't wake up. I left immediately. When I got there, I called an ambulance. He was breathing, but unresponsive. He was taken to the hospital where he died of a brain aneurysm at the age of 31. Now I was grieving my husband, my son, and my sister even though physically she was still with me.

As time went by, it was harder to go see Nancy, but I kept remembering what the doctor said. This was *our* hard time because she didn't know who we were anymore and our funny, quirky Nancy wasn't there. Eventually, she couldn't walk, talk or eat.

On June 2, 2022, at the age of 58, Nancy left this world and got a new body in heaven. God put me on a journey as a caregiver for my family and I wouldn't have had it any other way. I know God has a plan for each one of us. Jeremiah 29:11 says, *"For I know the plans I have for you," says the Lord. They are plans for good and not for disaster, to give you a future and a hope."* I know Alan, Nancy, and Caleb had the hope in Jesus that brings real joy.

Through all the laughs, trials, and tears, these two verses carried me through:

*"Do not be afraid or discouraged, for the Lord will personally go ahead of you. He will be with you; He will neither fail you nor abandon you."* Deuteronomy 31:8

*"You will keep in perfect peace all who trust in you, all whose thoughts are fixed on you!"* Isaiah 26:3

Peace isn't the absence of trouble; it is having the presence of God! This was my journey!

# THE PERFECT COMBINATION OF LAUGHTER AND LOVE

## BY PAULINE STANSEL

WHEN ELLEN ASKED me to write about being a caretaker, it really made me sit and think that I hadn't really thought of myself as a "caretaker" even though I was. To me, I was just taking care of my family member.

My mother-in-law started declining in the early 2000s but was still living in her house and that's when I stepped in to help with the normal chores, grocery shopping, doctor appointments, picking up her prescriptions and then, eventually, I had to start handing out her medicine. We often didn't see eye to eye on that. When someone has been on pain medication as long as she had, it makes life tough, and sometimes, I got upset with her.

Many times, I treated her as the enemy with my actions and words. But praise God, in 2003, I surrendered my life to Christ and God gave me many opportunities to extend mercy and grace to her that He had richly lavished over me.

As I look back now, I can see where the enemy tried to sabotage our relationship so many times. He will use anything he can to make us feel like we have "the right" to be angry at our loved ones or at anyone in our circle of influence, when they don't act or behave as we think they should. It wasn't our natural "go to" to run to or recall Ephesians

6:12: *"For we are not fighting against flesh-and-blood enemies, but against evil rulers and authorities of the unseen world, against mighty powers in this dark world, and against evil spirits in the heavenly places."* And anyway, who was I to expect perfection from her or anyone else when I can't deliver it? Martha needed me and God used her in my life to help me get over myself. Ouch!

Around 2009, she became wheelchair bound and soon after she was able to move into assisted living. She loved it there. She was loved and cared for by all the staff and was visited by her family and friends. Her three sons were the joy of her life until the grandkids and great-grand-kids came along. Overall, her being in an assisted-living facility was a huge plus for her and added to her quality of life.

I started talking to Martha about God every chance I could. She loved for me to read the Word of God to her, and we talked a lot about her relationship with Jesus. She loved me to pray for her and always told me how she could feel God when I did. Not too long after she moved into the facility, I convinced her to gather some people and start reading the Bible together and she did, and that study group is still meeting to this day.

In 2021, she had developed a cough and sore throat that wouldn't go away and she was diagnosed with lung cancer. Her doctor started radiation on her in April 2022 and she got a little tired, but no other symptoms. That was a blessing from God. Even though her health was declining, Martha kept, for the most part, that crazy, fun, sometimes sick sense of humor. Over the many years, she and I had more fun and laughter than most daughters-in-law and mothers-in-law ought to have had and, of course, our share of disagreements.

Well, the cancer took its toll and Martha passed January 1, 2023, two days before her 86th birthday and she had only been on hospice for a week. During that week, I prayed for the Lord to take her and to not let her suffer, and then He took her, and I was heartbroken...but not one without hope because I knew she was healed! For the Bible says in 2 Cor. 5:8: *"Yes, we are fully confident, and we would rather be away from these earthly bodies, for then we will be at home with the Lord."* In my heart, I knew she was healed, whole, and restored, and with her loved ones that went on before her that have trusted Christ as their Savior and Lord.

My biggest takeaway from being a caregiver is how important it is for us to love dearly the people that the Lord has entrusted us with. Give them your undivided attention, take time to hold their hand and hug them often, and to love them like our heavenly Father loves us.

# PART OF YOUR FAMILY

## BY SHIRLEY FONTENOT

MOM WAS DIAGNOSED with vascular dementia in 2014. So many thoughts of the future, the unknown, ran through my mind. What did the future hold for me and my siblings? We read, talked to doctors, and tried to prepare. Most importantly, we got legally prepared.

We secured power of attorney and ensured she had a will, and we added all three daughters' names to her checking accounts. Now, we (my two sisters and I) were caregivers.

Our schedules changed! On top of caregiving, there was also running the household, doctor visits, and more. Time went on and Mama's condition worsened. Now it was getting more challenging for all of us. We were trying to manage our homes, and jobs, and caring for Mama was getting exhausting, so we hired other caregivers.

They were a godsend. Take recommendations and interview thoroughly. We were blessed with most of ours. You still have to be an overseer which was mentally a strain, but with sitters in place, the physical strain on us was lifted. If finances are a little tight, take advantage of health care such as home health and then when needed, hospice.

Many days, as you watch your loved one go through these difficult changes, I found myself a quiet place, had a good cry and prayed, and believe me, I'm human and asked God, *"Why does this godly woman have to endure this?"* I might not have gotten a direct answer, but I had a peaceful feeling I could carry on for her. My favorite scriptures were Proverbs 3:5-6 and Romans 8:28. We listened to old gospel music all the time. It did help set the tone in the room.

Love your caregivers, and share your loved one's life past and present with them. Our caregivers talked to Mama and we shared our family pictures with them. They were like family to us. Encourage them, praise them. They were taking care of your loved one.

# MY MOTHER'S VOICE

## BY SUZY SHIPLEY

TRYING to clear messages from an old answering machine, I suddenly heard my mother's voice calling my name and leaving a message that instantly filled me with love. Her voice always did that when we had our long talks. I could not bring myself to erase that message.

Living hours from my mother, those phone calls were our continued connection until our next visit together. Dementia not only claimed my mother's fierce independence, but it also diminished her ability to communicate with her many children who lived out of town. I missed knowing her advice was a phone call away. I missed calling her with exciting news or sad disappointments. I missed the stories of her recent escapades or remembering the past. I missed passing the phone to my children as they waited excitedly to talk to their grandmother.

As the dementia progressed and phone calls were graciously facilitated by my sister, Ellen, the author of this book, it wasn't the same as before. However, it was always wonderful to hear my mother's voice. She was still full of joy and humor, but the recognition of who she was speaking to just didn't exist. I knew who she was to me and that had to be enough.

Ellen helped all the siblings living away from home realize there were other ways to stay in touch with our mother. Calls involved my sister holding the phone and giving Mama appropriate clues and guidance. The phone calls still existed but they were different and many times repetitive. Ellen also enabled us to communicate via Facetime and Marco Polo. No matter how uncertain her recognition was, maintaining some form of contact between visits was my lifeline to my treasured mother for as long as possible. It helped ease the incredibly long goodbye that dementia produced.

# TO HAVE NO REGRETS

## BY DAVID SHIPLEY

WHEN MY MOTHER died in 1996, I received a call late one night from my Episcopal rector. His words were kind and reassuring while I was dealing with a roller coaster of emotions. My mother was the first significant adult in my life to pass away, and I had never dealt with death as close up as this. I was in great need of a spiritual sign of some sort. But as C.S. Lewis once observed in the wake of his wife's death, God was silent.

What my priest told me that night was a source of comfort and a good lesson for all of us as our parents, aunts, and uncles age and face end of life issues. He said, "She cared for you when you needed her, and you cared for her when she needed you." My immediate reaction was that I hadn't done enough, having arrived at her bedside just 48 hours before she died. But maybe that was enough and just what she needed which brings me to another thing I learned thirteen years later when my aunt passed. Very often, you hear that someone has died "surrounded by family and loved ones." Very sweet. A peaceful end with those closest to you at your bedside. That was the atmosphere my family tried to create for my aunt, but a hospice worker visited us one day and shared her many years of experience and wisdom. It was something I had never heard before. She said some folks choose to go surrounded by loved ones, and some wait to be perfectly alone. It's as if some people want to make the transition to the next life by themselves, independently.

My time off from work had come to an end, and my wife and I had to leave my aunt's bedside to return home out of state. Other siblings and cousins had gone home for the night. Four hours after we had left, my aunt took that walk-through Death's Valley alone, on her own terms. My message to anyone who feels they let someone down because they weren't at their side when they passed is this: have no regrets about not being there. It might be that your relative or good friend wanted to take that walk on their own. And who knows, maybe they weren't alone at all, but walking with someone from the other side.

# GO THE DISTANCE

## BY KATHY HEDDINS

FOR YEARS, Brother Charlie, my father-in-law, struggled with Parkinson-like symptoms. A precious man who held so many titles, the most meaningful ones being father, grandfather, and spiritual mentor.

In 2010, he had a triple bypass. After surgery, he was required to recuperate in a nursing home. When we visited him six weeks later on Thanksgiving, we were saddened by his appearance and condition. He was simply not thriving. This 6'7" giant (physical and spiritual) of a man just wanted to come home. His wife couldn't do it alone, so we, as a family, told her that we would do whatever needed to be done so that Brother Charlie could come home. After weighing the options, my mother-in-law chose hospice for his end-of-life-care.

And so, it began... four sons and *no* daughters. This was where my role as a caregiver began. I was blessed to be in a position to be able to stay with him every other week while the oldest son stayed the opposite week.

My husband, David (son #2) drove me to his parent's farm on Friday, and assisted his Mama and brother for the weekend caring for Brother Charlie. On Sunday afternoons, David bid his farewells and headed back home to fulfill his work commitments from Monday to Friday. The routine repeated itself as he made the journey back to the farm every Friday night for another weekend shift. Every other Sunday, we made the 528-mile journey together, returning to our own cherished home. This cycle continued—528 miles one weekend and another 528 miles the following, etching our weekends with a sense of purpose and devotion.

My in-laws had prayed for us and spoke life and encouragement into us every day of our marriage. It was an honor to be able to play a role as one of Brother Charlie's caregivers in this season of his life. Saying that, I must add it was emotionally and physically tiring at times. I was missing my husband, my two and a-half-year-old grandson, friends, and my church, but my mother-in-law was so appreciative. She was even open to suggestions we made about her husband's care. This was a learning curve for everyone involved.

We moved the breakfast table and placed the hospital bed in the bay window area so that Brother Charlie had a beautiful view of his lake on their 90 acres of land he inherited. He thoroughly enjoyed seeing the fruit of his years of hard work and labor. *I often wondered what thoughts he was pondering as he gazed out the window.* I remember once as he stared outside, he said, "Darling, what's Hank's phone number?" Ms. Barbara replied, "Why?" Brother Charlie responded, "Oh, I just want to make something right with him."

He was a light even in the darkness of hospice, always kind to everyone who came through the doors to care for him and his wife. Even the small things like warming his blanket in the dryer and tucking it around him. He just loved it!

You could tell he was thinking about those that he would be leaving behind. While lying in his bed, he walked David and Roland through the location of where all the important papers were on the house and property while they videotaped the conversation. He told them details about the plumbing, electrical, and things only he knew, that would be needed after he was gone.

One day when Ms. Barbara had gone to an appointment, I asked Brother Charlie if he wanted to write a letter to Ms. Barbara. So, I sat next to his bed and wrote the letter as he dictated it to me for his wife of 50 years. The letter was given to her a year later on their wedding anniversary.

At one point, Brother Charlie requested physical therapy. A physical therapy student came to the house. As she worked with him, I could tell that all she saw was a dying old man. The next time she came and was preparing to leave, I asked her to come look at a video clip that I had set up for her.

The video was of my father-in-law in his prime, wrestling with the kids on the floor, full of laughter and life! I asked the young lady to try to see and think of THIS man, the man in the video, the next time she worked with Brother Charlie. I know from my own past experience I have had the same thoughts as this young lady. How would they know if we don't show them?

# RESOURCES

# Stages of Alzheimer's

## EARLY-STAGE ALZHEIMER'S (MILD)

IN THE EARLY stage of Alzheimer's, a person may function independently. He or she may still drive, work, and be part of social activities. Despite this, the person may feel as if he or she is having memory lapses, such as forgetting familiar words or the location of everyday objects.

Symptoms may not be widely apparent at this stage, but family and close friends may take notice and a doctor would be able to identify symptoms using certain diagnostic tools.

Common difficulties include:

- Coming up with the right word or name.
- Remembering names when introduced to new people.
- Having difficulty performing tasks in social or work settings.
- Forgetting material that was just read.
- Losing or misplacing a valuable object.
- Experiencing increased trouble with planning or organizing.

## MIDDLE-STAGE ALZHEIMER'S (MODERATE)

Middle-stage Alzheimer's is typically the longest stage and can last for many years. As the disease progresses, the person with Alzheimer's will require a greater level of care.

During the middle stage of Alzheimer's, the dementia symptoms are more pronounced. The person may confuse words, get frustrated or angry, and act in unexpected ways, such as refusing to bathe. Damage to nerve cells in the brain can also make it difficult for the person to express thoughts and perform routine tasks without assistance.

Symptoms, which vary from person to person, may include:

- Being forgetful of events or personal history.
- Feeling moody or withdrawn, especially in socially or mentally challenging situations.
- Being unable to recall information about themselves like their address or telephone number, and the high school or college they attended.
- Experiencing confusion about where they are or what day it is.
- Requiring help choosing proper clothing for the season or the occasion.
- Having trouble controlling their bladder and bowels.
- Experiencing changes in sleep patterns, such as sleeping during the day and becoming restless at night.
- Showing an increased tendency to wander and become lost.
- Demonstrating personality and behavioral changes, including suspiciousness and delusions or compulsive, repetitive behavior like hand-wringing or tissue shredding.
- In the middle stage, the person living with Alzheimer's can still participate in daily activities with assistance. It's important to find out what the person can still do or find ways to simplify tasks. As the need for more intensive care increases, caregivers may want to consider respite care or an adult day center so they can have a temporary break from

caregiving while the person living with Alzheimer's continues to receive care in a safe environment.

## LATE-STAGE ALZHEIMER'S (SEVERE)

In the final stage of the disease, dementia symptoms are severe. Individuals lose the ability to respond to their environment, to carry on a conversation and, eventually, to control movement. They may still say words or phrases, but communicating pain becomes difficult. As memory and cognitive skills continue to worsen, significant personality changes may take place and individuals need extensive care.

At this stage, individuals may:

- Require around-the-clock assistance with daily personal care.
- Lose awareness of recent experiences as well as of their surroundings.
- Experience changes in physical abilities, including walking, sitting, and eventually, swallowing.
- Have difficulty communicating.
- Become vulnerable to infections, especially pneumonia.

The person living with Alzheimer's may not be able to initiate engagement as much during the late stage, but he or she can still benefit from interaction in ways that are appropriate, like listening to relaxing music or receiving reassurance through gentle touch. During this stage, caregivers may want to use support services, such as hospice care, which focus on providing comfort and dignity at the end of life.

Hospice can be of great benefit to people in the final stages of Alzheimer's and other dementias and their families.

Late-stage care decisions can be some of the hardest families face. Connect with other caregivers who have been through the process on our online message boards.

As the disease advances, the needs of the person living with

Alzheimer's will change and deepen. A person with late-stage Alzheimer's usually:

- Has difficulty eating and swallowing
- Needs assistance walking and eventually is unable to walk
- Needs full-time help with personal care
- Is vulnerable to infections, especially pneumonia

*Source: Alz.org*

# HOSPICE AND HOME HEALTH

## HOSPICE VS. HOME HEALTH VS. PALLIATIVE CARE

You may not need hospice just yet, but you should ask about palliative care. It can be used when you are not quite ready for hospice, but you do require home healthcare.

## HOME HEALTH PROVISIONS

When a patient is on home health, the following items can be provided if needed: hospital bed, bedside commode, wheelchair, walker, oxygen, pull-ups, diapers, and any bed pads.

## HOSPICE PROVISIONS

Hospice offers the same medications as home health plus some of the medication costs are covered. In our case with our parents, heart medications as well as blood pressure meds were covered. Only medications covered by hospice would be delivered to your home or facility. For other necessary prescriptions, you will need to pick them up from your local pharmacy. Hospice covers medicine related to the **admitting** diagnosis and for comfort. Hospice offers what they call 'comfort measure' medications to help with shortness of breath, pain, sleep, anxiety, and depression.

## HOSPICE TEAM

A nurse visited the patient regularly. The patient need not go to a doctor. The nurse relayed all information to the group of doctors employed by the hospice company. The nurse checked vitals, medications, appetite, and noted any changes from week to week.The nurse came one to three times a week. The visits increased if the patient's condition worsened.

Patients are re-evaluated (re-certified) every 90 days for the first six months, then again every 60 days thereafter. During the 60-day time frame, a doctor or nurse practitioner visited the home or facility to see the patient.

Hospice nurses are on call 24 hours a day. You can contact your nurse from 8:00-4:30 daily. From 4:30 pm to 8:00 am, use the on-call triage and backup nurses. X-rays can be taken at the house, if necessary.

## HOSPICE SUPPORT STAFF

- A check-up with a doctor outside hospice is covered, but you must first call hospice to get permission.
- An air mattress for the hospital bed has to be approved. An egg crate topper is suggested.
- Blood work – Only if related to the primary condition of the patient.
- Catheter – Changed every 30 days
- Chaplain – Spiritual support
- CNA – Gives baths and provides shower support. They can come up to five days a week.
- Community Resources – Meals on Wheels
- Doctor – They utilized doctors in their hospice group. Every other week, the entire team met and reviewed cases.

- Hospital – If it's something hospice cannot handle, they direct you to the ER.
- Sitters are not provided
- Social Worker – Emotional support
- Physical therapy has to be approved by hospice.
- Volunteer Coordinator – Sets up help for haircuts, handicap ramps being built, etc.
- For other issues (not primary condition), they can draw and drop off blood, but it won't be covered by hospice.
- Wound care is available.

## OTHER HELPFUL THINGS

- Baby monitor (so you can be in the next room and still hear the patient).
- Bed extender for tall people
- Diffuser for essential oils
- Egg crate mattress
- Lift chair
- Sponge toothbrush
- Some hospice agencies now have their own hospitals. The patients go there instead of staying home. They could also go there for a crisis and at the end of life if the families don't want to or can't care for them when they are passing.

## ESSENTIAL OILS

I applied these oils on my mother and myself and always had my diffuser going in the special care apartment or the hospital. I prefer the Young Living essential oils brand. Of course, I do not use all of them every day. It depended on how I felt or what kind of support Mama needed. Staff and visitors loved coming into her room for the aroma. When my father-in-law was a frequent flier at the hospital, I put the diffuser on in his room. The staff, including the physicians, loved the aroma.

**Acceptance** – A blend of rose, lemon, and other oils to help with negativity.

**Bergamot** – Uplifting citrus blend that is calming and relaxing.

**Frankincense** – A grounding, woodsy aroma promotes spiritual awareness.

**Harmony** – Combination of 17 oils to create feelings of harmony and unity.

**Peace & Calming** – Tangerine, orange, and patchouli aid in restful sleep.

**Release** –Geranium and blue cypress provide emotional support.

**Stress Away** – Copaiba, lime, cedarwood, and other oils help stress levels.

**Surrender** – Lavender, lemon, and other oils promote feelings of peace.

**Trauma Life** –A combination of 10 oils offers support during difficult times.

**Valor** – Frankincense and more oils encourage bravery and confidence.

**White Angelica** – Bergamot and rose for a positive, peaceful environment.

**Ylang Ylang** – Fruity, flowery assists with anxiety and boosts your mood.

# PRAYERS FOR HEALTH AND HEALING

- I am healed by the stripes of Jesus. Isa. 53:5
- Jesus carried my sickness and infirmities. Matt 8:17
- I cast out all spirits of infirmity that would attack my body in the name of Jesus.
- I rebuke and cast out all spirits causing diabetes, high blood pressure, low blood pressure, heart attack, kidney failure, leukemia, blood disease, breathing problems, arthritis, lupus, Alzheimer's, or insomnia in the name of Jesus.
- I speak healing and strength to my bones, muscles, joints, organs, head, eyes, throat, glands, blood, marrow, lungs, kidneys, liver, spleen, spine, pancreas, eyes, bladder, ears, nose, sinuses, mouth, tongue and feet in the name of Jesus.
- I loose myself from high cholesterol rooted in anger and hostility and command these spirits to come out in the name of Jesus. I loose myself from all high blood pressure rooted in fear and anxiety, and I command these spirits to come out in the name of Jesus.
- I loose myself from a weakened immune system that is rooted in a broken spirit or broken heart, and I command these spirits to come out in the name of Jesus.

- I loose myself from all strokes rooted in self-rejection, self-bitterness, and self- hatred, and I command these spirits to come out in the name of Jesus.
- Forgive me, Lord, for allowing any fear, guilt, self-rejection, self-hatred, unforgiveness, bitterness, sin, pride, or rebellion to open the door to any sickness or infirmity. I renounce these things in the name of Jesus.
- I cast out any spirit of infirmity that came into my life through pride, trauma or accidents, rejection, or witchcraft in the name of Jesus.
- Give me a sound heart, which is the life of my flesh. Remove from my heart any evil or sinful attitude.
- Heal and deliver me from all my pains in the name of Jesus.
- I rebuke any sickness that would come to eat up my flesh, including cancer, in the name of Jesus. Ps. 27:2
- I break all curses of sickness and disease, and I command all hereditary spirits of sickness to come out. Gal 3:13
- I break all curses of premature death and destruction in the name of Jesus.
- I prosper and walk in health even as my soul prospers. 3 John 2.
- I receive the Word of God, which is health to my flesh. Prov. 4:22
- Let every tumor or evil growth melt at the presence of God. Ps. 97:5
- I will live and not die and I will proclaim the name of the Lord. Ps. 118:93
- Lord, you heal ALL my diseases. Ps. 103:3
- Heal me, O Lord, and I SHALL be healed. Jer. 17:14
- I release the fire of God to burn out any sickness or disease that would operate in my body in the name of Jesus.

*My thanks to John Eckhardt[1] for these prayers.*

---

1. *John Eckhardt, Prayers That Rout Demons (Lake Mary, FL: Charisma House, 2008), Used by permission.*

I loved to play music by Bethel, Maverick City, Brandon Lake, Elevation, Lauren Daigle, Zach Williams, Chris Tomlin, Kari Jobe, and Cody Carnes. I played them quietly in the background while I read these confirmations out loud every day. Sometimes I read just one, over and over.

# SITTERS

## Interviewing Sitters

- Before you interview anyone, you must figure out what time you want them there, the length of the shift, and precisely what you expect them to do. You have to be specific, so there are no misunderstandings.
- The applicant should interact with your loved one during the interview. Those who never even acknowledged Mama sitting nearby were written off immediately.
- There will be applicants who demand to be paid in cash. I was accountable to the government for how I spent Mama's money, and I needed to have a paper trail. My sitters were paid every week by check.

## Sitters Duties

- Have a central control board posted to keep everyone up to date. If Mama had constipation, I asked the sitters and aides to write on the board if she had a bowel movement. When we put her on oxygen, that was noted on the board. I

sectioned off a corner for sitters to write what supplies I
needed to purchase, i.e., diapers, wipes, soap, etc.

- I also posted a monthly calendar on the board so everyone
knew who was working and when. If I had some empty
shifts (I covered by default), then some could pick up an
extra shift.
- I had a blank shift calendar in the room about two weeks
before the first of the month. Sitters started choosing which
shift they wanted that month. Right before the first of the
month, I posted the completed or close-to-completed
calendar. I sent a copy of the calendar, especially if there
were empty shifts, to see if any of my siblings wanted to fill
in for me.

Mama should be in her recliner and dressed for the day when
you arrive. An aide will come between 7 am and 8 am to help
you bring her to the bathroom, dress her for the day, and place
her in the wheelchair. Please brush her hair and teeth, wash her
face, then wheel her down to breakfast. I usually move her place
setting in the dining room from in front of her so she won't play
with it.

Her oatmeal gets two pats of butter and two sugars. Salt and
pepper her eggs. Give her plenty to drink. Roll her back down
to her room and, with the help of the aide, put her back in her
recliner. The aides will come back around 11ish to potty her and
get her in the wheelchair for lunch at 11:30. If she's sleeping too
hard and skips lunch, no big deal. I always have snacks in the
cabinet.

After lunch, bring Mama back to her room to rest in the recliner.
The aides will return at about 4 pm to get her up, use the bathroom, and get ready for supper. Remember, she will take her
nasty-tasting medicine at the end of supper. Give her plenty to
drink to wash it down. Someone will help you put on her
pajamas and get her in bed. Please write in the notebook about

her eating, any changes in her breathing or bathroom, and cover her with her blue blanket while she is in the recliner.

Posted Information

AKA Norma Jean, Mamaw (MAM-AW), Mrs. Pettijohn

Shifts are 12-hour shifts, starting at 7 am or 7 pm

MAMA'S CURRENT STATE:

- Hospice
- Alzheimer's
- In a wheelchair
- 85%-90% blind
- Wears Depends
- Good hearing
- Her knees cause frequent pain
- Three recent falls
- Agitated easily by loud noises
- Does not know her own limitations
- Restless at night
- List the name of the hospice nurse
- List the name of the shower aide
- She loves music - Floyd Cramer, Fats Domino, anything with a beat or harmony, soul, country, etc.
- She is very loving and affectionate
- Great sense of humor

When asking her a question, she is better when you accept her answer. If she doesn't want to do something, then let it go. Try again in 15 to 20 minutes. Don't push her, or she gets agitated. You have to watch her constantly. She is a very high fall risk. She has fallen three times since February 28th, even from the wheelchair. She does not know her physical limitations and forgets how weak her legs are. She may want to walk, but should only be transported in a wheelchair. Inform her of what you're doing **before** you begin.

The right side of her face is very tender from her last fall.

Explain everything to her. Be kind and gentle. When using a wheelchair, go slow because she is a risk with that as well. Let me explain. If she decides to put her feet down quickly, it throws her. It is advised to pull her backward down the hallway.

It is not necessary to take her out on strolls. After breakfast and supper, you could take her to the TV room but stay with her. After lunch, you could take her back to her room for less distractions. She likes to stretch out on the hospital bed or her recliner. The couch has recliners on each end, too.

Please don't feel like you have to talk to her constantly. She is likely to tell you to "Shut Up!" She likes to listen to the TV or the radio. She enjoys being in the TV room. She is always listening, and there is absolutely nothing wrong with her hearing. She speaks French well.

According to the facility director, the aides are still supposed to do their regular duties with Mama. While you are here sitting, your job is to closely watch Mama and feed her at mealtime. If she needs assistance with the bathroom, do not try to toilet her by yourself. Get an aide to assist you. Pull the cord on the wall or look outside in the hallway for assistance. They will still get her dressed and change her diaper, etc.

She has a DNR, so no heroic measures are needed if/when she has an unresponsive event.

When feeding Mama, I move everything on the table away from her and put it in front of my seat to the side of her. She is very distracted by anything on the table. Watch her hands, because she is quick. Try to feed her protein first and cut her food into small bites. Salt and pepper the food. For breakfast, she loves oatmeal. She loves the biscuit with butter and jelly. Mama hardly ever eats bacon. She is picky about textures and vegetables. She will tell you if she likes it or not. If she's eating in the dining room and says she is full, give her about five minutes and talk small talk, then try again. She usually eats all her breakfast, except fruit and bacon. We have a special juice to make that has potassium and magnesium. I think one of the aides could make the drink for you if they aren't too busy. Get her to drink the juice first. She drinks from a straw. She enjoys the flavor of the drink. Try and get her to drink all of her juice by saying, "Here's your favorite juice," as opposed to asking if she wants some.

On days she stays in her room from exhaustion, you could request her meal be brought to her room. She will not eat/drink as well because she prefers to rest. Just try, but follow her lead. Also, watch out. When she gets little pieces of meat or something in her mouth she doesn't like, she will spit them out. Sorry.

I'm a big believer in speaking positive things, so I encourage Mama by telling her, "Here's your favorite juice," or how good her hair looks or anything uplifting. Doesn't it make you feel better when someone encourages you? She responds really well to that. Caution: Asking her too many questions could make her aggravated.

Her unresponsive episodes appear as periods of time when her head falls forward, she loses color, she is cold and clammy, and her body becomes limp. As she comes out of the episode, she will start to respond to you and begin regaining her color. She most likely would be much less active the next day, choosing to rest and not eat/drink. However, the last episode took four hours before she regained color and started responding to questions. The following day she was back to her normal self. When these episodes occur, notify the staff and Ellen ASAP.

Hospice aide comes on Monday, Wednesday, and Friday mornings. The aide has requested on those mornings after breakfast, we leave Mama in the wheelchair in her room until she gets there. It just makes things go more smoothly. Mama is typically spent after her shower. Under no circumstances leave her.

At supper time, she gets a medicine that makes her very sleepy. You have a 20-minute window after she gets the medicine to make sure she is in bed. The nurse typically waits until Mama is near the end of the meal before she administers the medicine. Make sure one of the aides knows you are about to need their assistance, and leave immediately after meds/water are given and bring her to the bathroom, then get her in bed.

Do not ever leave her. If you need the bathroom, take advantage of workers nearby and get them to watch her while you use the bathroom.

If you are sick, notify me immediately so I can find a replacement. That's the last thing Mama needs to deal with. Do not sit with her if you are sick. If you cannot come at your scheduled time, the sooner you let me know, the better. Twenty-four hours or more notice would be appreciated.

There is a sitter's notebook on the desk. Please note her eating/drinking, BMs/urination, and meds. Also note agitations, restlessness, etc. for me. There is no such thing as too many notes.

## Family Members Instructions

When you check in every morning, arrive between 6:30-6:40 AM because getting someone to answer the outside door could take a while.

I inquire about how Mama's night went, make sure the day sitter arrives, and then I help Mama get up (which could take three people) and to the bathroom and get her dressed. An aide or two will come and help you.

The sitters are fantastic with Mama. You have a great hands-on crew lined up. While the two aides are busy with Mama in the bathroom, I make her bed. Then when they get through with Mama's hair and teeth, we leave the room together. I'll go ahead of them and prepare the dining room table set up for Mama. I move the chair to the side in order for the wheelchair to go in its place, and move all Mama's place setting to the right so it is not in front of her. After they are settled, I leave.

I return about 6:30–6:40 PM, and Mama is almost always sleeping, so I chat with the day sitter about the day – eating, showers, BMs, sleepy or wakeful, agitated, and so on. I read over the notebook journal. I ensure the night sitter gets there and sometimes chat with them, too. I am usually home by 7:30, no later. I text the sitters and remind them of their shifts. I will give them your phone number. I also text the day sitter during the day, usually after lunch, to see how Mama's day was going.

Mama is starting to walk to her bathroom from her bed or recliner, but we've got to have two people plus the wheelchair close by. She is also beginning to push herself up to a standing position. I'm all for that as long as we keep a very close eye on her. Please don't hesitate to ask me questions if something comes up.

## SAMPLE CALENDARS

### MARCH

| SUNDAY | MONDAY | TUESDAY | WEDNESDAY | THURSDAY | FRIDAY | SATURDAY |
|---|---|---|---|---|---|---|
| | | | | 1 | 2 | 3 |
| | | | | VICKI | VICKI | DEB |
| | | | | CAT | ELLEN | CINDY |
| 4 | 5 | 6 | 7 | 8 | 9 | 10 |
| ELLEN | KATY | DEB | VICKI | VICKI | KATY | CINDY |
| PAT | CINDY | K.D. | CAT | CAT | PAT | DEB |
| 11 | 12 | 13 | 14 | 15 | 16 | 17 |
| CHRIS | KATY | BECKY | VICKI | VICKI | KATY | ELLEN |
| BECKY | PAT | CINDY | CAT | CAT | K.D. | DEB |
| 18 | 19 | 20 | 21 | 22 | 23 | 24 |
| ELLEN | CHRIS | KATY | VICKI | VICKI | BECKY | KATY |
| BECKY | K.D. | K.D. | CAT | CAT | ELLEN | PAT |
| 25 | 26 | 27 | 28 | 29 | 30 | |
| ELLEN | KATY | ELLEN | VICKI | VICKI | PAT | |
| BECKY | CINDY | DEB | CAT | CAT | CINDY | |

### MONTH and YEAR

| SUNDAY | MONDAY | TUESDAY | WEDNESDAY | THURSDAY | FRIDAY | SATURDAY |
|---|---|---|---|---|---|---|
| | | | | 1 | 2 | 3 |
| | | | | | | |
| | | | | | | |
| 4 | 5 | 6 | 7 | 8 | 9 | 10 |
| | | | | | | |
| | | | | | | |
| 11 | 12 | 13 | 14 | 15 | 16 | 17 |
| | | | | | | |
| | | | | | | |
| 18 | 19 | 20 | 21 | 22 | 23 | 24 |
| | | | | | | |
| | | | | | | |
| 25 | 26 | 27 | 28 | 29 | 30 | |
| | | | | | | |
| | | | | | | |

OCTOBER

| SUN. | MON. | TUES. | WEDS. | THURS. | FRI. | SAT. |
|---|---|---|---|---|---|---|
| | CINDY K.D. 1 | PAT COURTNEE 2 | VICKI CAT 3 | VICKI CAT 4 | VICKI COURTNY 5 | K.D. PAT 6 |
| PAT CAT 7 | CINDY COURTNEE 8 | K.D. KAY 9 | VICKI CAT 10 | VICKI CAT 11 | VICKI KATY 12 | PAT COURTNEE 13 |
| KAY CAT 14 | CINDY K.D. 15 | PAT COURTNEE 16 | VICKI CAT 17 | VICKI CAT 18 | VICKI KATY 19 | DEB COURTNEE 20 |
| DEB CAT 21 | CINDY K.D. 22 | K.D. KAY 23 | VICKI CAT 24 | VICKI CAT 25 | VICKI KATY 26 | K.D. Ellen 27 |
| Ellen CAT 28 | CINDY K.D. 29 | K.D. VICKI 30 | VICKI CAT 31 | | | |

**Contact Info:**

ELLEN STEPHENS
(452) 319-8827

JAMES STEPHENS
(452) 013-9178

*DO NOT GIVE PRN MEDS W/O CALLING FAMILY

**MOM HAS PRN MEDS FOR:
1. DIARRHEA
2. NAUSEAU/VOMITING (ZOFRAN)
3. E KIT AVAILABLE

Normal Angel's:
YOU'VE KEPT HER ALIVE FOR EIGHT MONTHS.
Thank you,
Elle

BM's:

VISITORS:

PAYDAY- MONDAY WEEKLY

Items Needed:
PUSH FLUIDS PLZ!
USE WATER BOTTLE IF NEEDED. ADD M10 DROPS
NEW MEAL TIMES
7:30 BREAKFAST
11:30 LUNCH
4:30 SUPPER

<u>New Requirements per the New Director:</u>

1. Help transfer Mama from recliner to wheelchair.
2. Help transfer Mama from the recliner to the bed.
3. Help transfer Mama to and from the toilet.
4. Help Mama walk to the toilet and back when she is able.
5. Help transfer Mama from wheelchair to bed.
6. Help turn Mama in the bed on her side.
7. Assist with diaper changes in the bed. Turn her, hold her, comfort her.
8. Continue feeding her.
9. Continue staying with her at all times.
10. Closely monitor her medications.
11. Assist the aide in everything she is doing.
12. Assist hospice shower aide.
13. If she has a soiled diaper, please close the bag and put it in the trash to take out at the end of the shift.

14. Please write on the board when supplies are low: toilet paper, shampoo, hand soap, shower gel, toothpaste, bed liners, diapers, etc.
15. Continue notating her BMs.
16. Continue writing everything that happens throughout your shift in the notebook.
17. If she wets the bed, please jump in and help with stripping sheets, wiping down the mattress, putting on new sheets, and helping to change Mama's clothes.
18. Ellen has PRN (as-needed meds) and an emergency kit.
19. If after hours (i.e. after 9 pm), please call Ellen if Mama requires something for gas, nausea, vomiting, diarrhea, or severe pain. * These items are directly from me, not the director.

Please sign and date your name below if you have read this and are willing to continue sitting with Mama. If you are unable to perform the duties, I completely understand.

Thank you, angels, for helping me with Mama. You are a huge blessing.

# FUNERAL PLANNING

- Call church organizations the deceased was a member of in the church.
- Suggested Scripture Readings – Proverbs 31:10-31; Ecclesiastes 3:1-8.
- Linens and paper goods for a meal after funeral.
- Choose burial outfit.
- Bring clothes to the funeral home.
- Daughters can style her hair (this was such an honor).
- Plenty of Kleenex.
- Soundtrack to play with pictures.
- Ask priest /pastor to come to see her before they pass. This is also a great opportunity for the family to share stories about their loved one with the priest/pastor.
- Provide mortician with photo asap to assist setting face correctly.
- Obituary with photo to local newspapers. Research deadlines for your preferred newspapers. Some cities do not run the paper everyday.
- Enlarge pictures for displays in funeral parlor and church.

Are easels needed at church for photos? Family members bring spare picture frames to use.

- Picture slideshow.
- Pallbearers
- Honorary pallbearers – perhaps older people who can't carry casket.
- Veterans need DD214 for the funeral home to get a flag.
- Consider Legacytouch.com for fingerprint keepsake, i.e., necklace, bracelets, etc.
- Appearance – Bring outfit. Paint nails. Put rings and earrings on, remove them before burial, and return them to specific family member. Bring underwear, socks or leggings, and a slip. Shoes are optional.
- Check prayer books for special notations.
- Update CaringBridge website if utilized.
- Bereavement Travel Services was one of the best things our funeral home offered at no extra cost if we pre-planned the service. The travel service was for one year for the children and grandchildren of the deceased. They give you an 800 number and you get discounts on rental cars, hotels, and airfare. Share with your family so they can take advantage of it when the time comes. It goes into effect the minute someone passes.

Please acquire updated pricing from your local funeral home.

- Inquire about cremation costs as another option.
- Basic services $6700
- Caskets range from $675 – $10,000
- 12" obituary runs $250-$300. Images were $20 each. Confirm costs and deadlines with each newspaper you want it printed in.
- Confirm previous arrangements with graveyard and whether it was prepaid.
- Adding name and date to the grave marker - $375
- Open and close vault - $1100

- Laminated Bible bookmarks for the family were $3-$5/each. Ask for a preview to make sure the print is readable.
- Honorarium for musicians and pastor
- Call life insurance
- In lieu of flowers – make donations to organization or church
- Casket flowers $400.
- Order five copies of the death certificate. Cost was $9 for the first one; $7 for each additional one.

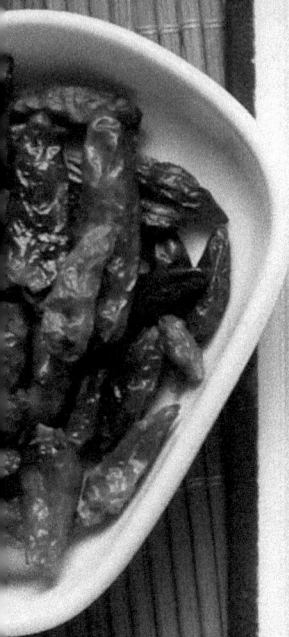

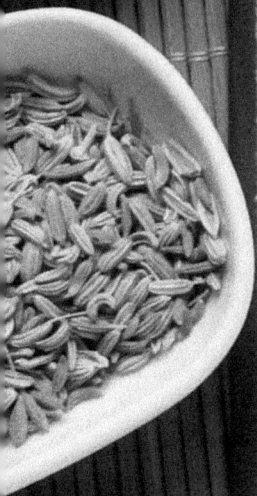

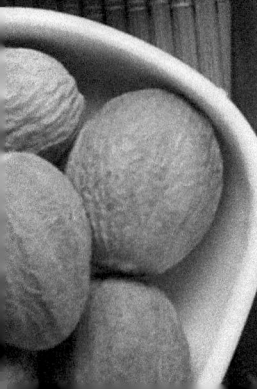

# NORMA JEAN'S RECIPES

## ITALIAN CREAM CHEESE CAKE

2 c. sugar
5 eggs, separated
1 stick butter
½ c. Crisco
2 c. flour
1 tsp. vanilla
1 tsp. baking soda
1 c. buttermilk
1 c. Angel Flake coconut
1 c. chopped pecans

### Frosting

8 oz. cream cheese
½ stick oleo
1 box powdered sugar
1 tsp. vanilla
Chopped pecans

Cream oleo, Crisco, and sugar. Add egg yolks one at a time, beat well. Add baking soda and buttermilk, alternating with flour. Add pecans and coconut. Fold in well beaten egg whites. Add vanilla. Grease and flour 3 (9-inch) pans. Bake at 350 degrees for 30 minutes. Frost when the cake is cool. May need to add milk to the frosting if desired. Sprinkle with chopped pecans.

~~∽⟨♋⟩∼~~

## Mama's Mexican Fudge (Pralines)

1 ½ c. sugar
¾ c. milk
1 c. pecans, chopped
1 c. brown sugar
2 T. butter

Cook mixture in a heavy saucepan and bring to a soft ball stage. Remove from heat and stir until mixture is creamy and begins to thicken. Drop by spoonfuls onto prepared buttered wax paper.

## Mamaw's French Toast (Pain Perdu)

2 eggs, beaten
1 t. vanilla
4 T. sugar
Milk
5 slices white bread

Mix first four ingredients. Dip bread in mixture letting it soak a few seconds. Place on hot oiled griddle, turning to brown each side.

## Norma Jean's Garlic Roast

1 medium/large sized rump roast
2-4 cloves of garlic, minced
1 small onion, diced small
Salt, pepper and/or Tony's Creole Seasoning to taste
Olive oil to coat the roast
*White vinegar

After the garlic and onions are minced, soak them in some *white vinegar. Cut an "X" all the way around the roast and stuff the minced garlic and onion in your roast. Don't worry if some falls out of the "X". Heat oil in a Dutch oven type pot and sear every side of the roast until nice and brown. (You may need tongs and a fork to hold the roast on its side). Once each side is brown, add about a cup of water to the pan, and deglaze any little bits that may be there. Close the lid and cook in the oven on 350 degrees or on the stove until the meat falls off the bone.

### Norma Jean's Sausage and Red-Eye Gravy

2 lbs. mixed sausage containing green onion and garlic from Market Basket.
Beef broth – 3 quarts
Water
Flour 1 T.
Rice – 2 to 3 cups

Cut sausage into 1-inch links. Place in a 5 or 6-quart pot. Add water to fill the pot halfway. All of the meat should be covered in water. Boil until water is almost gone. Refill the pot with 2 large cans of beef broth, enough to cover the sausage. Boil again until broth is halfway gone. Remove meat. Scrap the meat particles from the bottom of the pot and add another quart of broth to the pot. After the broth is heated, add flour to thicken the gravy to your liking. Place sausage back in pot, stir and season to taste. Serve over cooked rice. *Corn is an excellent side dish for this recipe. Serves 4-6 people.

# INDEX

# INDEX

# Acknowledgments

**With Sincere Thanks:** A high school friend called me and said God had given her a message to relay to me. He instructed her to tell me, "Tell my story." *What? Are you being serious? What a message!* Her message began the process of writing this book. Her obedience to God and delivery of His message is why you are holding this book in your hands. I pray I will always remember the impact obedience to the Father could have on one or perhaps thousands of other lives. Thank you, Elana.

**Gratitude** to friends and family who allowed me to bounce ideas off of them, offered critique and read and re-read my story. I am so thankful for Ethan, Chrissy, Cathy W., Eva, Cathy, Suzanne, Dave, Faith, Melissa, Alex, Heather, Terrie and all my Canyon Lake Writers Club members.

To receive notifications of book signings, speaking engagements or additional publications, please visit and subscribe to our website: www.thewritersporchllc.com

# About the Author

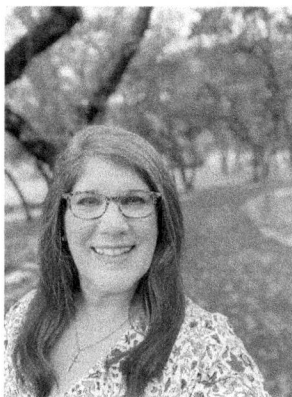

Ellen P. Stephens and her husband recently completed an 18-year consecutive journey caring for three parents. Ellen was compelled to share her story to help others after caring for her mother. The lessons learned, navigating all the decisions and more. When she is not writing, Ellen loves to travel, spend time with her four children, five grandchildren and friends. They retired to the Hill Country of Texas from their native Louisiana. She has served as Chair in the Canyon Lake Area Writers Club the past two years.

Her hobbies include photography, singing, attending concerts, and cruising.

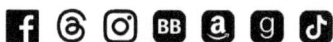